Human Movement

An Introductory Text

FIFTH EDITION

Edited by

Marion Trew
BA MSc MSCP DipTP

Head, School of Health Professions, University of Brighton, Eastbourne

Tony Everett
BA Med Dip TP MCSP

Deputy Director, Department of Physiotherapy, Cardiff University

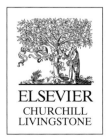

ELSEVIER
CHURCHILL
LIVINGSTONE

EDINBURGH   LONDON   NEW YORK   OXFORD   PHILADELPHIA   ST LOUIS   SYDNEY   TORONTO   2005

ELSEVIER
CHURCHILL
LIVINGSTONE

CHURCHILL LIVINGSTONE
An imprint of Elsevier Limited

© 2005, Elsevier Ltd
First published 1981
Second edition 1987
Third edition 1997
Fourth edition 2001
Fifth edition 2005

ISBN 0 443 07446 1

British Library Cataloguing in Publication Data
A catalogue record for this book is available from the British Library

Library of Congress Cataloging in Publication Data
A catalog record for this book is available from the Library of Congress

Note
Knowledge and best practice in this field are constantly changing. As new research and experience broaden our knowledge, changes in practice, treatment and drug therapy may become necessary or appropriate. Readers are advised to check the most current information provided (i) on procedures featured or (ii) by the manufacturer of each product to be administered, to verify the recommended dose or formula, the method and duration of administration, and contraindications. It is the responsibility of the practitioner, relying on their own experience and knowledge of the patient, to make diagnoses, to determine dosages and the best treatment for each individual patient, and to take all appropriate safety precautions. To the fullest extent of the law, neither the publisher nor the editors assume any liability for any injury and/or damage.

Printed in China

Contents

Contributors

Susan Corr PhD MPhil DipMedEd DipCOT SRPT
Reader in Occupational Therapy, Division of Occupational Therapy, University College Northampton Northampton, UK

Robert van Deursen PhD MSc MCSP MILTHE
Director of Physiotherapy Research Centre for Clinical Kinaesiology, Department of Physiotherapy, School of Healthcare Studies, Cardiff University, Cardiff, UK

Tony Everett BA Med Dip TP MCSP
Deputy Director, Department of Physiotherapy, School of Healthcare Studies, Cardiff University, Cardiff, UK

Bernhard Haas MSc BA(Hons) MCSP
Head of Physiotherapy, Department of Physiotherapy, Plymouth University, Plymouth, UK

Clare Kell MSc MCSP PGCHE MILT
Lecturer, Department of Physiotherapy, School of Healthcare Studies, Cardiff University, Cardiff, UK

Ann P. Moore PhD FSCP FMACP GradDipPhys CENT ED
Director, Clinical Research Centre, School of Health Professions, University of Brighton, Eastbourne, UK

Nicola J. Petty MSc MCSP SRP MMPA MMACP
Principal Lecturer, School of Health Professions, University of Brighton, Eastbourne, UK

Nicola Phillips MSc MCSP
Senior Lecturer/Manager, Postgraduate Studies, Department of Physiotherapy, School of Healthcare Studies, Cardiff University, Cardiff, UK

Valerie Sparkes PhD MCSP SRP
Lecturer, Department of Physiotherapy, School of Healthcare Studies, Cardiff University, Cardiff, UK

Marion Trew BA MSc MCSP DipTP
Head of the School of Health Professions, University of Brighton, Eastbourne, UK

Preface

For many years students hoping to enter the health professions have used this popular book as a means of developing an understanding of human movement. In addition, as the general population becomes more interested in physical activity, other groups have found the book to be of value and the range of readers has expanded. To meet the needs of this broad readership we have tried to take an eclectic approach to considering human movement but all chapters should be of interest to the serious student of human movement. Some chapters may appear to be profession specific but all chapters will still contain information that is of general interest.

This latest edition retains the features that previous generations of readers have indicated are most helpful but we have updated each chapter, incorporating new research where appropriate. We have increased the examples of how the scientific theory relates to movement and added more text boxes and case studies. These changes are most evident in the chapter on the musculoskeletal basis of movement.

The general presentation and format of the book remains unchanged as feedback from previous readers has indicated that it is well laid out and presented. We have also tried to maintain a 'plain English' approach to writing in order to uphold our reputation for providing information that is clear, understandable and easy to read.

We believe that human movement is a fascinating area of study. We hope that through these pages you will come to appreciate the complexity of what appears to most people to be simple activity and develop a passion for learning more about the miracle that is human movement.

Marion Trew
Tony Everett
Eastbourne and Cardiff 2005

Chapter 1

Introduction

Marion Trew   Tony Everett

LEARNING OUTCOMES

When you have completed this chapter you
should be:

1. Enthusiastic about the study of human movement

2. Aware of the range of factors that influence
   the initiation, production and control of human
   movement

3. Aware of the need to maintain a holistic
   approach to studying human movement whilst
   being conscious of the difficulties of
   simultaneously considering such a broad range
   of information

4. Beginning to develop awareness of your own
   body at rest and when moving

5. Starting to develop the skills of observation of
   human movement.

THE STUDY OF HUMAN MOVEMENT

The study of human movement is fascinating for
two main reasons. First, because it enables us to
understand our bodies and though most human
beings are surprisingly ignorant about themselves, they are also very curious. The science of
human movement explains how we are able to go
about our normal lives performing a vast range of

everyday functional activities, playing sport and taking part in other pastimes. The second reason for our fascination is stimulated by the complexity of human movement and the challenges we have to overcome when investigating exactly how we move.

The study of human movement inevitably leads to a sense of amazement at the wide variety of intricate tasks that we are able to perform with ease but there are still a surprising number of gaps in our knowledge. For example, whilst there have been a substantial number of scientific studies of walking and running, there are only a limited number of research papers on other major lower limb functions and a surprising lack of information on the everyday activities we perform with our upper limbs.

Observation of human movement reveals a complex and seemingly infinite variety of positional changes which involve or are controlled by a wide range of internal and external factors. To begin to understand how the systems of the body interact to produce finely controlled and purposeful movement, it is essential that some order is introduced into the study. It is necessary to know how human movement is initiated, performed and controlled and such knowledge forms the basis of those professions working in this area.

Human movement can be viewed from a number of different standpoints:

- *Anatomical*: describing the structure of the body, the relationship between the various parts and the potential for movement. Incorrect alignment or disruption of anatomical structures will clearly affect movement.
- *Physiological*: concerned with the ways in which the systems of the human body function. Physiology also informs us about the initiation and control of movement. In many cases incorrect functioning or failure of integration between systems will lead to movement abnormalities.
- *Biomechanical*: where the force, time and distance relationships in movement are investigated.
- *Psychological*: examining the sensations, perceptions and motivations that stimulate movement and the neurological and chemical/hormonal mechanisms which control them.

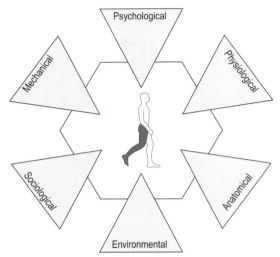

Figure 1.1 There are a number of ways in which the study of human movement can be approached; each approach is valid in its own right but, on its own, limited. For a holistic understanding of how the human body moves and why the component parts work as they do, a multidimensional approach has to be taken.

- *Sociological*: considering the meanings given to various movements in different human settings and the influence of social settings on the movements produced.
- *Environmental*: considering the influence of the environment on the way in which movement occurs.

This book primarily considers human movement from the perspective of anatomy, physiology and biomechanics. The psychological, sociological and environmental factors influencing movement are mentioned in some chapters but not dealt with in depth. This does not lessen the importance of these three approaches to understanding human movement but readers can familiarise themselves with this information from other well-recognised sources.

Studying the musculoskeletal basis of movement provides an anatomical framework on which movement can be referenced and described in an unambiguous manner. An intact musculoskeletal system is essential for correct movement to take place. Joints need to possess sufficient freedom of movement to perform the required activities and to be able to move in a smooth and unrestricted manner. Muscles provide the means of achieving this movement and they must possess the necessary strength, power and endurance to carry out this function. They must also be controlled in an extremely delicate and sensitive way and to do this, the efficient functioning and correct integration of the central and peripheral nervous systems are essential.

Most of the movements that adults undertake have been previously learned and, following months or years of practice, have become reflex and fluent. The neural processes that store, adapt and use these learned movements are complex and demonstrate the interdependence of all the systems of the body in the production of movement. However, no matter what our age, we have the potential to learn new movement patterns. Initially these new activities arise from a conscious decision to take action and require active thought processes. At the early stage of acquiring a new skill, considerable concentration is required and the movement may be clumsy. However, with practice, it will be converted into a learned sequence of movements that will be stored in the brain and can be reproduced with fluency and little thought.

Movement does not take place in isolation from the external environment. There is a complex interaction of forces acting on the body including the constant force of gravity and changing frictional forces. The force of gravity is a very important influence on movement because it is always present. It may have the beneficial effect of initiating or producing movement of body segments and it is always a force which the body has to counter to achieve and maintain an upright position. Friction, on the other hand, changes as the body comes into contact with a variety of surfaces, thus causing different reactions of the body's internal environment in response to these changing conditions.

Forces from many other sources such as wind, water, animate and inanimate objects all have their effect on the way movement is carried out. It is important that the physical laws of the external environment are understood so that the prediction of, and compensation for, these forces can be implemented by the controlling systems.

It is obvious that each of these aspects is inter-related and that between them they give a framework and a direction for the study of movement. However, any attempt to simultaneously consider all possible factors involved in human movement would result in a very lengthy, complex and expensive process. The impracticality of trying to understand all aspects of movement at one time inevitably means that research rarely encompasses

Case Study 1.1

A premier division soccer team were undergoing a series of tests of 'fitness' which, it was hoped, would provide information which could be used to build an improved training programme. These tests included anthropometric measurements, tests for elasticity of soft tissue, muscle length and the strength and endurance capacity of their lower limb muscles. Towards the end of the day one of the players, Mr F, was having the peak torque ratio of his knee and hip flexors and extensors tested on the isokinetic dynamometer.

When the results for the team were analysed, it was found that the torque generated by the non-dominant limb was always greater or equal to that of the dominant limb, except in the case of Mr F, where his dominant limb appeared to have generated substantially more torque than expected. There was concern that either there had been an error in the data collection procedure or that Mr F had an injury to his non-dominant limb which he had not mentioned to the laboratory staff and which was being reflected in abnormally low torque levels. It was decided to call him back in for review.

On reattendance, discussion with Mr F revealed that he had begun to lose interest in the testing procedures by the end of the day when his isokinetic test was scheduled. He speculated that he had not been putting as much effort as he might into the test until, just as the peak torque in his dominant limb was being measured, his team manager and coach walked into the laboratory. He clearly remembered trying to impress them with his keenness and fitness by working as hard as he could and as a consequence had distorted the data.

In this case the laboratory staff were looking for physiological or mechanical reasons why the data for Mr F should be aberrant. In the end, the reason was psychological.

more than one or two aspects. A serious student of human movement will have to go to many sources before the whole picture of what is happening can be revealed.

It is essential for you to remember that when considering human movement in the practical or clinical situation, you will only get a limited view of what is happening and this may give you a false or distorted picture of an individual's ability. Sadly, it is not possible to achieve the ideal situation and take simultaneous measurements of all components of a complex functional activity, but given awareness of the limitations of the way in which human movement is measured and assessed, the right conclusions about how an individual's performance may be corrected or improved may still be reached.

Self-awareness and observational skills

Case study 1.1 was used to illustrate how movement and performance can be affected by a number of factors, which may not always be those that are most obvious. Another interesting fact that became apparent during the testing procedures undertaken on these professional soccer players was that their balance and spatial awareness were surprisingly poor. This information came to light inadvertently during a plyometric testing procedure, when the players found the test hard to complete and lost their balance repeatedly. Despite the fact that their profession required a high level of physical ability, none of the players had a good level of awareness of the way in which their body moved and they all found it difficult to work out how to modify their approach to the plyometric test in order to remain in balance. This lack of consciousness of movement is common in the general population, with most people never considering how they are able to undertake everyday tasks until they lose that ability.

If you think about yourself, do you know exactly what movements occurred in the joints of your upper limb as you picked up this book and opened it? Were you even aware of the process or did it happen automatically? All people, during their waking hours, are constantly moving and yet they rarely stop to analyse these movements and have no idea of their level of complexity.

In the later chapters of this book, common activities such as walking or getting out of a chair will be considered and their complexity will become apparent. However, most people are oblivious to the way in which they perform tasks and many daily activities occur at a subconscious,

---

Task 1.1

You need to develop personal self-awareness and the skills of observation if you are to have a full understanding of normal movement. This can be done in a number of ways, all of which require you to put in some effort:

1. Try to become aware of all parts of your body. For example, think about the position of your shoulder girdle: is it elevated or depressed? Be aware of your vertebral column: are the various components flexed, extended or laterally flexed? Constantly reevaluate how your body is aligned and notice how your body changes the alignment of its parts for different activities. Become aware of the differing ranges of joint movement that can occur between individuals; compare yourself with others to see if your joints are more or less mobile. Notice what it feels like when you reach the limit of a movement. Is it the same feeling for all joints?
2. Think about what your body feels like when it moves in contrast to when it is still. If some movements cause discomfort, ask yourself why and try to work out exactly which structures are involved. Is it because you have moved too near to the limit of your normal range of movement or because you are working a muscle particularly hard?
3. Notice the difference in feeling when a muscle is contracted or relaxed by making a very tight fist and holding it tight for 30 seconds. Then relax and notice the changing sensations as relaxation occurs: is the process of relaxation instantaneous?
4. Try to become aware of the way in which your body weight is distributed during activities which require balance ability. Is your weight equally distributed between both feet or is it more on one foot than the other? Consider whether your weight is distributed across the whole foot evenly or if there is more taken through the ball of the foot than the heel. What advantages come from different alignments of body weight across one or both feet?

reflex level. This frees the brain to undertake other tasks at the same time; for example, it becomes possible for a musician to play a guitar, sing and move about the stage simultaneously.

If a detailed analysis of everyday activities is carried out, it is clear that there are patterns of joint movement and muscle action which are common to several activities. For example, going up stairs uses the same basic pattern of movement as standing up from a chair or walking up a slope. Swinging the upper limbs in walking is similar to taking food to the mouth, though the range of movement is different. The brain works in terms of patterns of movement rather than movement of individual joints and contractions of individual muscles. It is probably because of this that tasks performed frequently become reflex. As long as the ability to perform tasks automatically exists, most familiar movements can be undertaken in a smooth and efficient manner. When this ability is lost, perhaps through injury or disease, movement becomes noticeably slower and less coordinated.

Anyone whose work involves the moving human body needs to become aware of the way normal movement occurs and which patterns of movement are frequently used. The best way to do this is to start by increasing personal self-awareness and then backing this up with theoretical knowledge from research papers. Once understanding and awareness of normal movement are acquired, it becomes possible to recognise deviations from normal and to plan rehabilitation or training programmes with precision.

Knowledge of human movement through direct experience

Few people consciously explore their full potential for movement, but students of human movement must become very aware of themselves and the way they move before they can consider others. It is as important to be aware of movement and to 'feel' or consciously experience joints moving and muscles contracting as it is to observe others.

In addition to developing self-awareness, it is also essential to learn observational skills, as these are the mainstay of work with the human body. Every opportunity should be taken to observe the movements of other people. Look at the different

---

Task 1.2

Do elderly people move differently from the young; or women from men? If you think the answer is yes, then you should try to identify the differences.

---

ways in which they walk or stand and try to identify exactly what makes one person move differently from another. Be precise in this, observing not only which joint moves but by how much or how fast. As you develop the skills of observation you should try to compare groups of people and analyse any differences you may see.

Understanding human movement and its clinical application

To develop the skills of human movement analysis, it is first important to become more self-aware and this, combined with a knowledge of relevant research, will lead to an understanding of many of the factors of 'normal' movement. This needs to be combined with the ability to observe, in a structured and purposeful manner, the way other people perform everyday activities. In the professional setting it is possible to use the senses of hearing, sight and touch to collect information about an individual and their problems. The skills of interviewing, listening with understanding, looking and seeing, palpating and testing all contribute to a pool of qualitative knowledge. This can then be enhanced by using modern measurement equipment to obtain quantitative data.

When working with patients or clients, it is necessary to identify the skills they require to perform activities of daily living and to analyse the way in which they actually try to undertake these activities. With this knowledge it becomes possible to consider how certain tasks might be made more efficient or how a person with a disability might be helped towards greater independence. Specific problems can be identified, goals set and a realistic programme designed. Finally, the individual's progress will need to be regularly evaluated and goals altered when necessary. By systematically approaching each person's movement problems in this way, clinical judgement will be developed and clinical practice enhanced.

USING THIS BOOK

For practical reasons, research into human movement has to be broken down into small parts and this book reflects the same approach. In the initial chapters some of the different theoretical approaches to studying human movement are considered. This is followed by an overview of the qualitative and quantitative ways in which human movement is measured. Finally, in the later chapters there is a more holistic evaluation of some common everyday activities and consideration of how movement can be affected by factors such as ageing or stress.

Use the early chapters, in conjunction with other specialised textbooks, to gain a grounding in the theories underpinning how human movement is planned, initiated and controlled. This basic knowledge is essential to understanding what is happening when movement occurs. Use the later chapters as introductions to the way in which various parts of the body contribute to functional movement and to how complex movements are analysed. These chapters will also consider some of the common factors that lead to deviations from normal movement patterns.

Throughout the book there are case studies which form the link between theory and real life. If you are already working with patients or clients, then you should try to see how the content of the chapters relates to your experience.

In all the chapters there are tasks that are designed to encourage thought or help you develop skills. If you are to benefit fully from the learning process you should undertake each task, attempting to fulfil all its requirements. Some of the tasks are short but a number will develop into skills that you will use for the rest of your working life. Most of these tasks are easy and do not require answers to be provided within the book; if you are unsure of any of the answers then reread the relevant parts of the chapter, discuss the problem with your colleagues and talk to more experienced staff.

When you use this book you must be aware that it is a basic text designed as an introduction to the study of human movement. It is not a definitive repository of all knowledge in the subject area but should help in your understanding of more advanced research. If you are to become an expert in human movement then you must constantly strive to further your knowledge through reading and enquiry. This should not be a burdensome task because human movement is a fascinating subject, intriguing in its complexity and of direct interest to every one of us.

Chapter 2

Musculoskeletal basis for movement

Marion Trew

LEARNING OUTCOMES

At the end of this chapter you should be able to:

1. Understand how the skeletal system is able to fulfil several different roles

2. Understand how the design of the skeletal system facilitates movement

3. Describe the structure and function of muscle

4. Discuss the physiological processes for the different types of contraction

5. Explain the role of the muscle in different activities

6. Discuss the different types of muscle activity.

INTRODUCTION

The majority of animals have evolved as specialists; for example, the greyhound is a dedicated running machine with limited precision, whereas the elephant is power personified. In contrast, the human body is a marvel of versatility, having the ability to move with precision, power and speed. The human limbs, unlike the limbs in most other mammals, can be moved into a wide range of positions, leading to the ability to perform an infinite variety of tasks on all aspects of the body. The anatomical structure that gives humans such versatility also enables the grace and precision that we see in an ice dancer or the power of a weight lifter; it can give the dexterity of a neurosurgeon or the speed of an Olympic free-style swimmer.

How the skeletal system facilitates this versatility is considered in the first section of this chapter. In addition, we look at the anatomical 'defence mechanisms' that enable the body to cope with unexpected forces and trauma. The second section of the chapter addresses the structure and role of skeletal muscle in human movement. Throughout the chapter examples of human movement will be used to show how the design of the human body enables it to function magnificently.

To understand human movement and to be able to analyse the range of activities that are possible, it is essential to have a good understanding of anatomy, biomechanics and muscle function. This chapter does not attempt to reproduce this basic information as it can be found in great detail in specialist textbooks. Our aim is to address some of the important factors that explain how human movement is able to take place and through this, enable you to make sense of the more theoretical information provided in anatomy or biomechanics textbooks. Before commencing this chapter, you should make sure you have a basic knowledge of human anatomy and the terminology relating to movement. Figure 2.1 acts as a reminder.

THE SKELETAL SYSTEM

The skeleton has a number of purposes related to movement:

- providing shape to the body
- facilitating movement through a network of different types of joints
- providing attachments for muscles, ligaments and joint capsules
- protecting the vital organs and delicate structures
- absorbing or dissipating stress generated by movement or external forces.

The design of the skeletal system is closely related to its function. The rigidity of the bones ensures that the body has a constant form and the shape and alignment of the individual bones dictate the overall shape of the body. Whilst, theoretically, it might seem desirable to have a body like an amoeba so that we could change shape and mould round or between structures, there would be a major drawback. Animals without a rigid skeleton have little ability to manipulate their surroundings; they can respond to their environment but fail to make a large impact upon it.

The human skeleton has a large number of bones, the rigidity of which gives the body shape; however, by having many bones connected by joints, the human body has a wide range of movement options (Fig. 2.2). Some of the joints, such as the ball and socket arrangement of the shoulder joint, allow a massive range of movement. Other joints are designed to give great stability with only small amounts of flexibility. This is seen in the pelvis where the two sacroiliac joints and the pubic symphysis have very little movement, but their rigidity allows substantial forces to pass safely through the bones during weight bearing. One of the functions of the pelvis is to support the weight of the trunk over the moving lower limbs; by having joints rather than being a continuous ring, it also provides some capacity for shock absorption and a small amount of flexibility to cope with compressive forces applied to the rim of the pelvis.

The shape of the bones is closely related to function. Protuberances and spiny processes increase the amount of bone surface available for soft tissue attachment. For example, the transverse and spinous processes on the vertebrae greatly enhance the surface area of each bone. Without these processes, the muscles and ligaments would

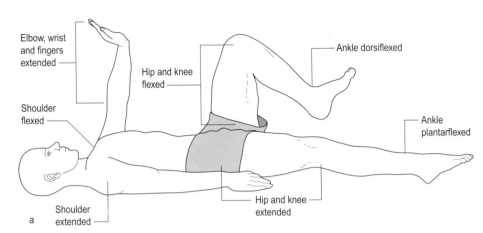

Elbow, wrist
and fingers
extended

Hip and knee
flexed

Ankle dorsiflexed

Shoulder
flexed

Ankle
plantarflexed

Shoulder
extended

Hip and knee
extended

a

Figure 2.1   (a) Some of
the major joints in
positions of flexion and
extension. (b) Hip and
shoulder joints in varying
degrees of abduction.

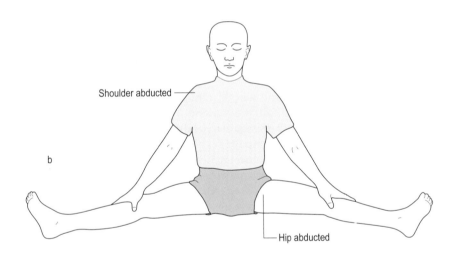

Shoulder abducted

b

Hip abducted

be competing for space and would have to manage with much smaller areas of attachment. This would weaken them and increase the likelihood of soft tissue avulsion at times of physical stress.

The shape of bones also affects the mechanics of movement by altering the line of force of muscles and their tendons. The processes of the vertebrae not only extend the area of bone available for soft tissue attachment but also facilitate the turning moments produced by muscles by lengthening the lever arm. The organisation of the spinous and transverse processes of the vertebrae is ideal for this purpose and is mimicked in many everyday objects where a turning force is required. A good example of this can be seen in the design of taps and is illustrated in Figure 2.3. Just as bony protuberances are valuable, so are the grooves that are found in many bones. Within the grooves lie tendons, often held in place by transverse bands of fibrous tissue such as retinaculae. These grooves ensure that tendons are held in a fixed position regardless of whether they are contracting or relaxed. This means that the direction of force produced by a muscle is consistent.

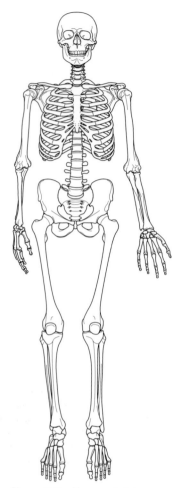

Figure 2.2   Human skeleton.

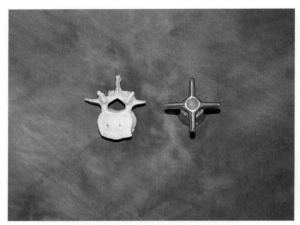

Figure 2.3   Similarity between structure of a vertebra and a tap. This arrangement lengthens the lever arm between the point of force application and the axis of movement, providing a mechanical advantage over structures where the turning force is applied closer to the axis. In the human, the force is applied at the point of muscle attachment and the axis of movement is located within the joint.

The skeletal system plays a major role in protecting vulnerable structures and its effectiveness means that humans can undertake quite extreme movement activities with the reasonable expectation that important organs such as the brain, heart and kidneys will be safe. Protection occurs through the provision of bony cavities in which vital structures are housed. The three major bony cavities of the skull, thorax and pelvis are good examples of this.

Forces and stresses

There are always forces acting on the body and it is therefore important to be aware of their effects and the way in which these forces can be used to facilitate movement or, conversely, where defence mechanisms are needed to ensure that they do not cause damage.

The basic structure of the body is a series of long and short bones connected at joints. Each joint has a specific design that allows for movement in certain directions. Movement at joints is produced by either internal or external forces. Internal forces are generated by muscle contraction, whereas external forces are produced outside the body. Both these forces impact on the body and need to be precisely controlled. Gravity is perhaps the most important external force as it is always present and must be taken into account when considering the factors responsible for movement. Other external forces could be manual pressure, as seen when a physiotherapist pushes against a patient's limb, or a mechanical force produced by a door swinging into someone. Even the wind, as a variable external force, can have a substantial effect, producing or altering movement.

Some external forces are desirable and can be used to replace muscle activity, thus reducing energy expenditure. Normally muscle contraction produces movement but whenever a movement takes place in the direction of gravity, the prime factor in producing movement will be gravity itself and the only role for muscles will be to control or enhance the effect of gravity so that the required movement takes place. All downward movements such as sitting down, stepping down and bending down are primarily produced by gravity, the muscles only being used to initiate the activity and control the speed of movement.

Some external forces are not particularly desirable as they may have the potential to cause injury. Each time we take a step and the heel strikes the floor, a 'ground reaction force' is transmitted through the whole body. As the speed of walking increases so do the ground reaction forces, leading to greater forces through the lower limb and an increased likelihood of injury. If fast movement is to occur but injury be avoided, it is essential to have mechanisms to attenuate the effects of the ground reaction forces so that the body is not damaged by their sudden and repeated application. At heel strike the relatively soft heel pad on the sole of the foot initially absorbs some of the force. Simultaneously the knee flexes as the limb takes the load of the body and this movement of approximately 40° of knee flexion has a shock absorption effect (Payne 1998). Further small movements at the hip and spine will absorb residual forces so that by the time the forces reach the skull and brain, there is a minimal effect.

Forces are transmitted in straight lines. Every time they meet an interface between tissues, some are absorbed by the soft tissues and bone and others are reflected. Close inspection of the skeleton shows that there is no single, straight structure running the length of the body and thus there is no direct route of force transmission. All the long bones in the body are curved, as is the vertebral column. As externally applied forces are transmitted through the bones, the curvatures will cause the forces to repeatedly meet tissue interfaces and on each occasion some of the force will be absorbed or deflected. By the time the forces have reached the cervical spine and the skull, much of the effect has been removed and jarring at the junction of the skull and the vertebral column is kept to a minimum.

There is a second advantage to having curved bones. When a force is applied longitudinally to a

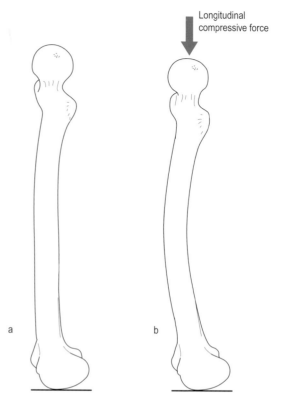

Figure 2.4   The femur is slightly curved, giving a posterior concavity. (a) When a compressive force is applied longitudinally to the femur, the curvature increases, absorbing some of the force in the process. (b) Longitudinal compressive forces will cause a small increase in the curvature.

curved structure such as the femur, the bone will deform and the magnitude of the curve will increase, absorbing some of the forces rather than transmitting them to the more vulnerable structures such as the cervical spine and skull (Fig. 2.4). The absorbed forces form elastic (potential) energy which is released as kinetic energy as the bone returns to its resting shape. This energy transfer is used to benefit many human movements. For example, a higher jump can be achieved if compressive forces are applied to the long bones in the lower limb immediately before take-off. This is one of the effects utilised by plyometric exercise.

The influence of bone shape on movement

Dissipating longitudinal forces is a major function of the curved long bones but there is another

---

Task 2.1

To do this task you will need to work with a friend.

   Stand still and then jump up as high as you can, touching the wall at the peak of your jump. Get your friend to record where you touched.

   Then stand on a low stool. Jump off it, immediately rebounding to jump up as high as you can, again touching the wall. You should be able to jump higher on the second attempt because the small jump off the stool will have caused a compressive force to pass through your lower limbs and the potential energy caused by this will be released simultaneously with your muscle contractions to produce the main jump. This will enable you to jump higher.

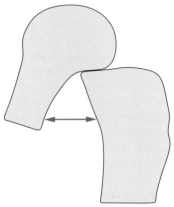

Figure 2.5   The curved nature of the lower limb bones provides space for housing the bulk of the hamstrings and calf muscles, thus facilitating a large range of joint movement.

benefit to having bones that are not entirely straight. Curved bones provide a 'cave' in which muscles may lie. All joints are surrounded by the muscles that produce movement, but these muscles are often bulky and can get in the way of the desired movement. Where a joint permits movement that brings two bones closely together, for example in knee flexion, the muscles attached to the posterior aspect of the femur and the tibia and fibula will come into contact as flexion nears its limit. The larger the muscles, the sooner they will come into contact with each other and thus halt the movement before the physiological end of joint range has been reached. The range of movement can be slightly increased by the curvature in the long bones. Both the femur and the tibia are concave posteriorly and as full knee flexion is reached these concavities provide some additional space in which the major muscles can lie (Fig. 2.5).

   Apart from the bulk of the muscle preventing full-range joint flexion, there is another factor that could restrict joint movement if it were not for the bony architecture. Consider a hypothetical femur and tibia where the bones are straight and the joint surfaces are set centrally at the end of each bone (Fig. 2.6). On flexion, the posterior articular surface of the tibia would impinge on the femoral shaft before a reasonable range of flexion had been achieved. To avoid this problem, the distal articular surface of the femur is set posteriorly. This enables a greater excursion of the tibial articular surface before contact with the femur occurs. In addition,

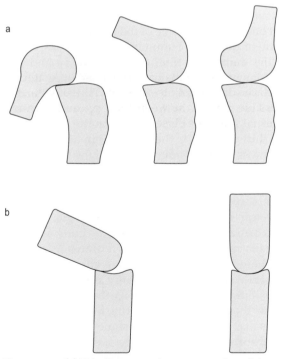

Figure 2.6   (a) This diagrammatic representation of the femur and tibia shows how the design of the articular surfaces facilitates a large range of movement. (b) A hypothetical, simple design for the femur and tibia shows that the range of movement would be substantially restricted.

Task 2.2

Look at the skeleton and decide whether there are any other joints that have articular surfaces offset from the line of the bones.

this structural arrangement increases the space between the two bones in which the muscles can lie.

Joints

All joints where significant movement occurs are synovial in structure. The joint surfaces are covered with hyaline cartilage and surrounding the joint is a strong fibrous capsule lined with a synovial membrane that produces synovial fluid. The combination of fluid and the shiny cartilaginous surfaces produces an almost friction-free environment that enables the muscles to direct their energies to moving the bones, rather than to overcoming friction. However, when the joint surfaces become worn with age or disease, the loss of the low friction environment impedes movement, which becomes increasingly difficult and tiring.

All synovial joints have one position where the surfaces fit precisely together and there is maximal possible contact between the opposing surfaces. This is called the close packed position and when in this position the ligaments and surrounding soft tissue are at their tightest, compressing the two joint surfaces together. In some joints, as the surfaces approach the close packed position one of the bones may rotate in relation to the other and this twisting action further tightens the surrounding soft tissue. These mechanisms mean that in the close packed position, the joint is at its most stable. When not in this position, the joint is said to be in the loose packed position and accessory movements may occur. Each joint has a least packed position in which the capsule is at its most lax. Joints tend to assume this position when there is inflammation in order to accommodate the increased volume of synovial fluid.

The open and closed kinetic chain concept

It has become fashionable to consider the human body in engineering terms and whilst this often helps with understanding biomechanics, it can sometimes lead to problems. The term 'kinetic chain' is used in engineering to describe a series of rigid segments linked to each other by hinge joints and fixed at each end to form a closed system. When one of the segments is moved, it always causes stereotypical movement of the adjacent segment and that in turn affects the next segment and so on. The human body functions in a similar way and so it has been found useful to apply the kinetic chain concept.

The long bones represent the chains and they are linked by joints, though not necessarily hinge joints. The kinetic chain concept explains why movement at one joint will have an effect on nearby joints; for example, flexion at the hip joint will cause flexion at the lumbar spine while full shoulder flexion leads to thoracic extension. Knowing how the human body can act as a kinetic chain can be important in circumstances when it is necessary to move one joint but keep nearby joints motionless, for example in exercise following localised injury. Conversely, when one joint is stiff or inhibited from moving, knowledge of the kinetic chain leads us to move an adjacent joint in order to cause desirable, secondary movements at the affected joint.

Despite its usefulness, care must be taken when using the kinetic chain concept because the human body is not an engineering structure and does not always function stereotypically. In engineering the chain is fixed at both ends but in the human it could be argued that the ends of the chain are not fixed as they comprise the hands, the feet and the head. In biomechanics, the term 'closed kinetic chain' is used when at least one end of the human chain is temporarily fixed; for example, in squatting the weight of the body keeps the foot fixed to the supporting surface, technically closing the chain at that end. For the upper limb, if the hands are firmly gripping onto a fixed structure such as an overhead bar and the body weight is raised towards the bar, this could be described as a closed chain activity. The term 'open kinetic chain' is used when the hands, the feet or the head are not attached to a fixed structure during limb movement. Sitting on a high chair and extending the leg against a weight would be described as an open chain exercise.

Unfortunately the concept is not easily applied to human movement. For example, a true chain system requires that the chain is fixed at both ends, but there are very few human activities that conform to this rule. A modified kinetic chain concept has been adopted but the versatility of human movement still gives rise to problems; not least is the uncertainty about where the chain ends. Some authorities state that the pelvis or shoulder girdle constitutes the fixed end to the chain but both these girdles are capable of movement and the kinetic chain effect can be transmitted beyond them. When used in engineering, the chain concept tells us that movement of one segment will cause a predictable movement in all the other segments. In human movement such predictability is not possible as voluntary muscle activity can hold a joint still despite movement in adjacent joints and this will prevent the chain effect.

UPPER LIMB CONSIDERATIONS

The upper limb consists of the shoulder girdle, humerus, radius, ulna and the bones of the wrist and hand. The primary functions of upper limb are to:

- enable grasping and manipulation of objects
- play a role in communication
- provide major sensory input
- support the body weight in a limited way
- act as a weapon or a means of transmitting force.

The shoulder girdle

The shoulder girdle is quite different from the pelvic girdle in terms of its structure, weight and capacity for movement. Upper limb weight bearing is not a major function and whilst some of the body weight can easily be taken on the hands, it is uncommon for the upper limb to carry the whole weight of the body. As weight bearing is not a major consideration, the bones of the shoulder girdle are relatively lightweight in comparison with their pelvic counterparts.

Whilst the pelvis forms a strong bony ring in order to support the body weight, the shoulder girdle is better described as half a ring. The anterior part of the girdle consists of the acromion processes of the scapulae, the clavicles and the manubrial part of the sternum, all joined to each other. Posteriorly the scapulae are loosely connected to the ribs through the muscles and, in the absence of ligaments, a large range of movement is possible. The anterior part of the shoulder girdle gains most of its stability through the involvement of the sternum, a robust bone with little movement. The sternoclavicular and acromioclavicular joints provide a moderate amount of mobility that enables the position of the glenohumeral joint to vary over about 50°.

The shoulder girdle is a compromise between rigidity and mobility. When movements of the shoulder girdle and shoulder joint are combined, the upper limb has a high degree of mobility, an essential attribute if the hands are to have access to all areas of the body and surrounding space. Unfortunately this mobility can leave the shoulder complex vulnerable to injury when powerful forces are applied, and dislocation of the glenohumeral joint is common.

For effective upper limb activity, the visual field and the range of movement of the upper limb and hands must correspond. The scapula, rather than lying on the posterior aspect of the thorax, is displaced anteriorly in order to facilitate the hands working in front of the body where the eyes can see them. This position of the scapula ensures the shoulder joint muscles are working in their stronger, middle range when the hand is performing activities within the visual field. If the scapula was to be positioned posteriorly then the shoulder flexor and extensor muscles would have to function in a less optimum and weaker part of their range when the hands were brought together. There is limited need to have hands behind body other than for a small number of toileting and dressing activities and so it is of little consequence that these movements utilise the end of joint and muscle range.

Feeding is an important function of the upper limb and the relationship between the humerus and the scapula facilitates this activity. In its resting position the humerus is rotated slightly medially, a position that means that simple elbow flexion will bring the hand directly in front of the

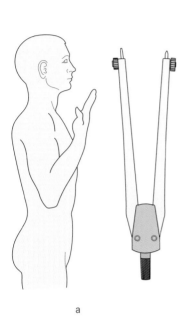
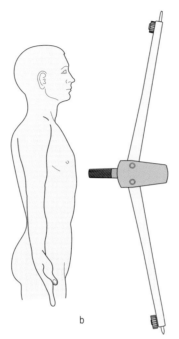

Figure 2.7   A comparison of compass and elbow joint showing how a simple hinge design can bring two points close together.

a

b

face, rather than to the anterior aspect of the shoulder. This anatomical arrangement ensures that getting the hand in front of the mouth or eyes requires minimal muscle activity at the shoulder. When the natural movement is disrupted, for example by holding an implement such as a spoon, the effective length of the forearm is changed and getting the spoon into the mouth requires an increased range of shoulder joint abduction. This immediately increases energy expenditure.

The function of the shoulder girdle/joint complex is to position the upper limb anywhere in the space surrounding the body. The role of the elbow joint is mainly to convert the upper limb from a long grasping unit to a short limb, bringing the hands close to the body. To do this the elbow works like the joint in a pair of compasses, with the humerus and the forearm acting as the limbs of the compass. As the 'compass' closes or opens up so the limb appears shorter or longer and the hand moves towards or away from the body (Fig. 2.7). If the elbow joint is injured and held rigidly in extension then it becomes impossible to get the hand to the face or indeed to any part of the upper body.

The forearm and wrist

The more distal joints have an increasingly important role in the precise placement of the hand. The superior radio-ulnar joint lies in very close proximity to the elbow joint, but its function is quite different. Whilst the elbow joint is responsible for the gross movement of shortening or lengthening the limb, both radio-ulnar joints have a major function in positioning the hand with precision. This they do in conjunction with the wrist joint. The radio-ulnar joints allow pronation and supination to take place and it is this rotation that enables the hand to be placed in the ideal position for grasping any object. The wrist joint is then responsible for final adjustments to enable the hand to correspond exactly with the object to be gripped. That leaves the fingers and thumb to produce the precision activity of grip. The muscles that lie most distally in the limb take responsibility for precise movements and it is for this reason that there are many more muscles between the elbow and the hand than between the scapula and the elbow.

The hand

For humans, the combination of a large brain and a hand with an opposable thumb has without doubt led to advanced abilities. However, having a thumb that is set at right angles to the other digits to allow opposition is not the sole reason for the hand's success. The secret lies in the hand's versatility. The anatomy of the hand enables it to convert instantaneously from a means of communication to a weapon, a power tool or a precision instrument. An examination of the structure of the hand reveals how this is all possible.

The hand has a substantial number of muscles to control the fine and power movements that are necessary for normal function. If all these muscles were to be located within the hand it would become excessively bulky and delicate movement would be impossible. To avoid the bulkiness that would interfere with function, many of the muscles that control the digits are located more proximally within the forearm and the forces that they generate are conveyed through long, slender tendons to the appropriate digits. As these tendons cross the wrist before reaching the fingers, they influence wrist as well as finger movement and it is possible that their dual role facilitates very precise adjustments of position. Having long tendons crossing a fairly mobile joint like the wrist introduces a potential problem. When the muscles contract to produce flexion and extension there is the potential for a bow-stringing effect to take place (Fig. 2.8). This is undesirable but simply avoided by placing a fine bracelet of connective tissue, called a retinaculum, around the wrist to hold the tendons in close contact with the bones. A similar arrangement is found at the ankle.

The carpal bones, the metacarpals and the phalanges of the hand are all concave anteriorly, giving the hand an arched structure. The arches of the hand provide some protection for the soft tissues when the hand is weight bearing, but they also enable the hand to mould round different shaped objects. There are three arches:

- a longitudinal arch from finger tips to wrist
- a transverse arch from medial to lateral side of hand and wrist
- an oblique arch running diagonally across the hand.

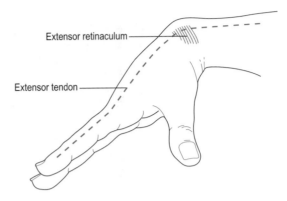

The extensor retinaculum of the wrist holds the finger extensors in place during movements of the wrist

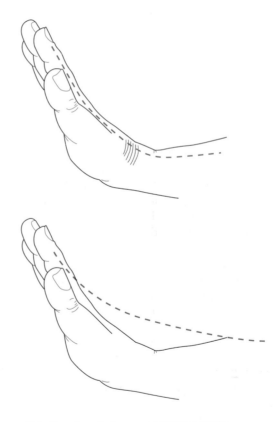

If the finger flexor tendons were not held against the bones, on wrist extension they would act like a bow string. To compensate for this there would need to be very loose skin around the wrist and fingers, and a loss in mechanical efficiency of the muscles.

Figure 2.8 The tendons of the finger extensor muscles held in place by a retinaculum.

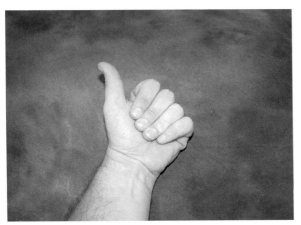

Figure 2.9 Convergence of the fingers to the thenar eminence enhances the ability to grip objects in the palm of the hand.

Task 2.3

Flex your fingers in the same way as shown in Figure 2.9. Note how the finger tips come to rest on your thenar eminence. Now try to perform the same movement so that your fingers lie straight rather than obliquely across the palm of your hand. With considerable effort, it is nearly possible – but not quite. As a second task, allow your flexed fingers to rest on your thenar eminence and then try, whilst maintaining this position, to separate them. You will find this abduction impossible. Start to allow your fingers to extend at the metacarpophalangeal joints and note how much extension needs to occur before you can abduct the fingers.

These arches are flexible and can, to an extent, be flattened by muscle action or by the pressure exerted by objects held in the hand, making the hand a very pliant structure.

The ability to grip effectively is also enhanced by the direction of finger flexion. The structure of the metacarpophalangeal joints results in the combined movements of flexion and adduction so that as the fingers flex, the adduction brings the fingers together and ensures that small objects cannot fall between them. The size and alignment of the metacarpal bones also cause the finger tips to converge diagonally towards the thenar eminence as the joints flex (Fig. 2.9). The angulation of the fingers causes a deep groove to form between the metacarpal heads and the thenar eminence overlaying the oblique arch of the hand. This ensures that cylindrical objects such as the handle of a hammer can be held extremely securely in the hand. It also enables the middle, ring and little fingers to grip an object, freeing the thumb and index finger to perform simultaneous precision activities.

The functional components of the hand

To understand the multiplicity of movement functions that the hand can perform, it is helpful to consider that the hand can be divided into three functional components.

First there is the thumb, which is positioned at right angles to the other fingers and is therefore able to wrap around objects held in the hand and produce an effective grip. When the thumb works in synergy with all the other fingers, a power grip is produced. If a precision grip is required then only the thumb and one or two other fingers are involved.

The second functional component consists of the index and middle fingers, including their metacarpal bones. These two fingers have longer, thicker and stronger bones than the other fingers, and stronger ligaments. When a fist is formed, the heads of these long metacarpal bones are more prominent than the rest and well designed to transmit forces. If the hand is used to punch then the force of the blow should be transmitted through the second and third metacarpal bones. The strength of their ligaments lends rigidity to their structure which ensures that longitudinal forces will not drive the two metacarpals apart. The strength of these two fingers also helps the formation of a powerful tripod grip, using the thumb, index and middle fingers. Indeed, it is mainly these two fingers that work in conjunction with the thumb in all precision grips. They have the ability to perform in a very precise manner but, if required, can exert considerable force onto the object they are holding or absorb large external forces.

The third functional component comprises the ring and little fingers, and is distinguished by its

Task 2.4

You can test the flexibility of the medial side of your hand quite easily by gripping the metacarpal heads of your index and middle finger of your left hand and attempting to move them anteriorly and posteriorly. You will find that they feel quite stiff. Now grasp the metacarpal heads of your ring and little fingers and try to move these. In this case you will notice how much more freely they move, in particular the little finger.

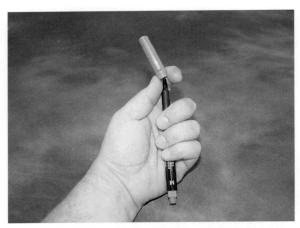

Figure 2.10 The hand is so well designed that it is able to perform complex grips simultaneously involving power and precision activities.

flexibility. The role of this medial component of the hand is to give a flexible grip, enabling the hand to mould around different-shaped objects, pulling the object into the centre of the hand and towards the opposed thumb. These two metacarpal bones are shorter and more delicate than the others and the shape of their joint surfaces results in the flexed fingers moving diagonally across the palm towards the thenar eminence. This facilitates a number of grips but in particular enables the combination power/precision grip to occur. An example of this is found when a pen is gripped in the hand using a power grip. The pen naturally lies diagonally across the hand with the medial fingers wrapped round it while the position of the pen means that the thumb and index finger can be released from the power grip and used to manipulate the cap off the pen (Fig. 2.10). If all the metacarpal bones were of the same length then the pen would be held horizontally across the palm and the thumb and index finger would not be able to oppose to manipulate the cap. The only way the pen cap could be removed would be to involve the contralateral hand.

Carrying angle

One of the major functions of the upper limb is to carry objects, some of which may be heavy. The most energy-efficient way of carrying an object in one hand would be to allow the upper limb to lie in its natural relaxed position of shoulder adduction and medial rotation and elbow extension and with the forearm in the mid position between pronation and supination. In this position, the only significant muscle activity would come from the finger flexors

and the energy requirements would be low. Unfortunately, in this position, unless the object being carried is very thin, it will catch on the lower limbs during walking and to avoid this annoyance, the shoulder has to abduct slightly to move the object away from the body. This causes a considerable increase in muscle activity and energy expenditure and can become uncomfortable after a short period of time. The solution lies in the carrying angle of the elbow. The trochlea and the trochlear groove of the humerus are slightly offset from the horizontal and vertical respectively. When the elbow is extended and the forearm supinated, the radius and ulna are angled laterally, so that the hand lies several centimetres away from the thigh. In this position the supinated forearm can rest on the lateral border of the iliac crest, transmitting some of the load through the pelvis, and the hand holding the load is angled away from the lower limb (Fig. 2.11). This angulation also means that on elbow flexion the radius and ulna do not come to lie directly over the humerus, but are deviated medially towards the mouth.

LOWER LIMB CONSIDERATIONS

A simple observation of the upper and lower limbs shows that they are very similar in structure. The pelvic girdle forms a strong, rigid union with

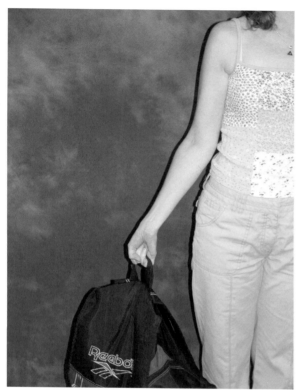

Figure 2.11 The skeletal structure of the upper limb produces a 'carrying angle' at the elbow. This arrangement gives an energy-efficient way of carrying objects without them catching on the lower limb.

the trunk and has a more mobile union with the lower limbs. The largest and most proximal lower limb bone is the femur; distal to that are the tibia and fibula and then the tarsal bones, metatarsals and phalanges. The hip joint functions to position the limb in space, the knee enables the limb to shorten or lengthen using the compass principle and the foot–ankle complex ensures full contact with any supporting surface.

The main functions of the lower limb are to:

- support the body weight
- enable locomotion to take place
- provide supplementary force during pushing or lifting.

To fulfil these it needs to be both strong and relatively mobile, but unlike the upper limb it has little requirement for precision activity.

The pelvic girdle

The pelvic girdle has to transmit considerable forces between the trunk and the lower limbs and to perform this task effectively it consists of a continuous ring of bone. To reduce the weight of the pelvis, there are two large holes in the bone (the obturator foramina) and the majority of the rest of the bone has a lightweight cancellous structure. The hip, knee and ankle joints need to be sturdy in order to survive the forces generated in weight bearing but must have a good range of movement in order to cope with everyday activities. As the main requirement is for stability rather than detailed and precise movements, the tibia and fibula are solidly united with only sufficient movement between them to adapt to transmitted forces and prevent mechanical injury.

To provide stability, the hip joint is firmly supported by ligaments that also tend to restrict the range of movement available. For example, there are only a few degrees of extension available at the hip joint. To compensate for this, when extra hip extension is needed, the kinetic chain effect means that supplementary movements occur in the lumbar spine.

Generating force over a large range of movement

In most activities the hip joint has to bear considerable loads whilst the surrounding muscles generate substantial force. It also has a relatively large range of movement. For example, in climbing, the hip may pass through 120° of movement, raising the full body weight with some force.

Task 2.5

Look in a book or on the Internet to find images of female ballet dancers performing the arabesque (standing with one lower limb extended backwards parallel with the ground). Observe that at first glance, they appear to have up to 90° of hip extension. Now look very closely at the images and you should observe that the degree of hip extension is not as great as first appeared and that a large compensatory lumbar extension gives the illusion of substantial hip extension.

Bearing in mind the length–tension relationship in muscles (see p. 28), it can be reasoned that in the initial position of a climbing action, the major hip extensor muscle – the gluteus maximus – will be at full stretch and therefore least able to generate force. However, the hip joint has a second, important extensor muscle group in the hamstrings. The hamstrings are long muscles crossing both the hip and the knee joints. In the step-up phase of the climbing movement, both the hip and knee joints are flexed and in this position, whilst the gluteus maximus muscle is fully stretched, the hamstring muscles are in mid range and in the optimum position for generating force. As the climbing action continues and the hip and knee both extend, the hamstrings become shorter and less able to generate force but gluteus maximus is now in mid range and ideally positioned to contract strongly (Fig. 2.12). A similar arrangement is seen at the knee where, to facilitate movement, there are both long and short muscles. The rectus femoris muscle passes over both the hip joint and the knee joint, whereas its counterparts in the quadriceps group only cross the knee. This ensures that for different combinations of hip and knee joint movements, there is always one muscle that is at its optimal length for generating muscle force.

In the upper limb the combined movements of shoulder rotation and of pronation and supination enable the hand to be positioned anywhere in space. This degree of precision is not required in the lower limb but to move effectively it is important that the foot can make good contact with the supporting surface, no matter how uneven. The body relies on the combination of movements available at the ankle joint and the small joints of the foot to achieve this. All these joints lie closely together and when working in combination, give the effect of a single, very mobile, but very strong joint.

The foot

The foot is an arched structure, considerably stronger than the hand but having a degree of flexibility that enables the arches to flatten and mould to underlying surfaces. There are two main arches in the foot.

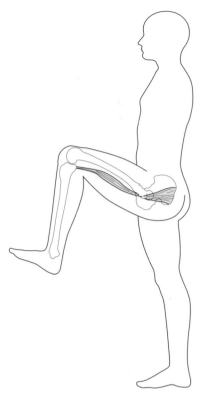

Figure 2.12 When stepping up, the gluteus maximus muscle is initially working in its outer range and therefore weak; however, the hamstrings are kept in their strong, middle range because of the concurrent knee flexion. Towards the end of the step up, the hamstrings will be working in inner range and therefore weak, but the gluteus maximus muscle will be in middle range and able to supply the necessary force.

The longitudinal arch runs from the calcaneus to the metatarsal heads and is subdivided into a medial and a lateral arch, with the calcaneus forming a posterior pillar common to both. The medial arch terminates at the head of the first metatarsal and the lateral arch goes to the head of the fifth metatarsal.

The transverse arch is often described as half an arch because it runs medially from its lowest point, at the head and shaft of the fifth metatarsal on the lateral side of the foot, to its high point at the shaft of the metatarsal of the great toe on the medial side of the foot. When standing with the feet together these two half-arches make one complete arch.

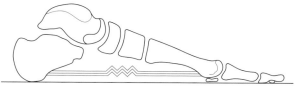

Figure 2.13 The longitudinal plantar structures, such as the plantar aponeurosis, firmly bind the calcaneus to the metatarsal bones and act to maintain the longitudinal plantar arches. These structures have a small degree of elasticity, imparting flexibility to the arches and storing elastic energy.

The arched shape of the foot serves several purposes related to movement. First, the flexibility of the arches means that the foot can mould itself to a variety of supporting surfaces, thus helping the balance process. The benefit of this is noticeable in people with inflexible, prosthetic feet. When a prosthetic foot is placed on an uneven surface, perhaps on a small stone, it acts like a see-saw, the area of contact between the foot and the stone becoming a fulcrum around which the prosthetic foot rotates. This results in significant instability and affects balance. The living foot is able to re-position itself if the supporting surface is uneven and can even mould itself to the surface in order to maintain as much contact with the ground as possible. Second, the strong plantar structures that bind the pillars of the longitudinal arches together impart elasticity to the foot and serve as a shock absorber and energy store (Fig. 2.13). As weight is taken through the foot, the longitudinal arch compresses slightly and the non-contractile plantar structures are stretched, absorbing some of the forces and later imparting these forces as the body is propelled forwards. These are the structures that literally put a 'spring in the step'. Finally the arched structure of the bones provides a shelter in which the more delicate soft tissues such as muscle, nerve and vascular structures can lie, protected from the crushing forces that occur when weight-bearing bone contacts forcefully with the ground. Without this protection the types of locomotion seen in humans would be restricted by the need to avoid soft tissue damage.

The forefoot has both a flexible and a rigid component, similar to those seen in the hand. The metatarsal bones on the medial side are strong and sturdy and firmly bound together by strong ligaments, giving a good degree of rigidity. In normal locomotion most force is transmitted through the great toe and the medial side of the foot. There is a need for substantial rigidity to enable effective power activities such as the 'push-off' phase in walking and running. The lateral side of the foot is less rigid; the metatarsals are more delicate and are loosely supported by ligaments. This gives them the flexibility to mould to uneven surfaces during weight bearing. This anatomical arrangement enables the foot to perform effectively in a range of very different situations.

TRUNK, HEAD AND NECK

The vertebral column runs the whole length of the trunk, connecting the skull to the pelvis and forming the core of the body. The ribs, attached posteriorly to the vertebrae and anteriorly to the sternum, form a protective thoracic cage for the vital organs and provide a relatively firm base of attachment for the shoulder girdle and its muscles.

The functions of the skeletal system of the trunk and head include:

- protecting the vital organs and delicate structures
- providing attachments for muscles, ligaments and joint capsules
- facilitating respiration
- providing attachments for the upper and lower limbs
- absorbing or dissipating stress generated by movement or external forces.

The arrangement of the bones of the trunk and head has resulted in the formation of bony cavities that are well designed to protect the vital organs that they enclose. The bones that form these protective cavities are then utilised as firm bases to which the strong muscles of the trunk and limbs attach. The skull completely encloses and protects the brain and its curved shape ensures that most of the force from trauma to the head will be deflected, rather than being transmitted through the bone and causing fracture and potential brain damage.

The brain is an essential organ and needs to be totally encased in bone for effective protection. There are other essential organs that need effective protection, but it is not functionally possible to encase all of them in a rigid bony shell. If the whole of the trunk were constructed like the skull, it would give excellent protection to vital organs such as the heart, kidneys and lungs but movement of the spine and ribs would not be possible which would leave the human being with limited lung function and the movement ability of a tortoise. The thoracic cage is a compromise of anatomical design that offers a good level of protection to vital structures whilst allowing trunk and rib movement. By having a cage rather than a solid structure, each individual rib can be articulated with the vertebral column posteriorly and can move slightly to facilitate spinal movement. The rib movement is also utilised in respiration. The ribs offer effective though incomplete protection to internal organs but the sternum, lying anteriorly, ensures that the heart is safe from most trauma. Posteriorly the ribs extend down to the level of the 12th thoracic vertebra, but anteriorly their borders and the costal cartilages are angled upwards so that there is no bone below a level of approximately the fifth thoracic vertebra. Similarly the pelvic ring is quite high posteriorly, but has a very shallow anterior border. This bony arrangement facilitates the movement of trunk flexion. Because the majority of the anterior abdomen comprises soft tissue it is able to compress when trunk flexion is required. The more substantial bony structures on the posterior aspect of the trunk tend to limit extension but as this movement is not a major functional necessity, the restriction is of little importance.

The lack of bony protection across the anterior aspect of the abdomen leaves that area of the body vulnerable; however, the most vital structures are placed within the thorax, deep inside the pelvis or nestling safely against the bodies of the vertebrae. The less vital structures such as the intestines are able to withstand considerable trauma before fatal injury occurs and so can be safely placed where bony protection is least effective.

The vertebral column plays a major role in giving shape and support to the trunk and provides the joints at which trunk movement occurs. Of equal importance is its role in protecting the spinal cord and the nerve roots. In order to allow trunk movement without damaging stretch on any one point of the spinal cord, it has evolved as a structure consisting of 33 bones. Between each pair of bones in the cervical, thoracic and lumbar regions is a complex set of joints that permit movement small enough not to damage the spinal cord but when summated between all the vertebrae, the overall movement is sufficient to provide good function. (see Chapter 12 for more detail).

Absorption of forces within the vertebral column

The majority of vertical forces pass through the vertebral column. The column demonstrates four anterior/posterior curves that have a function similar to the curves in the long bones of the limbs. When compressive forces are applied longitudinally to the vertebral column, such as in landing heavily on the feet or having a heavy load fall onto the head, the effect of these forces is attenuated as each of the curves increases in magnitude (Fig. 2.14).

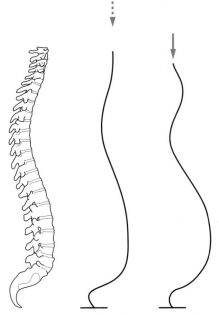

Figure 2.14 The effect of longitudinal compression of the vertebral column is to cause an increase in the cervical, thoracic and lumbar curves. Force is absorbed throughout the length of the column so that the effect on the skull and brain is reduced.

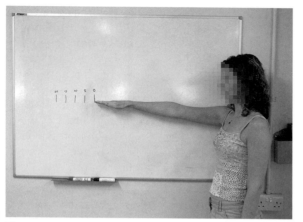
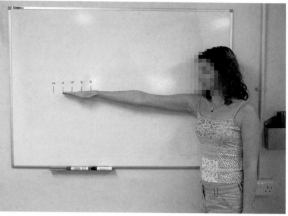

a   b

Figure 2.15   The effect of trunk rotation on increasing the length of reach.

This defence mechanism is enhanced by the intervertebral discs that also deform under compression and absorb some of the force. Without these mechanisms, the incidence of mechanical trauma to the structures at either end of the vertebral column would be greatly increased.

Whilst the joints of the vertebral column do not produce large ranges of movement, they make a valuable contribution to movements taking place in the limbs. For example, when reaching high above the head, shoulder movement can be enhanced by extension of the whole spine; when reaching forwards, reach can be increased by trunk rotation (Fig. 2.15). In the lower limb the effective range of the hip joint is supplemented by associated movements in the lumbar spine.

THE ROLE OF MUSCLES IN MOVEMENT

The skeletal system provides the rigid framework for the body and the joints at which movement can occur, whereas the role of muscles is to cause or control movement. There are three major types of muscle: skeletal (striated), cardiac and smooth muscle. It is beyond the scope of this book to consider cardiac and smooth muscles, found in the heart and the walls of blood vessels and gut, as they have no direct role in human movement. Skeletal muscles, as their name implies, are predominantly attached to bone and their functions are to produce movement of one bone on another, to control movement produced by external forces or to hold bones still in order to maintain posture and balance. Skeletal muscles are under both voluntary and reflex control and their activity is central to human movement.

Muscle attachments

The vast majority of muscles attach to bone, there being only a few that take one or more attachments from soft tissue. Traditionally in anatomy, the more proximal of the two muscle attachments is called the muscle origin and the distal attachment is called the insertion. The proximal attachment is usually the more stationary, in that the proximal bone may be held still and the distal bone will move towards or away from it. For example, the biceps brachii muscle attaches proximally to the scapula and humerus and distally to the radius. In the action of drinking, the scapula and humerus as the proximal bones are kept still whilst the radius and ulna are moved towards them. However, there are instances where this arrangement may change and the roles may be reversed. In this case the distal bone is fixed, often by the hands holding onto something, and the proximal bones are drawn towards it. If neither of the bones is held stationary, then on contraction both bones will move closer together but in normal human movement this is not common. It is more usual for one of the bones to

Task 2.6

When a glass is raised to the lips, the proximal attachment of biceps brachii on the humerus and scapula is held still and all the force is transmitted through the distal attachment on the radius. The effect is to draw the radius towards the humerus, thus flexing the elbow.

If gymnasts hold onto an overhead bar and raise themselves up towards the bar by flexing their elbows, the fixed attachment would be the radius and the humerus becomes the moving bone as the elbow flexes and draws the body up towards the bar.

Now think of two examples using the elbow extensor muscles that would demonstrate how the muscle can produce an activity first with the proximal attachment fixed and then with the distal attachment held still.

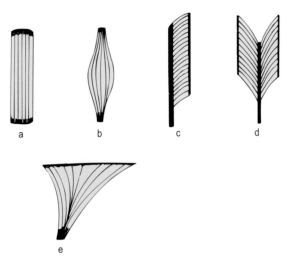

Figure 2.16 Some of the common arrangements of muscles. Strap (a) and fusiform (b) muscles have a tendon at either end and relatively long muscle fibres which run between the tendons. The muscle fibres are arranged in parallel to or are very similar to the angle of pull of the tendon. Unipennate (c) and bipennate (d) muscles have a central tendon into which short muscle fibres are inserted. The fibre direction is different to the angle of pull of the tendon. Triangular muscles (e) display mixed characteristics.

which the muscle is attached to be held still, giving the muscle a fixed base from which to work and the other bone will move.

Skeletal muscle structure

The function of skeletal muscle is to produce or control movement and to fulfil this function it must have components that are capable of contraction. Muscle is not entirely composed of contractile elements – there are parts that are non-contractile, though they may have a small degree of elasticity. Filaments of actin and myosin make up the contractile components and they are responsible for the generation of active force (tension). The non-contractile components include tendons, connective tissue sheaths and structural proteins which, whilst not able to produce contraction, are slightly elastic and contribute to the development of passive tension within the muscle.

An understanding of how skeletal muscle works requires knowledge of its structure from the level of gross anatomy to molecular organisation. Gross muscle structure can easily be observed and the most obvious example of this is the contour of a muscle visible under the skin.

Examination of a dissected specimen shows that most muscles are connected at each end to bones, either through direct attachment or there

may be a tendon or aponeurosis that forms the actual point of attachment. At this stage visual inspection will also reveal that each muscle is encased in an external connective tissue sheath. Through the sheath it is possible to see groups of muscle fibres organised into bundles called fascicles and observation of different muscles will show that the fascicles are arranged in several different ways. The way the fascicles are arranged is often referred to as the muscle architecture and this has an impact on muscle function (Fig. 2.16).

Some muscles have their fibres arranged parallel to the underlying bone and to the direction of force of the whole muscle. This arrangement has two subdivisions, 'strap' and 'fusiform' (L. *fusus* = spindle), the terms being descriptive of the muscle architecture. But in both examples the muscle usually inserts into the bone by a tendon at one if not both ends of its belly. In these muscles the fibres may be many centimetres long and may even run the full length of the muscle. Other muscles may have much shorter fibres that run

Table 2.1   The hierarchy of muscle organisation

Whole muscle	Bundles of fascicles	Surrounded by connective tissue sheath (epimysium)
Muscle fascicles	Groups of muscle fibres	Surrounded by connective tissue sheath (perimysium)
Muscle fibres	Bundles of myofibrils (about 2000) arranged in parallel	Surrounded by connective tissue sheath (sarcolemma) 10–100 µm diameter, multinucleated
Myofibrils	String of sarcomeres arranged in series	Surrounded by sarcoplasmic reticulum and T tubules about 1 µm diameter
Sarcomeres	Functional unit of muscle contraction	Composed of myofilaments and structural, non-contractile proteins
Myofilaments	Actin (thin) and myosin (thick) filaments	

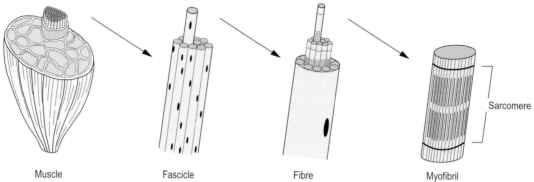

Muscle   Fascicle   Fibre   Myofibril

Figure 2.17   Representation of the relationship between muscle, muscle fibres and myofibrils. The striations in the myofibrils are the result of the arrangement of the actin and myosin filaments. Each myofibril consists of adjacent sarcomeres connected to each other in series. These run the length of the fibre.

diagonally to a central, longitudinal tendon. Whilst the central tendon lies parallel to the direction of force produced by the muscle, the fibres lie at an angle to it. This arrangement is described as pennate (L. *penna* = feather) because the architecture of the fibres bears a strong resemblance to a feather. Pennate muscles can have a simple arrangement or can be bipennate or multipennate. Finally there are some muscles whose fibre architecture is reminiscent of a fan and these are often called fan-like or triangular. They have some long strap-like fibres and some shorter pennate fibres.

Muscle fibres and cells

Moving from gross to microscopic anatomy, a series of subdivisions of muscle can be identified (Table 2.1; Fig. 2.17). Within the whole muscle, groups of muscle fibres are bundled together. The muscle fibres are long, multinucleated muscle cells that may extend over the whole length of the muscle or may be much shorter, depending on the muscle architecture. The muscle fibres require a good blood supply and are surrounded by a network of capillaries. When the muscle is not working most of the capillaries close down but as soon as the muscle becomes active, the capillaries open sufficiently to allow the blood flow to increase to meet the muscle's metabolic demands.

The muscle cells contain many mitochondria that are responsible for aerobic metabolism. The mitochondria enable the muscle to function continuously in the presence of oxygen and their number varies according to fibre type and also endurance training. The cells also contain glycogen and lipid droplets.

Myofibrils

Within the muscle fibre, and running along its length, are bundles of fibrils called myofibrils encased in a sheath called the sarcolemma. Within the myofibril (and also running along the axis of the muscle) are two sets of filaments (thin and thick) which give a striated appearance. The thin filaments primarily consist of the proteins actin and tropomyosin and the thick filaments are mainly formed from a thick protein called myosin.

A membranous network called the sarcoplasmic reticulum surrounds each myofibril. The interior of the sarcoplasmic reticulum is quite separate from the contents of the fibre and contains the calcium that is necessary for the interaction of actin and myosin and the generation of force. The signal for calcium release from the sarcoplasmic reticulum is the arrival of the action potential from the nerve via the neuromuscular junction. This travels over the surface of the fibres and is transmitted into the interior by a series of invaginations in the surface membrane called the T (tubular) system. The sarcoplasmic reticulum is in close proximity to the T tubules and ensures effective calcium release. Once the action potential has passed, calcium is pumped back into the sarcoplasmic reticulum and the muscle relaxes.

The sarcomere

Sarcomeres are the structural units for muscle and many sarcomeres lie in series along the length of each myofibril. To understand them, the arrangement of the thin and thick filaments within the myofibrils needs to be considered in more detail (Fig. 2.18). The thin filaments are arranged as a lattice and attached to a structure that runs transversely across the myofibril, called the Z line. The Z line is attached to the sarcolemma to give it stability. The thick filaments also form a lattice work within the myofibril and their size gives a dark appearance called the A band. Whilst the thick filaments interdigitate with the thin filaments they do not attach to the Z line; instead they are maintained in place by a number of structural proteins. These proteins include some whose purpose is unclear whilst others have an identified role. An example of the latter is dystrophin which is absent or reduced in muscular dystrophy.

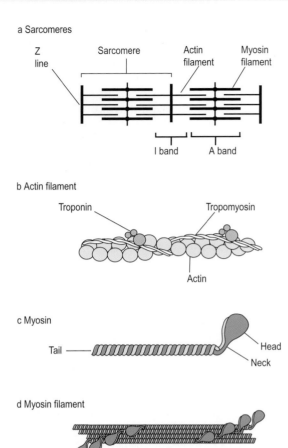

Figure 2.18 (a) Two adjacent sarcomeres. This pattern is repeated along the length of the fibre. The actin (thin) and myosin (thick) filaments give the striations to skeletal muscle. The A band contains both types of filament, while the I band contains only actin filaments. (b) A section of an actin filament, showing the relationship between the actin, troponin and tropomyosin. (c) Myosin molecules consist of two identical chains. The globular head combines with actin and the extensible neck region (S2 fragment) is connected to a long tail or backbone. (d) The myosin molecules are packed together to form the thick filaments. They are rotated so that the heads are arranged around the filament.

The area of myofibril containing only thin filaments and Z line is called the I band as it is light in colour (isotropic). Each area of a myofibril found between two Z lines is called a sarcomere. A sarcomere therefore contains two half I bands and a complete A band. In the centre of the A band there is no overlap of thin and thick filaments so the A band looks paler and this area is called the H zone. Running down the H zone (at right angles to the filaments) is the line of proteins which link the thick filaments together. This line of proteins is called an M line.

The actin filament is a globular protein that appears as double helical strands with tropomyosin and three troponin (Tn) subunits: TnC, TnT and TnI (see Fig. 2.18). The regulatory protein tropomyosin blocks the myosin-binding sites until it is caused to move and uncover them by the binding of calcium to TnC. TnT binds troponin and tropomyosin and TnI inhibits tropomyosin in the absence of calcium.

Myosin filaments are two identical chains arranged in an antiparallel fashion. They have a globular head, called the S1 fragment, that is attached to a flexible 'neck' called the S2 fragment. In turn, the flexible neck region connects to the long tail of the molecule. It is the S1 fragment that forms a crossbridge with the actin filament and causes force generation.

Individual myosin molecules pack together to form a thick filament; the myosin heads project out around all sides of the filament but there is a central area that is entirely free of crossbridges.

Muscle contraction – the sliding filament mechanism

Figure 2.19 is a diagrammatic representation of a muscle contraction. It shows that when a muscle contracts, the actin and myosin filaments do not change length. However, there is a change in the overall length of the sarcomeres caused by changes in the amount of overlap between actin and myosin filaments and this gives the impression of the filament changing length (Huxley & Simmons 1971). The myosin heads attach to binding sites on the actin filaments, forming crossbridges. The myosin heads then rotate, pulling the actin filaments towards the centre of the sarcomeres and exerting a passive extension force on the S2 fragments. This increases the overlap between the actin and the myosin, causing shortening of the sarcomere. The myosin heads are then released and attempt to attach to another binding site and the whole process is called the crossbridge cycle. The crossbridge cycle continues as long as the

muscle is activated and the energy requirements are met.

Factors affecting force generation

Studies on isolated muscle preparations have shown that the force generated by a fully activated muscle fibre, or even a single sarcomere, is affected by a number of factors. These are intrinsic properties of skeletal muscle and also apply to intact human muscles. The factors affecting force generation include:

- muscle length
- type of contraction
- velocity of contraction
- frequency of stimulation
- motor unit recruitment
- muscle fibre type
- muscle fibre alignment.

Length of the muscle

The length of each individual muscle varies depending on whether it has contracted to its limit

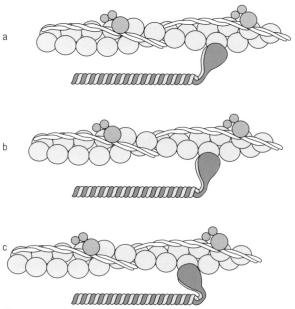

Figure 2.19   During a muscle contraction, the crossbridge of the myosin molecule attaches to a binding site on the actin filament (a), the myosin head rotates (b, c) and pulls the actin filament to the left.

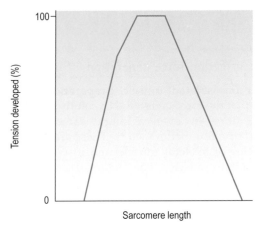

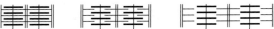

Figure 2.20 The length–tension curve was produced from measurements from a single sarcomere. The sarcomere was stimulated to produce isometric activity at different lengths. The tension developed at each length was recorded. When the sarcomere was short, the force generated was low but when the sarcomere was lengthened, the force increased. The optimal length for force generation was found when the sarcomere was at mid length and the force then declined as the length increased.

and is at its shortest or whether it has been stretched out to its maximum length. How long the muscle is when it is contracting will affect the force it can generate. The active and passive tension that is generated within a muscle will affect the force that is produced.

Active tension is the force generated by cross-bridge activity and is illustrated in Figure 2.20. This figure shows what happens when a muscle is moved from its shortest position to its longest position (moving through full range) and stimulated electrically at numerous different lengths. The electrical stimulation causes activation of the crossbridge cycle and the subsequent increase in overlap between the actin and myosin causes force to be produced. The tension generated in the muscle at each of the different lengths is recorded and a graph can be produced. The contractions measured in this experiment are all isometric. It can be seen that there is an optimum length for force generation. If the muscle is activated when it

is either at its longest or shortest then the force it produces is reduced (Gordon et al 1966); in fact, at the very extremes of length no force is generated. The muscle generates the greatest force when activated in its middle range, in other words when it is neither fully lengthened nor fully shortened.

The explanation for this lies in the amount of overlap between the actin and myosin filaments and underlies the sliding filament theory of contraction (Huxley & Simmons 1971). When the muscle is in its middle range it is in the optimal position for overlap of the actin and myosin filaments and the maximum number of cross-bridges are able to form. This gives greatest force generation. At lengths shorter than optimal, the actin filaments from the two ends of the sarcomere come closer together, causing a disruption in the lattice arrangement of the filaments and the thick filaments collide with the Z line. Fewer cross-bridges are able to form, thus reducing force generation. At lengths longer than optimal, the amount of overlap between actin and myosin filaments decreases, reducing the number of cross-bridges that can be formed and thus the force that can be generated.

Muscles in intact animals and humans do not reach the extremes of length shown in Figure 2.20 because of anatomical constraints. However, a number of intact human muscles demonstrate a length–tension relationship which clearly shows an optimal length and decreasing force as length changes in either direction. Other muscles show flatter curves and this is probably due to bio-mechanical changes and also orientation of fibres within the muscle.

Some muscles in the intact human body develop maximal active tension at approximately the mid-point of joint range, but relatively few muscles have been studied systematically in this respect.

Passive tension develops in the non-contractile elements of muscle and is found whenever a muscle is stretched. The non-contractile elements include the tendons that lie in series with the muscle belly and the connective tissue that surrounds the various components of muscle (lying in parallel). The connective tissue is not totally inelastic; if it were it would seriously hinder movement. It has a small amount of elasticity and if it is stretched, tension develops. Passive tension

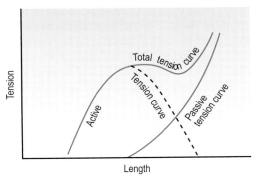

Figure 2.21 The effect of length on total tension, taking into account the force developed as the actin and myosin overlap and the passive tension that develops in the contractile components. The non-contractile components start developing tension at approximately mid length.

develops in the surrounding non-contractile structures when a resting muscle is stretched and when the muscle is active. The location of the non-contractile elements means that passive tension will develop both in series and in parallel with the myofilaments.

Total tension can be calculated when active and passive tensions are both measured, as illustrated in Figure 2.21. This calculation is taken from laboratory experiments on isolated muscles. Initially when a muscle contracts from its shortest position, the connective tissue is not stretched and generates no tension. All the tension produced within the muscle comes from the crossbridge cycle. However, when the muscle is at mid length or longer the connective tissue is stretched and passive tension develops, which adds to the tension generated actively by the crossbridge cycle. Further increases in length cause a rapid increase in total tension and can eventually be sufficient to cause muscle rupture.

In the living body most muscles that cross a single joint cannot be stretched to the point where passive tension contributes significantly to total tension. However, muscles acting over more than one joint may be stretched sufficiently for passive tension to take effect.

It is important to remember that the length–tension relationship discussed here describes the effect of muscle length on the force generated by isometric muscle activity. Where joint movement takes place it is necessary to consider the effect of the type and velocity of contraction.

Types of muscle activity (contraction)

The word 'contraction' means to draw together or shorten, but active muscles do not always succeed in shortening and so it is better to use the term 'muscle activity' rather than muscle contraction when considering how muscles produce or control movement. The sliding filament theory dictates that an active muscle will attempt to shorten. The relationship between the force generated internally by the muscle and external resistance to the moving part will determine whether or not the length of the muscle changes. There are commonly used terms that provide information about the length changes in muscle fibres when the muscle is activated:

* *Isometric* (static) activity occurs when the muscle is active but there is no visible movement of the bones. The internal tension generated by the muscle is equal to the external force and so balance is achieved.
* *Isokinetic* activity occurs when the muscle produces movement of one or more of the bones to which it is attached and that movement appears to occur at a constant velocity. It is accepted that

at the beginning of a movement there is usually a period of acceleration, followed by a period of constant velocity before the movement is decelerated. During the period when the velocity of movement remains constant, the muscle activity is described as isokinetic. The force produced by the muscle during isokinetic activity may vary as the length of the muscle changes.

- *Isotonic* activity occurs when there is movement of one or more of the bones to which the active muscle is attached. This is a dynamic process and the muscle may become longer or shorter. Both the velocity of length change and the force produced may vary during the activity.

Isotonic activity can be subdivided using the terms 'concentric' and 'eccentric' (pronounced *ek-sen-tric*). Concentric activity occurs when the active muscle generates an internal force that is greater than the external force and shortening takes place. Eccentric activity occurs when an active muscle generates less force than the external load and is lengthened by it.

The characteristics of isometric, concentric and eccentric contractions and the forces generated by each type of activity are very different, as shown in Table 2.2 (Jones & Round 1990, Lieber 1992).

Isometric activity occurs when there is no visible movement of bones or joints and thus, in mechanical terms, the muscle does no external work. An example of this would be holding a glass of water with the elbow joint held at 90° by activity in the biceps brachii muscle. The external forces acting on the muscle include the weight of the forearm and hand, and the weight of the glass of water. In order for the glass to be held still, the force generated by the muscle must exactly match the external forces acting on the limb. Although in

an isometric activity the muscle does not visibly change length, there is some internal shortening as the actin and myosin filaments slide past each other until they have taken up all 'slack' in the muscle. In the intact body, the elastic components of the tendons are slightly stretched by this activity. The maximal force that can be generated and the energy cost required for a given amount of force are intermediate between concentric and eccentric contractions.

Isotonic-concentric activity occurs when the muscle shortens; movement of bones and joints occurs and, in mechanical terms, external work is done. An example of this would be in raising a glass to the lips. The biceps brachii muscle becomes active, generating sufficient internal force to overcome the external load that comprises the weight of the forearm, hand and glass. Because the internal force is greater than the opposing external force, movement occurs and the glass is raised to the lips. The maximum force a muscle can generate concentrically will always be less than the maximum force produced by isometric activity. During concentric activity the myosin heads are repeatedly moving onto the next actin binding site and it takes a certain amount of time for crossbridges to form and re-form. During this repeated activity the number of crossbridges that are formed at any one moment, and thus the force generated, is less than during an isometric contraction where repeated cycling of crossbridges is not a feature. This rapid cycling of crossbridges has a high energy cost and, therefore, the highest oxygen demand and heat production occurs during concentric contractions.

Isotonic-eccentric activity occurs when the external load exceeds the internal force generated by the muscle and as a consequence the active

Table 2.2   The characteristics of the three types of muscle contraction. The determining factor for movement is whether the internal force generated by a muscle is the same, lower or higher than the external forces

Type of contraction	Function	External force (relative to internal)	External work by muscle	Force generated	Energy cost (oxygen demand)
Concentric	Acceleration	Less	Positive	Lowest	Highest
Isometric	Fixation	Same	None	Intermediate	Intermediate
Eccentric	Deceleration	Greater	Negative	Highest	Lowest

muscle is lengthened. Mechanically, work is done on the muscle, rather than by it, and this is sometimes described as negative work. Eccentric activity can be illustrated by lowering an empty glass from the lips to the table. Whilst drinking is taking place, the glass is held in contact with the lips by isometric activity in the biceps brachii muscle. When the time comes to lower the glass to the table, the biceps brachii muscle will reduce the number of active crossbridges until the combined force of the forearm, hand and glass exceeds the force being generated within the muscle. As the external forces now exceed the internal forces, the muscle is unable maintain the crossbridges and they 'break' and re-form with reduced overlap. As this continues the muscle gets longer, resulting in elbow extension and the glass is returned to the table. The biceps brachii muscle does not relax during this process because that would result in the elbow extending at the speed of gravity and that would definitely result in a broken glass.

Eccentric activity is therefore used to control movements produced by external forces such as gravity. During eccentric activity the maximum force a muscle can generate is higher than under isometric or concentric conditions. This is thought to be partly because the tension generated by crossbridge formation is increased by the additional component of elastic force caused by the stretch of the neck of the myosin molecule (S2 fragment). The crossbridges remain attached to the actin binding site until ripped away by the external stretching force.

Curiously, in view of their high force generation, eccentric contractions are performed at a very low energy cost. This is thought to be for two reasons. First, the external force causes the myosin head to be mechanically pulled from the binding site, rather than requiring adenosine triphosphate (ATP) to cause joining as in other types of contraction. Second, when the myosin head is pulled away from the actin filament, it is in the correct position for subsequent reattachment to another binding site and does not require energy to move into the attachment position.

The high force generation and low energy cost of eccentric exercise are often seen as beneficial in training, but there are accompanying problems. The performance of unaccustomed, high force eccentric activity will cause muscle fatigue, pain and mechanical damage in excess of that caused by isometric or concentric contractions (Clarkson & Newham 1995). In subjects unused to eccentric exercise, the incidence of delayed-onset muscle soreness is always high.

Isokinetic/isotonic controversy

Within the last 30 years machines have been introduced that allow muscles to be exercised at a constant velocity. Whilst it is not possible for a muscle to change length at a constant velocity, the term 'isokinetic activity' has been introduced to cover the form of exercise where the exercise machine functions at a constant velocity. Prior to the introduction of isokinetic dynamometers, the term 'isotonic' was used to signify any muscle activity that involved a change in muscle length, regardless of the velocity or the force generated. It is regrettable that since the introduction of iso-kinetics the term 'isotonic' has been redefined by some authorities to mean a contraction in which the force remains constant throughout. This is an incorrect interpretation of the original concept, as an active muscle will vary in both the velocity of contraction and the force it generates throughout its range of movement. It is therefore incorrect to describe isotonics as a constant force activity. These terms are considered in more detail in Chapter 13.

Functional activity

Most activities performed by humans are complex and it is rare for a muscle to act in only one way in any particular activity. In the example of drinking given above, it was shown that the biceps brachii muscle first acts concentrically to raise the glass to the lips, then maintains the position of the glass through isometric activity and finally changes to eccentric activity as the glass is lowered to the table. All muscles have the ability to change the way in which they work according to functional need.

When eccentric activity occurs, the stretch on the non-contractile components of muscles results in the storage of potential energy. If eccentric activity is immediately followed by concentric activity, the release of the potential energy increases

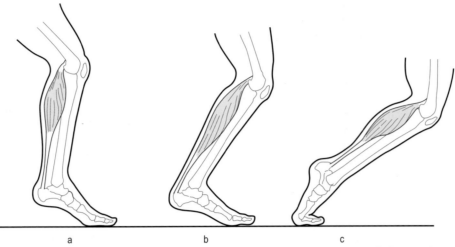

Figure 2.22 The stretch–shortening cycle of the calf muscles illustrated here during running. (a) Just before the toes strike the ground, the calf muscles become active in order to resist the forces of impact. (b) As the weight transfers onto the foot, the still-active calf muscles are stretched (eccentric activity). (c) On push-off the calf muscles shorten (concentric activity). The stretch prior to shortening enables the storage and then release of kinetic energy.

the overall mechanical efficiency of the activity (Komi 1986). This is referred to as the 'stretch–shortening' cycle and a common example is seen in the calf muscles where the active muscles are stretched prior to shortening during the push-off phase of walking, running and jumping, as illustrated in Figure 2.22.

Velocity of contraction

The amount of tension that a fully activated muscle can generate also varies with the velocity of contraction. If a muscle is active either concentrically or eccentrically and changes length at a range of different velocities, the force generated can be measured at each velocity and the force–velocity relationship can be determined (Fig. 2.23). This also shows the effect of contraction type on force as discussed above. It can clearly be seen that the velocity of change in muscle length has a marked and different effect on the two types of dynamic contraction. The greatest force that can be

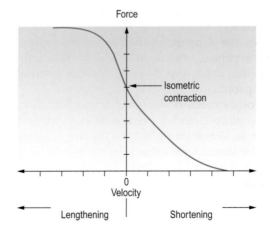

Figure 2.23 The force–velocity relationship of a maximally activated muscle. The force that can be generated when the muscle is shortening (concentric activity) increases as the velocity of contraction reduces. More force can be generated during an isometric activity than during a concentric activity, when the muscle is not changing length. Eccentric force is always greater than isometric; it initially increases with velocity, then remains relatively constant.

developed occurs during eccentric activity, when the muscle is lengthening. Maximum isometric activity occurs at zero velocity and produces a force that is less than that generated eccentrically, but more than the maximum generated concentrically. Concentric force decreases as the velocity of muscle length change increases, but conversely the force generated eccentrically increases with velocity. In concentric activity, the higher the velocity of shortening, the shorter the time available for the myosin heads to attach to the actin binding sites that are moving past them. The proportion of myosin heads that manage to attach to the actin filament and form crossbridges decreases as velocity increases. Therefore, the number of crossbridges that are successfully formed decreases with increasing velocity and as force generation is dependent on crossbridge formation, then force must also reduce.

Eventually a velocity is reached at which no force can be sustained; this is the maximal velocity of shortening (V_{max}). The V_{max} differs between individuals and also in different muscles in the same person. It is largely determined genetically by the fibre types within muscle and is little affected by physical training (Jones & Round 1990).

In contrast, during eccentric activity the force increases with increases in velocity. It is only when the eccentric activity has generated a force about 1.8 times the maximum isometric force that it reaches a plateau. As the velocity of stretch increases, the extensible S2 portions of the crossbridges produce more passive, elastic force. The plateau of the eccentric force–velocity relationship suggests that skeletal muscles are relatively resistant to stretch and this is useful in many normal movement patterns.

Activities of daily life frequently demonstrate the practical consequences of the effects of velocity on force generation. The heavier a weight, the more slowly we are able to move or lift it using concentric muscle activity. However, eccentric activity, for example in lowering heavy weights, becomes faster as the load increases.

Frequency of stimulation

When an individual muscle fibre is electrically stimulated at intensities above the threshold for

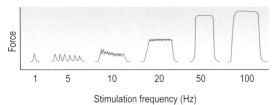

Figure 2.24 The relationship between force and the frequency of external electrical stimulation. Note that increased frequency initially increases force and reduces oscillations. However, increasing the frequency above that which produces a fused tetanic contraction does not increase force.

motor activation, it will generate force. The force generated is strongly influenced by the frequency of stimulation. A single impulse will result in a mechanical response called a twitch. If stimulation frequency is increased, the force initially increases and then remains relatively constant despite further, substantial increases in frequency, as shown in Figure 2.24.

As the electrical stimulation frequency initially increases, two observations can be made. The first is that the contraction becomes smoother because the muscle fibre has less time to relax between consecutive stimuli. The second observation is that the force increases with stimulation frequency because the next impulse arrives before the muscle fibre has completely relaxed and the impulse is superimposed on the remaining tension. This is known as the summation of force. When stimulated at a sufficiently high frequency (termed the fusion frequency), there is no relaxation between individual stimuli. The outcome of this is that the muscle fibre will produce a smooth, tetanic force. The frequency at which this occurs depends on the fibre type and is discussed later in this chapter. An increase in stimulation frequency above the fusion frequency does not increase the force of contraction.

Recordings from muscles during voluntary contractions have shown that the physiological firing rates are usually at a frequency lower than the fusion frequency found when muscles are stimulated electrically (Binder-Macleod 1992). In normal movement the neurological firing rates are at a frequency which, if mimicked by electrical stimulation, would result in marked oscillation;

the muscle would appear to have a tremor. However, it is quite clear that during movement most people do not demonstrate visible muscle tremor when contracting a muscle voluntarily. This is because during external, electrical stimulation the muscle fibres affected by the stimulus will all contract simultaneously (synchronous contraction of fibres) and a smooth contraction will be seen until the muscle is allowed to relax. In voluntary activity the nerves fire asynchronously, so whilst some fibres are contracting others are relaxed and recovering. As the contracting fibres start to fatigue, they will relax and different fibres will be stimulated in order to take their place. This cycling and recycling of muscle fibre contraction smoothes out force oscillations and the contraction, which may be quite prolonged, appears smooth.

The motor unit

Each individual muscle fibre generates a force so small as to be impractical for even the most delicate movements. Therefore, the system is designed so that a group of muscle fibres share common innervation from a single alpha motor neurone (gamma motor neurones innervate the intrafusal fibres within the muscle spindle). This functional grouping is called a motor unit and is composed of the cell body of the alpha motor neurone (the anterior horn cell in the spinal cord), the motor neurone itself and those muscle fibres that it innervates (Fig. 2.25). If a motor neurone fires, all the muscle fibres in that unit will contract at the same time, producing a synchronised electrical discharge (action potential) which can be measured by electromyography. This will result in the generation of force. The size of both action potential and force are proportional to the number of muscle fibres within the motor unit. There is a range of motor unit sizes within a single muscle and also between muscles. Muscles requiring the precise regulation of small forces, such as the small hand muscles, have many small motor units that may contain only 10 fibres. Large postural muscles, such as the quadriceps, have much larger motor units that may contain several thousand fibres.

The fibres belonging to an individual motor unit are scattered throughout a muscle, thus adjacent fibres are unlikely to belong to the same motor unit. All the fibres within a single unit are the same fibre type.

Gradation of muscle force

It is clear that both voluntary and reflex muscle force can be precisely controlled. There are two ways in which force can be varied: motor unit recruitment and rate coding. Both have been shown to be used in voluntary contractions of human muscle, but it is unclear to what extent they are employed. It is possible that large postural muscles, which do not require fine control of force, predominantly use motor unit recruitment. Those needing fine control, such as the hand muscles, may rely more on rate coding.

Motor unit recruitment

Activating more motor units will increase the force generated and this is termed 'motor unit recruitment'. The smaller motor units have the most excitable motor neurones and therefore are recruited first. As more force is required, the larger, and progressively less excitable, motor neurones are recruited in an orderly fashion. This has become known as the size principle (Hennemann et al 1974).

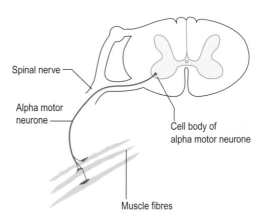

Figure 2.25 A single motor unit is composed of the motor neurone and the muscle fibres which it innervates. The cell body of the motor neurone is in the anterior horn cell in the spinal cord and its axon is one of the motor nerves in a mixed peripheral nerve.

Table 2.3   Examples of differences between fibre types. Note that different terminology exists for types of muscle fibre and motor unit

Property	Type I	Type IIa	Type IIb
Muscle fibre type	Slow oxidative (SO)	Fast oxidative glycolytic (FOG)	Fast glycolytic (FG)
Motor unit type	Slow (S)	Fast fatigue resistant (FR)	Fast fatigable (FF)
Motor unit size	Small	Medium	Large
Twitch tension	Low	Moderate	High
Mechanical speed	Slow	Fast	Fast
Fatigability	Low	Low	High
Mitochondrial enzyme activity	High	Medium	Low
Glycogenolytic enzyme activity	Low	Medium	High
Myoglobin content	High	Medium	Low
Capillary density	High	Medium	Low

Rate coding

The force of active motor units can also be varied by the frequency of stimulation of the motor neurone and by utilising the force–frequency characteristics. Recordings from single motor units have shown that the firing rate varies considerably even within a constant low force contraction. Initially, a short burst of firing may be used to generate relatively high forces by the motor unit, but rapidly decreases to maintain force.

Fibre types

The observation that some muscles are dark and others light, as in the leg and breast muscle of a chicken, is an indication that not all muscle fibres are the same. It was thought previously that discrete fibre types existed, but it seems that there is a spectrum of fibre types with considerable variations in histochemistry, contractile properties and the type of metabolism. This is shown in Table 2.3.

The colour differences exist because of the different amounts of the red-coloured myoglobin within different muscle fibres. It can be seen from Table 2.3 that type I fibres are specialised to use oxidative (aerobic) metabolism and are resistant to fatigue. They have high levels of myoglobin and are relatively slow to contract and relax. They are recruited early in low force muscle activity due to their small axon size. The number of muscle fibres in slow motor units is small and so motor unit recruitment can result in fine gradations of force.

Type II fibres are subdivided into types IIa, b and c. The type IIb fibres contrast sharply with type I fibres in almost all respects. They are fast to contract and relax and rely on anaerobic metabolism and intramuscular stores of fuel. Due to the large axon diameter, they are recruited only during high force activity and fatigue rapidly. This is illustrated in Figure 2.26. The motor units contain relatively large numbers of fibres and so recruitment of additional motor units causes relatively large force increases.

Type IIa fibres and their motor units are intermediate between types I and IIb and span a broad range of the characteristics of both. The subgroup IIc is found mainly in regenerating fibres and in the embryo.

Functional activity and the different fibre types

During a low force contraction only the type I fibres are recruited. Therefore, they are used mainly for normal everyday activities that do not

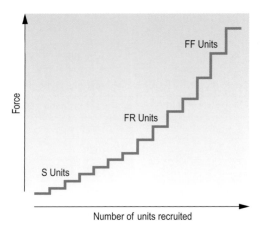

Figure 2.26   The regulation of force by recruitment of motor units. At low forces only the small, slow (S) units are recruited. As force increases, the larger, fatigue-resistant (FR) and then the largest fast, fatigable (FF) units are recruited. The S units have relatively few muscle fibres and the FF units have the most. Therefore the increment in force as a new unit is recruited also varies.

require maximal or high force contractions. Their resistance to fatigue makes them well suited to this role. As the force generated by the muscle increases, the type IIa and then IIb fibres are progressively recruited and during maximal activity, all the motor units are involved. However, maximal force rapidly declines due to the high rate of fatigue in the fast-contracting type IIa and IIb fibres.

There is wide variation in the proportion of the different fibre types between muscles and between people. All muscles have a mixture of fibres but some have a higher proportion of one type than others. So, for example, the gastrocnemius muscle has a higher proportion of type II fibres than the neighbouring soleus muscle. As a consequence soleus, with its preponderance of type I fibres, will function mainly in everyday activities which rely on endurance, whereas gastrocnemius plays a major role when power and speed are required. Each person has a unique proportion of type I to type II fibres and as the fibre type is largely determined genetically, it is unlikely that training with voluntary activity will change the relative proportion of type I and type II muscle fibres in an individual.

Effect of fibre alignment on muscle performance

Muscles fulfil two functions: one is to cause and control movement, the other is to generate sufficient force to hold the body still, as in the maintenance of static posture. Most muscles can fulfil both functions, but the fibre type and alignment may reflect habitual usage. Muscles that predominantly function in postural activities are likely to have a different fibre alignment to those that often produce quick, large-range movements. The different ways in which muscle fibres can be aligned were described earlier in this chapter. On the whole the muscles that produce large-range movement tend to have a predominance of long, parallel type II fibres whereas pennate arrangements are seen more in muscles that need to generate large or continuous forces during postural activities.

Determinants of force

The force a muscle can generate in any given situation is proportional to its cross-sectional area, i.e. the number of sarcomeres that lie in parallel to each other. The force generated is not related to the length of the muscle fibre. Along the length of a fibre the tension generated by adjacent sarcomeres is equal and opposite at the central Z line and therefore they cancel each other. The only forces transmitted through the muscle attachments are those generated by the sarcomeres at either end of the muscle. Therefore, force is independent of fibre length (Fig. 2.27).

Muscles that are mainly required for isometric activity tend to have a large cross-sectional area. A pennate structure has the advantage that more fibres can be packed into the same cross-sectional area. The disadvantage is that the force transmitted to the tendon is the cosine of the angle between the angle of pull of the tendon and the fibres and therefore some of the generated force is lost.

Muscle cross-sectional area can be increased by strength training (see Ch. 13) and this increases force generation. However, in pennate muscles with a large angle between the line of pull and fibre alignment, an increased cross-sectional area may result in an increased angle of pennation and therefore a relatively small increase in force.

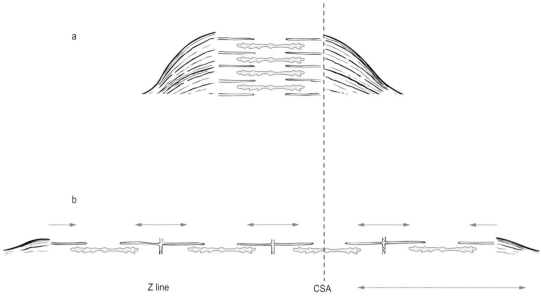

Figure 2.27 Illustration of four sarcomeres arranged in parallel (a) and in series (b). When they are arranged in series, the forces from adjacent sarcomeres at each Z line are equal and opposite. Therefore the only force transmitted by the muscle is that from the outside half of the two sarcomeres at the end of the fibre. The same force is generated by each fibre, irrespective of its length. With a parallel arrangement the force of each sarcomere is transmitted to the tendon. Therefore the same four sarcomeres will generate four times as much force as when they are arranged in series. Note that the cross-sectional area (CSA) is proportional to the force that is produced.

Determinants of velocity

The maximal velocity at which a muscle can contract is determined by its length, i.e. the number of sarcomeres arranged in series, and is independent of the cross-sectional area. At the start of muscle activity, all the sarcomeres begin to contract at about the same time and velocity. If a muscle contained only one sarcomere which shortened by 1 mm in 0.1 seconds (s), the shortening velocity would be 10 mm/s. If the muscle contained 100 sarcomeres in series, each would shorten at the same time and velocity, so the total velocity of shortening of the whole muscle would be 1 mm/s.

The maximal velocity of shortening of a single crossbridge and sarcomere is governed by the fibre type and activity of the enzyme myosin ATPase and appears to be relatively unaffected by training.

Muscle length, strength and power

We have already seen that strength is proportional to the cross-sectional area and velocity to length of a muscle. Therefore, a short, fat muscle will generate more force and have a lower velocity of shortening than a long, thin one. However, as power is the product of force (cross-sectional area) and velocity (length), it is proportional to volume.

Roles of muscles

An individual muscle rarely works alone. Usually many different muscles are active simultaneously in even the simplest movement. The forces generated by the active muscles may vary considerably throughout a movement and each muscle can fulfil several roles in different movements or patterns of movement. These roles are discussed below.

The *agonist* or *prime mover* is the term used to refer to the muscle(s) that plays the major role in initiating, carrying out and maintaining a particular movement. For example, the psoas major is the agonist for hip flexion because it is the main muscle responsible for producing the movement.

Antagonists are muscles that act in a direction that is opposite to the agonist. So if the psoas major muscle is the agonist for hip flexion then the antagonists would be gluteus maximus and the hamstring group, as they normally produce hip extension. Normally when a prime mover is working, the antagonistic muscle is relaxed. The antagonists are often inhibited by a reflex mechanism originating from the agonist and this is known as reciprocal inhibition.

Assistant movers are those muscles which perform a movement similar to the agonist, but that play a less significant role in a particular movement. This is the role played by sartorius or rectus femoris in hip flexion.

Stabilisers or *fixators* are muscles that contract to control the position of a bone so that it can act as a steady base from which the agonist can contract. They provide a fixed attachment for another muscle. For example, during hip flexion the pelvic girdle will be held still by most of the trunk muscles acting as fixators, thus giving the hip flexors a steady base from which to contract.

A *synergist* is a more difficult concept. The term means to act together or to produce combined action. A muscle that is working synergistically acts simultaneously with one or more muscles to produce a movement. There are two types of synergists: true and helping.

True synergists can be demonstrated when the long finger flexor muscles grip an object in the hand. The long finger flexor muscles are the agonists for finger flexion but because they cross the wrist joint, they also produce wrist flexion. This is an unwanted action and needs to be controlled or opposed by the simultaneous contraction of the wrist extensors. In this example the wrist extensors are acting as true synergists.

Helping synergists are also groups of muscles acting simultaneously. Flexor carpi radialis and extensor carpi radialis longus are usually antagonistic to each other in that one produces wrist flexion and the other produces extension. If they contract simultaneously the combined effect of the force they produce will result in radial deviation at the wrist, rather than flexion or extension. In this case they would be described as helping synergists.

Range of movement

During a dynamic contraction or when a muscle is being stretched, the muscle involved will change length. When a muscle starts contracting from its most lengthened position and continues contracting until it is as short as possible, it is said that the muscle has moved through full range. Movement through the full range will be from long to short length for the agonist during a concentric contraction. Conversely, during eccentric activity the agonist will move from short to long length.

The full range of muscle excursion is subjectively described using the three subdivisions shown diagrammatically in Figures 2.28 and 5.4. In *the outer range* the muscle length moves between its longest length and the midpoint. The *inner range* is between the shortest length and the midpoint of range. In the *middle range* the muscle changes its

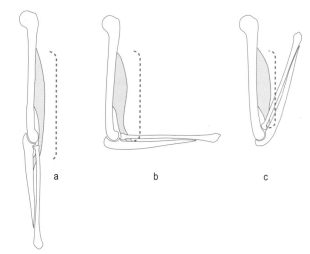

Figure 2.28 The term 'range' is used to describe the length of a muscle. (a) When the muscle is working and the fibres are near their longest position, it is said to be working in outer range. (b) When the working muscle is neither fully lengthened nor shortened it is said to be working in middle range.(c) When the muscle fibres are short, the muscle will be working in inner range.

length from the middle positions of the inner and outer ranges.

It is important not to confuse this terminology with that of the range of joint motion, since muscle and joint range may not be the same, particularly in muscles acting over more than one joint. Whilst muscle range is described subjectively using the terms 'inner', 'middle' and 'outer', joint range is normally measured in degrees. An understanding of whether a muscle is contracting in outer, middle or inner range will help formulate expectations about how much force the muscle will be able to generate (see earlier in this chapter).

Active and passive insufficiency

Every muscle has a structural limit to how much it is able to shorten or be stretched; its range is defined and not infinite. If it is required to shorten beyond its ability then as the muscle approaches the limit of inner range, it reaches a point when it is no longer able to generate force and the movement will cease (see the section on p. 28 on active tension). If it is stretched beyond its natural limit then tension within the muscle will restrict the movement, there will be pain and eventually muscle fibres will tear. Muscles which cross only one joint are usually capable of shortening and lengthening sufficiently to allow full range of joint movement, but this is not necessarily the case for muscles crossing several joints. When multiple-joint muscles are actively shortening they can cause simultaneous movement at all the joints they cross. This sometimes places the active muscle in a position where, to achieve the full potential range of movement at each joint, the muscle would have to shorten to beyond its natural length. When this happens the muscle reaches a length which represents the limit of inner range, the active muscle can no longer generate useful force and the movement stops. At this point the muscle is said to demonstrate active insufficiency.

A functional example of active insufficiency can be easily demonstrated in the hamstring muscles that cross both the hip joint and the knee joint. If this muscle group actively contracts to simultaneously flex the knee and extend the hip, then in most people the muscle will reach its limit of shortening before both joints have reached the end of their ranges of movement. The hamstrings will demonstrate active insufficiency because, whilst actively changing length, they will be unable to complete the two required movements.

If the antagonist is considered, a similar situation arises. If the antagonist to a movement is a muscle that crosses a number of joints then initially, as the movement starts, the antagonist will be relaxed and will be passively stretched as the agonist moves increasingly through range. If the antagonistic muscle crosses several joints then it is quite likely that it will be unable to stretch sufficiently to allow all the joints to achieve their full anatomical range. As the antagonist nears the limit to which it can be stretched pain will be generated and any further motion will be inhibited. In this situation the antagonistic muscle is being passively stretched throughout the activity. When the antagonistic muscle causes the movement to stop, the term 'passive insufficiency' is used.

The hamstrings can also provide an example of passive insufficiency. This muscle group will be stretched if other muscles actively contract to flex the hip joint and extend the knee joint. As the hip and knee joints move towards their anatomical limits of flexion and extension respectively, the hamstrings, as the antagonistic muscle group, will have been stretched to their natural limit. Many of us have experienced this when trying to touch our toes whilst standing with extended knees, as it is not always possible. The limiting factor for those of us who are not very flexible is the failure of the hamstrings to stretch sufficiently.

Passive insufficiency occurs when the passive tension in a multiple-joint muscle reaches its limit and prevents further movement from occurring. There are examples where a joint movement called tenodesis may occur as a solution to increasing passive tension in an antagonistic muscle group (Greene & Roberts 1999). An example of tenodesis can be seen if the fingers are relaxed and the wrist joint is moved from full flexion to full extension. As the wrist reaches full flexion the fingers automatically start to extend due to the passive tension in the long finger extensor muscle; conversely during wrist extension, passive tension in the long finger flexors causes the fingers to flex as the limit of movement is reached. This is illustrated in Figure 2.29 and you can easily demonstrate it on yourself.

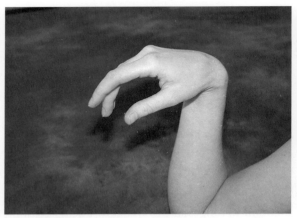 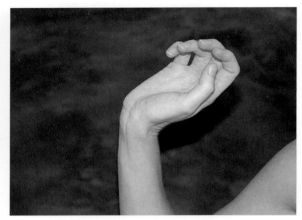

Figure 2.29   When a relaxed hand is moved into full wrist extension, the tenodesis action of the long finger flexors causes finger flexion to increase. Conversely, as the wrist is flexed the relaxed fingers will slightly extend.

Task 2.8

Sit on the floor, flex your hip and knee joints and then note two things. First, whether you can rest your head on your knees and second, how near you can get your heel to your bottom. To test active insufficiency, now lie prone so that your hip joints are in full extension. In this position use your hamstrings to flex one knee as far as possible. The chances are that you will be unable to match the range of knee flexion that you achieved in sitting. Unless you are extraordinarily flexible, your heel will be nowhere near your bottom. Now get a friend to gently press on your leg to see if it is possible to gain more knee flexion when the active force is your friend, not your hamstrings. If your friend is able to produce an increase in range then it shows that the movement was originally limited by active insufficiency of the knee flexor muscles. Note: if you use a friend to help you in this activity, instruct them to be very gentle.

To demonstrate passive insufficiency, sit on the floor again but this time with both knees fully extended; you must keep your knees extended throughout the task. With your arms by your side, lean forwards, flexing at the hip to see if you can produce sufficient hip flexion to get your head onto your knees. In this position, with your knees extended, you will probably be unable to flex your hips sufficiently to get your head onto your knees. You will also be likely to feel pain in your hamstring muscles as they reach their limit of extensibility and prevent the full movement occurring. This is passive insufficiency.

REFERENCES

Binder-Macleod SA 1992 Force-frequency relation in skeletal muscle. In: Currier DP, Nelson RM (eds) Dynamics of human biologic tissues. FA Davis, Philadelphia

Clarkson PM, Newham DJ 1995 Associations between muscle soreness, damage and fatigue. In: Gandevia SC, Enolta RM, McComas A et al (eds) Advances in experimental medicine and biology. Fatigue – neural and muscular mechanisms. Plenum Press, New York

Gordon AM, Huxley AF, Julian FJ 1966 The variation in isometric tension with sarcomere length in vertebrate muscle fibres. Journal of Physiology 184: 170–192

Greene DP, Roberts SL 1999 Kinesiology, movement in the context of activity. Mosby, St Louis

Hennemann E, Clamann HP, Gillies JD, Skinner RD 1974 Rank order of motorneurons within a pool, law of combination. Journal of Neurophysiology 37: 1338–1349

Huxley AF, Simmons RM 1971 Proposed mechanism of force generation in striated muscle. Nature 233: 533–558

Jones DA, Round JM 1990 Skeletal muscle in health and disease. Manchester University Press, Manchester

Komi PV 1986 The stretch shortening cycle and human power output. In: Jones NL, McCartney N, McComas AJ (eds) Human muscle power. Human Kinetics, Champaign, Illinois

Lieber RL 1992 Skeletal muscle structure and function. Williams and Wilkins, Baltimore

Payne CB 1998 Biomechanics of the foot in diabetes mellitus. Some theoretical considerations. Journal of the American Podiatric Medical Association 88(6): 285–289

Chapter 3

Biomechanics of human movement

Robert W.M. van Deursen, Tony Everett

LEARNING OUTCOMES

At the end of this chapter you will be able to:

1. Describe the concept of force and its relevance
   for human movement

2. Discuss the general kinematics and kinetics of
   human movement

3. Apply your knowledge of kinematics and kinetics in specified situations

4. Describe the graphical and mathematical analysis of force systems and use this knowledge in the analysis of solid and fluid mechanics

5. Integrate the above knowledge to perform simple biomechanical movement analyses.

INTRODUCTION

Biomechanics can be defined as the study of the structure and function of biological systems, such as the human musculoskeletal system, by application of (Newtonian) mechanics. Newtonian mechanics refers to Sir Isaac Newton who laid the foundations for the field of mechanics as currently used. The scope of biomechanics is both wide and deep. Therefore, a choice has been made to highlight the aspects considered most relevant for the study of human movement. (For a complete discussion of biomechanics, see Further Reading suggestions at the end of this chapter.) The main focus of this chapter is understanding *forces and their effects*. Principles of *kinematics* (the description of motion) and *kinetics* (the description of motion including the consideration of forces as the cause of motion) will also be discussed.

A first step in understanding human movement is knowledge of the anatomy and physiology of the human body, the musculoskeletal system in particular. However, anatomy books describe movement as though it occurred in a state of weightlessness and only using the anatomical position as the starting point. It is important to realise that movements cannot be considered out of context but occur in an infinite number of body configurations and within a mechanical environment. A biomechanical analysis is required to unravel these influences to determine which muscles (if any) are required to produce a given movement. In addition, such an analysis can quantify the amount of loading occurring on different anatomical structures. Although biomechanical analyses can be very powerful in providing information about movement, it should be noted that the environment within which the movement occurs is generally a lot richer than mechanics

Table 3.1 SI units, their names and imperial equivalents

Quantity	SI unit	Conversion
Mass	Kilogram (kg)	1 kg = 9.807 N 1 kg = 2.2 lbs 1 stone = 6.35 kg
Time	Seconds (s)	
Length	Metre (m)	1 m = approx. 39 inches 1 ft = 0.305 m
Angle	Degrees (deg)	1 rad = 57.3 deg 1 deg = 0.0175 rad

alone. Therefore, it is best to consider this field of study as a set of tools in a toolbox that contains various other methods used to learn more about human movement.

Basic concepts

It is important that before any calculations are attempted, the basic elements of trigonometry are revised and some basic mathematical conventions are explained.

SI units

By convention, the international system of units is used for the dimensions of biomechanical quantities. Table 3.1 gives the basic SIU (Systeme International d'Unites) units and their equivalent values in other systems.

Trigonometry

The most basic concept of trigonometry is that of the triangle with its three sides and three angles. The three angles of any triangle will always add up to 180°. If one of these angles is 90° (the right-angled triangle) and the dimensions of the sides of the triangle are known, then the value of the angles can be calculated. If an angle and a side or two sides are known then it is possible to calculate all the remaining unknown parameters. This is possible by the use of the *sine, cosine* and *tangent* rule. Figure 3.1 shows a right-angled triangle where angle ABC is the right angle. Side b is known as

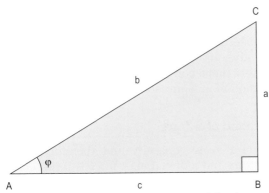

Figure 3.1 A right-angled triangle is used for the definition of the sine, cosine and tangent of the angle φ.

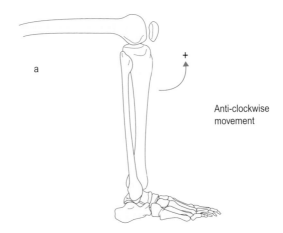

Anti-clockwise movement

the hypotenuse, side c as the base or adjacent and side a as the perpendicular or opposite. Mathematically the value of the angle CAB (φ) can be found using the formula:

$$sin\ \varphi = \text{opposite/hypotenuse or } sin\ \varphi = a/b$$

$$cos\ \varphi = \text{adjacent/hypotenuse or } cos\ \varphi = c/b$$

$$tan\ \varphi = \text{opposite/adjacent or } tan\ \varphi = a/c$$

It is also possible to calculate the lengths of the sides of the triangle by using Pythagoras' Theorem, which states that the square of the length of the hypotenuse is equal to the sum of the squares of the lengths of the other sides. In this case:

$$b^2 = a^2 + c^2 \text{ or } b = \sqrt{(a^2 + c^2)}$$

Scalar and vector quantities

In biomechanics two types of quantities are discussed. The first are those that have magnitude only, such as mass, temperature, work and energy. These are called *scalar* quantities. The second are those that have both magnitude and direction, such as force. These are called *vector* quantities. Scalar quantities can be added, subtracted, multiplied or divided without any problems. To manipulate vector quantities, trigonometry is used because those quantities may have varying directions.

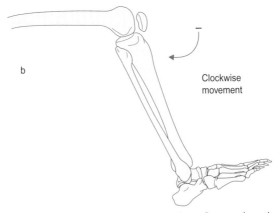

Clockwise movement

Figure 3.2 In describing the direction of a rotation, the convention is to call anti-clockwise rotation positive and clockwise rotation negative.

Rotations

Figure 3.2 shows that rotations in biomechanical terms can occur in one of two directions: anti-clockwise, as illustrated in Figure 3.2a, which is defined as positive rotation, and clockwise, as illustrated in Figure 3.2b, which is defined as negative rotation. In this example the thigh is fixed and the leg is moving. The arrow indicates the direction of movement and it is important that this direction arrow is added to any diagrammatic representation of movement.

Newton's laws of motion

Although not the first to study movement, Sir Isaac Newton (1642–1727) provided a major breakthrough in the understanding of the causes of movement of objects. He explained this in 1687 by addressing the relationship between force and one of its effects, namely *motion*. As a result of his studies Newton formulated three statements known as the *laws of motion*.

1. Law of Inertia

Every body continues in a state of rest or uniform motion in a straight line except when it is compelled by external forces to change its state.

2. Law of Acceleration

The rate of change of momentum of a body is proportional to the applied force and takes place in the direction in which the force acts.

3. Law of Action/Reaction

To every action there is an equal and opposite reaction.

These three laws still play a major role in the study of biomechanics and their implications will be considered and explained later in the chapter.

FORCE

Definition of force

A force is not a tangible object and should therefore be considered as a concept. It can be thought of as an entity that is generated by an action, a push or a pull for example, or imparted as in a kick. The above examples will probably result in movement but the object to which the force is imparted may remain stationary while it deforms, as with the force imparted to a soft chair when somebody sits down.

With this in mind, a force can be defined as: *An influence that changes the state of rest or motion of a body or object.* This is essentially what Newton describes in the Law of Inertia, stating that a body/object which is at rest will remain at rest unless some external force is applied to it and a body/object which is moving at a constant speed in a straight line will continue to do so unless some external force is applied to it. Similarly, inertia of a body/object (or mass) can be defined as the resistance that a body/object offers to any changes in its motion. It is measured in kilograms (kg).

Description of a force

Force is a vector quantity and therefore has a magnitude and a direction. A force is represented graphically as an arrow with the following three descriptors:

- *Magnitude*: the longer the arrow, the greater the magnitude.
- *Direction/line of action*: the arrow points in the direction of the force.
- *Point of application*: the point of the arrow is located at the point of application.

Equation of force

Encapsulated in Newton's Second Law or the Law of Acceleration is the equation:

$$\text{Force} = \text{mass} \times \text{acceleration} \ or \ F = m \times a$$

where mass (m) is the quantity of matter that makes up a body/object measured in kilograms (kg) and acceleration (a) may be the acceleration due to gravity measured in m/s^2.

The unit of force is the newton (N) whilst the dimensions of force are $kg.m.s^{-2}$ or $kg.m/s^2$.

Force systems

It is unusual for forces to act singularly, since there is usually a combination of forces acting together. For convenience these forces can be described as *force systems* which are defined as two or more forces acting together. Force systems can be described as follows:

- *Co-linear* (one-dimensional): this is where the forces are acting in the same plane and along the same line of action. They either point in the same or opposite directions. This is shown in Figure 3.3.
- *Co-planar* (two-dimensional): this is where the forces are acting in the same plane but not

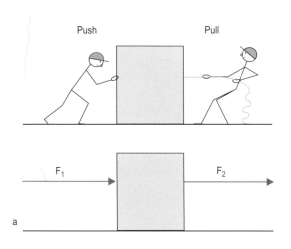

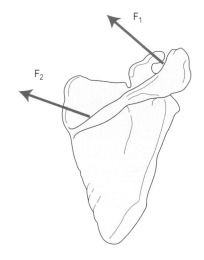

Figure 3.4 Two examples of co-planar force systems.

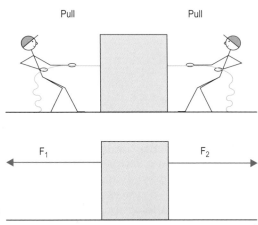

Figure 3.3 Two examples of co-linear force systems: (a) two forces acting in the same direction along the same line of action and (b) two forces acting in the opposite direction along the same line of action.

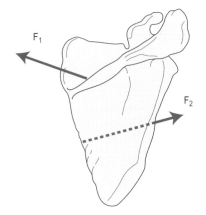

along the same line of action, as shown in Figure 3.4.

Special cases include the following:

- *Parallel forces*: the directions of the forces are parallel in the same or opposite directions (Fig. 3.5). Parallel forces in opposite directions may produce a *force couple,* as in a steering wheel.

- *Orthogonal forces*: the directions of the forces are perpendicular to each other.
- *Concurrent forces*: two or more forces originate from the same point of application or their lines of action intersect at a common point (Fig. 3.6).
- *Three-dimensional force systems*: forces are acting in more than a single plane. Although this represents the situation most often encountered in everyday examples, this is more difficult to analyse. In this chapter examples will be used of one- or two-dimensional force systems only.

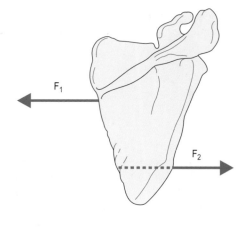

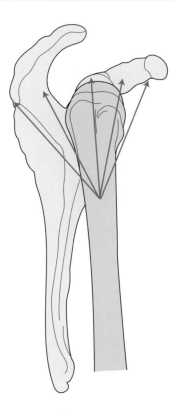

Figure 3.6   An example of a concurrent force system. The deltoid muscle is made up of multiple components that can act together.

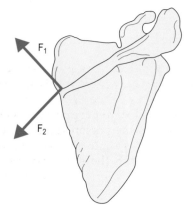

Figure 3.5   Two examples of co-planar force systems: (a) two forces acting in parallel and (b) two forces acting perpendicular two each other (orthogonal).

Force analysis

Because forces are vector quantities, the analysis of force systems will involve trigonometry. Two basic techniques for manipulating vector quantities are important. These are *summation* and *resolution* of forces. Summation involves adding the force vectors to find the *resultant* or the force that could replace the combined effect of all the forces acting on the body. Splitting a force into its *components* to establish its effects in two or three principal directions is called *resolution* of forces.

Simple force systems can be analysed using a graphical method. In a vector diagram each force vector is represented by an arrow drawn to scale. The resultant of two forces is determined by completing a parallelogram and joining the diagonally opposing corners (Fig. 3.7). This diagonal is then measured and the magnitude determined by using the scale.

In the case of more complex force systems, the more useful method of force analysis is by means of trigonometry. Each force is first split into its orthogonal (x and y) components (in three dimensions there is also a z-component) as illustrated in Figure 3.8:

$$F_x = \text{Force} \times \text{cosine } \varphi$$

$$F_y = \text{Force} \times \text{sine } \varphi$$

where F_x is the force component in the x direction and F_y is the force component in the y direction.

All the x-components are then added up or subtracted to obtain the resultant on that axis. The

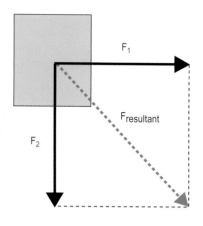

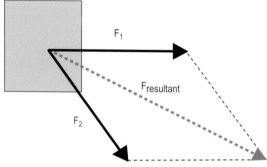

Figure 3.7 Two examples of obtaining the resultant force of a simple force system by means of the graphical method.

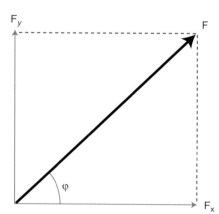

Figure 3.8 Resolution of a force: the angled force is resolved into two orthogonal components, F_x and F_y. The magnitude of the two components can be calculated by means of trigonometry.

same is done with the y-components. The resultant x and y are then added up by means of the following equation:

$$F_{resultant} = \sqrt{(F_x^2 + F_y^2)}$$

Types of forces

Force due to gravity

There is a force of attraction of the earth to any object on or near to its surface. The acceleration due to the gravitational pull of the earth is seen as the acceleration any mass has when it is allowed to freely fall to earth and has the value of 9.81 m/s². The weight of an object is the force exerted by the earth on the mass of the object or weight = mass × 9.81 (acceleration due to gravity). Weight is expressed in newtons.

Ground reaction force

Newton's Third Law is demonstrated when considering the forces that are involved when standing on the ground. In this situation a force is applied by the feet to the ground which is equal to the weight of the person standing. This force is reflected back up into the feet through the same action line with the same magnitude. This is the *ground reaction force* and is shown in Figure 3.9.

Centripetal force

As stated earlier, a body/object which is moving at a constant speed in a straight line will continue to do so unless some external force is applied to it. Therefore, if an object is to move in a circle, such as during a hammer throw, a force will have to be applied to make the object change direction continuously. This force is called a *centripetal force*. In the hammer throw this centripetal force is produced by the thrower. The thrower will, however, perceive himself as being pulled by the hammer, which is often called the *centrifugal force*. In a biomechanical analysis it is better to consider the centripetal force only. As soon as the thrower lets go of the hammer, it continues moving in a straight line since the centripetal force is no longer operating.

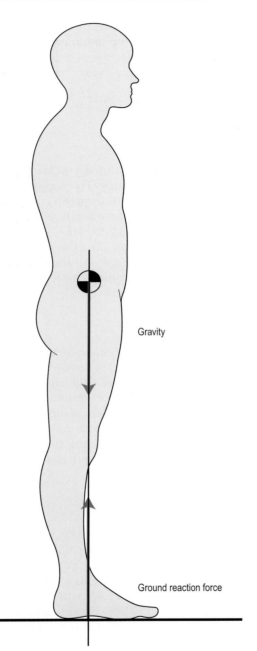

Gravity

Ground reaction force

Figure 3.9   The ground reaction force is the force of the floor acting on the body opposing the effect of gravity.

Frictional forces

When two objects move, or tend to move, over each other they experience a resisting force. This is referred to as *frictional force* and occurs if the objects are solid, fluid or a combination of both. Friction can occur between two surfaces moving over each other: between a wheel and the ground (rolling resistance) or between air/water and an object (drag).

If a force is applied to an object that does not move over a surface then there must be a frictional force (f) that is equal and opposite to the applied force (Newton's Third Law). As the applied force increases so will the resistance until it reaches a critical value (F_{max}). At this point the object will move. Until the object moves the friction is referred to as *static friction* but when the object is moving the friction is referred to as *dynamic or kinetic friction*.

The *coefficient of friction* (μ; *mu*) is dependent upon the conditions under which the friction is occurring (static or dynamic), the condition of the surfaces of the material and the type and direction of the applying force.

The frictional force can be calculated by multiplying the coefficient of friction and the force perpendicular to the contact surface of the two objects (also called *normal force*).

In some instances frictional forces are useful as they allow controlled movement to take place (as in walking) or they may be a hindrance as they require energy to overcome them (as in some types of exercise). Friction can produce heat and wear and tear to the surfaces that are moving over each other; this may be detrimental to the system (either machine or human body) and there may be a need for a lubricant to decrease these adverse effects.

Elastic forces

Elastic forces will be discussed in more detail in the section below about deformation of materials.

External and internal forces

Forces that act from outside the body, for example gravity, moving objects, ground reaction force and wind or water resistance, are called *external forces*. Forces can also be generated inside the body by a muscle or be transmitted between body parts by, for instance, ligaments or bone-on-bone contact. These are examples of *internal forces*. It is important to realise that muscle forces that are under voluntary control are just one aspect of the force system acting on our body. Movement of the body depends on the resultant of the force system, which includes external and internal forces, and not only on muscle forces.

Pressure

Pressure is the manifestation of force when the surface area over which the force is acting is taken into consideration. Pressure can be defined as the force per unit area (in m^2) or $P=F/A$. The official unit of pressure is the pascal (N/m^2) although the kilopascal (kPa; 1000 Pa) is more useful for human application.

It can be seen from the equation above that if a force remains the same and the surface area increases then the pressure exerted by the force will be less. Conversely, if the surface area is decreased whilst the force remains the same, greater pressure will be felt from the force. This is important when considering the pressure felt on the human body when lying in a bed. If the force is being channelled through a small surface area, like a bony point, then the pressure over that area will be much greater than if the force from the body were acting on a large surface area. In the latter case pressure sores would be less likely to occur.

Moment of force

When application of a force produces a turning or rotary effect, the force is said to be producing a *moment*. The twisting effect of a force, however, is often referred to as *torque*. There are no real differences between rotation and twisting so the words 'moment' and 'torque' cannot be considered separately. To calculate the magnitude of the moment of force, the equation of moment/torque is used:

Moment = Force × moment arm *or* M = F × d

In the above equation, d stands for distance, representing the moment arm. The moment arm is the shortest distance (perpendicular) from the line of action of a force to the axis of rotation. In Figure 3.10 the moment arm is shown for a weight on a see-saw (a) and the muscle moment arm is shown

for the elbow flexor (b). A line is drawn perpendicular to the force line of action and through the axis of rotation. The moment arm is the distance between the two. The unit of moment/torque is the newton.metre or N.m whilst the dimensions of moment/torque are $kg.m.s^{-2}$ or $kg.m/s^2$.

Internal and external moments

When forces act from outside the body, gravity, ground reaction force, wind or water resistance for example, and produce rotatory effects, they are called *external moments*. When the forces are acting inside the human body they produce *internal moments*. These are often muscle forces acting on the various segments of the body but they can also be forces acting from one segment to the next by means of the ligaments.

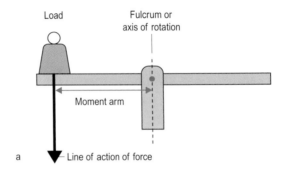

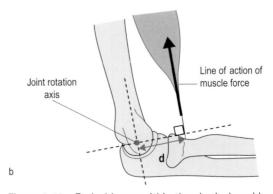

Figure 3.10 Typical levers within the physical world and the body are shown. In (a) the moment arm is shown for a weight on a see-saw and in (b) the muscle moment arm is shown for the elbow flexor. A line is drawn perpendicular to the force line of action and through the axis of rotation to determine the distance between the two.

Task 3.1

Moment arms during strength testing.
When testing the maximum muscle strength of the knee extensor, placement of the hand on the leg is important because of the effect on the moment arm of the resistance. The muscle moment arm of the knee extensor will not change during an isometric strength test. If the left knee test produces a maximum resisted force of 300 N at a distance of 25 cm distal from the knee joint axis and the right knee test produces a maximum resisted force of 250 N at a distance of 30 cm distal from the knee joint axis, can you calculate which side is stronger?

Levers

When levers are considered, the moment of force is an important factor. A lever is defined as: *a rigid bar that rotates around a fixed point or fulcrum*. The rigid bar may be represented by a crowbar in the physical world or a bony segment inside the human body, whilst the fulcrum may be the point about which the crowbar turns or it may be a joint.

Figure 3.10 represents a typical lever within the physical world and the body. The resistance has to be met by a force on the other side of the lever to balance or lift the load. In Figure 3.11, the moment arms of a lever system are shown. The moment arm between the fulcrum and the load or resistance to be moved is also called the load/resistance arm ($d_{resistance}$). The moment arm between the fulcrum

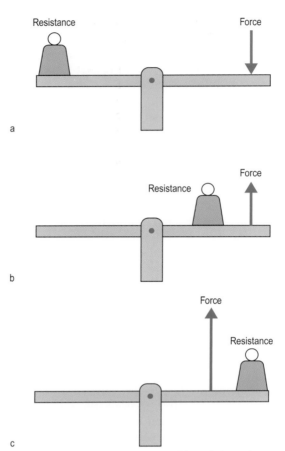

b

c

Figure 3.12   Depending on the position of the resistance, the force and the fulcrum relative to each other, levers are divided into (a) first-order, (b) second-order and (c) third-order levers.

and the effort or force is also called the force/effort arm (d_{force}).

As can be seen from Figure 3.12, there are three distinct forms that the lever can take, the formation of which depends on the relative position of the fulcrum to the resistance and the force. The form that the lever takes decides its function. A lever is often used to make work easier (as in the case of the crowbar). This does not always happen, however. Figure 3.12a represents a lever where the fulcrum lies between the force and the resistance, as in a see-saw. This is called a *first-order lever*. In this example the moment arms are equidistant. If the resistance lies between the fulcrum and the force (Fig. 3.12b) this is referred to as a *second-order*

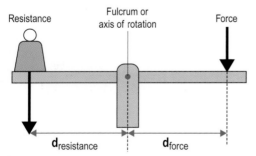

Figure 3.11   The moment arm is the distance between a force and the fulcrum. In this system, the resistance has to be met by a force on the other side of the lever to balance or lift the load. The moment arms for both are shown.

lever. The lever is helpful for lifting a load, as in a crowbar or wheelbarrow. The final combination can be seen in Figure 3.12c where the force lies between the fulcrum and the resistance. This is called a *third-order lever* and at first it appears quite difficult to see any advantage in this. However, this arrangement frequently occurs inside the body where the muscle insertion lies closer to the joint axis than the load. The advantage for the muscle is that the distance and velocity of shortening during contraction are smaller. The tissue loading is obviously large.

Mechanical advantage

The explanation of why some levers help (*mechanical advantage, MA*) and others do not is mathematical. The equation to calculate the MA is given as:

$$MA = \text{force arm}/\text{load arm} \; or \; MA = \text{load}/\text{force}$$

where force arm is the distance from the fulcrum to the force and the resistance arm is the distance from the fulcrum to the resistance (Fig. 3.13).

From the example of the see-saw in equilibrium, it can be seen that the MA will be 1. This means that there will be no advantage or disadvantage. If the example of the wheelbarrow is taken where the force arm is greater than the load arm then the MA is always going to be less than 1. Therefore any lever with an MA of less than 1 will have a true advantage. This advantage is sometimes called a *force advantage* which distinguishes it from a lever where the load arm is always greater than the force arm, giving an MA of more than 1. This last lever has a *speed advantage* over the other two types of lever. This is because, despite requiring a greater force to overcome the resistance, once this is achieved the load end of the lever will move with a greater velocity than the point at which the force is applied. Thus it has a speed advantage.

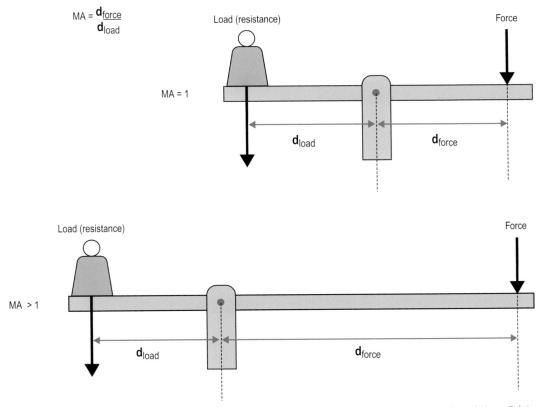

Figure 3.13 The mechanical advantage of levers can be calculated to determine whether the lever is beneficial in assisting to lift a load. A mechanical advantage greater than 1 indicates that the lever makes lifting easier.

Task 3.2

Are there situations where a muscle in the body has an arrangement different to a third-order lever? For shoulder flexion, consider the position of the fulcrum (joint), the resistance (for instance, weight of the arm) and the force (point of application of the muscle force). What type of lever is operating and has it got a force or a speed advantage?

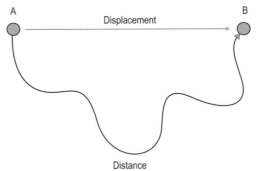

Figure 3.14   When moving from A to B the displacement between the two positions does not have to be the same as the distance travelled.

Effects of force and moment of force

It has already been said that a force can be described by its effects and there are two main effects, namely motion and deformation. Deformation will be described later in the chapter. Motion can be categorised as either *linear* or *angular*.

Linear motion

Linear motion is also referred to as translation. During a linear movement all the particles of the body describe equal and parallel paths. If the trajectory of the linear movement is a straight line it is called *rectilinear* movement and if the trajectory is curved, it is called *curvilinear* movement.

Displacement is the shortest distance between two points, as opposed to *distance* which may be travelled by a more circuitous route. This is shown in Figure 3.14.

Velocity can be defined as the *rate of change of position* (displacement) and is expressed in metres per second or m/s. Acceleration is defined as the *rate of change of velocity* and is described in metres per second squared or m/s². Figure 3.15 shows the linear displacement, velocity and acceleration of a person running and stopping. The velocity was between 2 and 3 m/s at first and then rapidly declined as the person decelerated (see Fig. 3.15b). Maximum deceleration was over 15 m/s² (see Fig. 3.15c). The velocity then gradually declined to zero. The total displacement during this period was almost 2 m (see Fig. 3.15a). It is obvious from this example that velocity and acceleration can vary from one moment to the next. The graph

therefore represents the *instantaneous* velocity and acceleration.

Angular motion

Angular motion of a body is also known as rotation. The displacement of angular motion (φ) is measured in degrees (one circle = 360°). In biomechanical calculations this is often expressed in radians (1 radian = 360°/2 pi = 57.3°).

Angular velocity (ω) is defined as the *rate of change of angular displacement*. It is measured in degrees per second or radians per second. *Angular acceleration* (α) is the rate of change of angular velocity and is expressed in degrees per second squared ($°/s^2$) or radians per second squared (rad/s^2). Figure 3.16 shows the angular movement of the right knee during the same activity of a person running and stopping as displayed in the previous figure. Peak knee flexion is close to 70°, peak knee angular velocity (towards knee flexion) is well over 500°/s and peak angular acceleration (towards knee flexion) is more than 10 000°/s².

Linear and angular motion resulting from a single force

A single force can result in a variety of effects depending on where the force is applied to the object. Once the force analysis of a system has revealed what the magnitude, direction and point of application of the resultant force are, the movement resulting from the force system can be

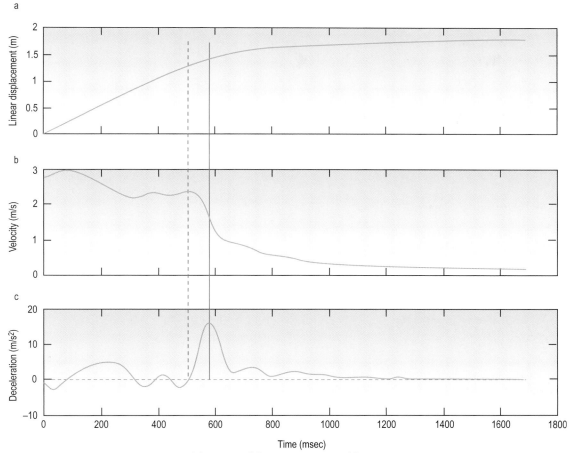

Figure 3.15 The linear displacement (a), velocity (b) and deceleration (c) of a person jogging and then stopping. In all graphs the point at which deceleration was started is indicated by the first vertical line. The second vertical line indicates where the subject was decelerating the most, which is at the peak in the bottom graph.

determined. If the line of action of a (resultant) force travels through the centre of gravity of an object/body and is parallel to the direction of movement, the force will result in linear acceleration (Fig. 3.17). Obviously, if the force is applied in the direction opposite to the direction of movement, a deceleration will occur.

If the line of action of a (resultant) force does not travel through the centre of gravity of an object/body and is parallel to the direction of movement, the force will result in linear and angular acceleration (Fig. 3.18).

If the line of action of a (resultant) force does not travel through the centre of gravity of an object/body and is not parallel to the direction of movement, the force will result in linear and angular acceleration and a change of direction (Fig. 3.19).

Linear and angular motion combined

Human movement often involves a combination of linear and angular movement. For instance, during gait, rotation of the lower limbs is used to achieve curvilinear movement of the trunk represented by the dotted line in Figure 3.20. At the start of Figure 3.20 (left side), the first rotation occurs around the ankle (a) resulting in trunk linear movement (b). In the middle, the second rotation occurs around the hip, resulting in

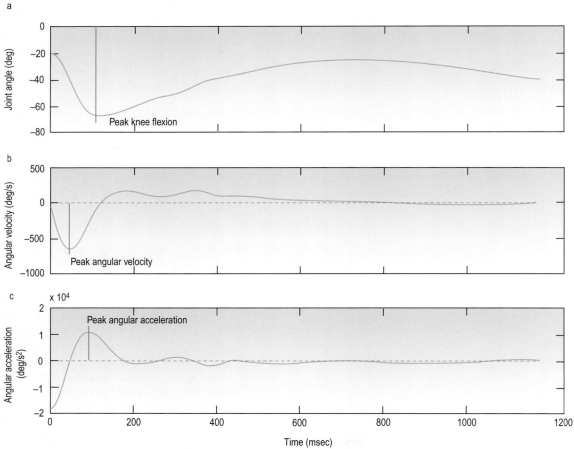

Figure 3.16 The knee angular displacement (a), velocity (b) and acceleration (c) of the same person jogging and then stopping as in Figure 3.15. A vertical line in each graph indicates the peak angular angle, velocity and acceleration. It is obvious that these peaks do not occur at the same point in time.

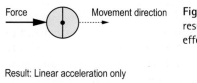

Figure 3.17 A force resulting in a linear effect only.

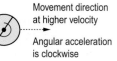

Figure 3.18 A force resulting in a linear and angular effect.

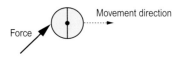

Force

Movement direction

Result: Linear and angular acceleration
(including direction change)

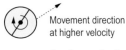

Movement direction
at higher velocity

Angular acceleration
is clockwise

Figure 3.19   A force resulting in a combined effect.

First rotation   Third rotation

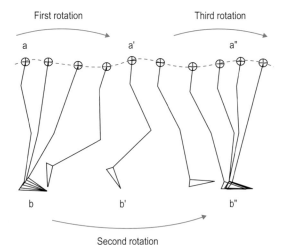

a   a'   a"

b   b'   b"

Second rotation

Figure 3.20   Gait involves rotation of the limbs to achieve curvilinear motion of the trunk (dotted line) through space. A single step is shown where a sequence of ankle (a), hip (a') and ankle (a'') rotation provides for the forward progression of the body.

curvilinear movement of the ankle (b'). The trunk continues to move forward because of the effect of the other lower limb. At the end, rotation occurs again around the ankle (b'').

Angular motion and moment of inertia

As discussed above, objects offer resistance to any changes in motion. For linear motion this is termed inertia. The tendency for an object to resist changes of angular motion is termed its *moment of inertia* or I. It can be represented by the equation:

$$I = m \times r^2$$

where m = mass of the object and r is the distance of the mass from the axis of rotation.

As the mass of the body increases so does its moment of inertia but as the mass distribution moves away from the axis of rotation, the radius increases and the moment of inertia increases in proportion to the square of that increased distance. The human body has different moments of inertia depending on the direction of rotation considered. Rotation about the longitudinal axis is easier to generate than rotation about the frontal axis because, in the latter case, the mass of the body will be located at greater distances from the axis of rotation.

CENTRE OF GRAVITY AND BASE OF SUPPORT

Theoretically mass is distributed throughout the segment and gravity (weight = mass × acceleration due to gravity) acts on every particle of mass of the segment. It would be almost impossible to perform any calculation if this were to be considered in calculations so instead the *centre of mass* (COM) of the segment is used. It is defined as the point about which the mass of an object is evenly distributed. The COM is closely associated with the *centre of gravity* (COG). The COG is sometimes explained as the point at which the force of gravity is said to act. The COM of an object is the geometrical centre of that object if it is symmetrical and regular (cube, cylinder or cone). The body segments do not fit exactly into these descriptions but can be approximated in this way. The percentage weight of the body segments and the position of the COM for each body segment can be seen in Tables 3.2 and 3.3.

Body COG, line of gravity (LOG) and centre of pressure (COP)

The COG of the body as a whole can be thought of as the point about which the mass of all body segments is evenly distributed. In the anatomical position it is thought to be at the level of the second sacral vertebra, inside the pelvis. However, as soon as the configuration of the body differs from the anatomical position, the COG will shift

Table 3.2 Mass of each body segment as a percentage of total body mass

Segment	% of body mass
Trunk	49.7
Head and neck	8.1
Arm	2.8 each
Forearm	1.6 each
Hand	0.6 each
Upper limb	5.0 each
Thigh	10.0 each
Leg	4.7 each
Foot	1.4 each
Lower limb	16.1 each

Table 3.3 Location of the COM of each body segment as a percentage of segment length (after Winter 1990)

Segment	Location
Trunk	50% between greater trochanter and glenohumeral joint
Head and neck	At the point of the ear canal
Arm	43.6% from proximal joint
Forearm	43% from proximal joint
Hand	50% from proximal joint
Thigh	43.3% from proximal joint
Leg	43.3% from proximal joint
Foot	50% between lateral malleolus and MTP5 joint

and can even be located outside the body. For instance, if both arms are elevated to a horizontal position, the COG moves forward and upward relative to its location in the anatomical position. This change of the COG location is an important consideration when discussing balance and equilibrium and the different human postures. See Chapter 13 for a full discussion on body posture and balance.

The line of gravity can be said to be the projection of the centre of gravity on the ground, represented by a line perpendicular to the ground through the COG. In Figure 3.21, the COG is represented by the target and the dotted line represents the line of gravity. Although the position of the LOG is given relative to the different joints, it should be realised that there is a wide variation in posture between different people. The LOG is not very useful for biomechanical calculations.

The *centre of pressure* is the point of application of the ground reaction force. This force reflects Newton's Third Law, the Law of Action/Reaction, in that the force exerted by the body onto the ground is reflected back at the centre of pressure. On average, during quiet standing, the ground reaction force and gravity pulling on the COG will be co-linear but this is not necessarily the case during movements.

Base of support

Every object, unless it is floating in space, has to rest on a supporting surface. The surface area of the part which is involved in support of the object, be it inanimate or a human body, is known as the *base of support* (BOS). The shape and size of the base of support depend upon the posture that the body adopts (lying, sitting or standing, for example), the position of the feet and hands and the use of extra support (crutches or a chair, for example). When standing upright unsupported, the BOS is in between and underneath the feet (see Fig. 3.22).

Balance, equilibrium and stability

These terms are often used interchangeably but they are all slightly different paradigms. If the line of gravity is within the base of support then the body is said to be in *balance*. When all the resultant forces and moments acting on a body are equal to zero then *equilibrium* is said to occur. If the body is stationary when all the forces add up to zero then the body is said to be in *static* equilibrium. If, on the other hand, the body moves with a constant linear velocity it is said to be in *dynamic equilibrium*. If, after a displacement by a force of short duration, the body tends to return to its original starting position then it is said to be *stable*.

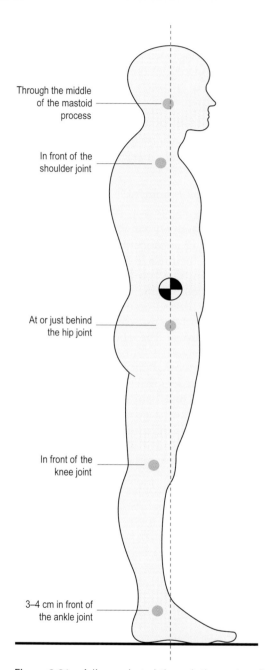

Through the middle of the mastoid process

In front of the shoulder joint

At or just behind the hip joint

In front of the knee joint

3–4 cm in front of the ankle joint

Figure 3.21   A line projected through the centre of gravity onto the floor is called the line of gravity. In the picture this line is shown on a person standing upright. Some anatomical landmarks give a better indication of where the line is located.

Types of stability

If an object tends to return to its original starting position after a force of short duration is applied or if the object is placed such that an effort to disturb it would require its COG to be raised then the object is said to be *stable*. In other words, the LOG remains well within the BOS when the object is tilted.

In the situation where an object tends to continue its displacement under the influence of gravity after a force of short duration is applied then it is said to be *unstable*. When the relationship of the LOG to the base and the height of the COG are the same after displacement (rolling of a tube, for example) then the stability is said to be *neutral*. The stability of a body depends upon:

• the surface area of the BOS
• the location of the LOG within the BOS
• the height of the COG above the BOS
• the mass of the body.

Base of support, stability limit and centre of pressure

In Figure 3.22, quiet standing with the feet parallel and slightly apart, the BOS is the area within a line drawn around the outer edges of the feet and the area in between. In theory, a person should be able to move their line of gravity to the edge of the BOS and still be stable. However, this is very difficult to do because it would require a lot of muscle force at the ankle joint. There is therefore a limited area within the BOS within which a person can move their line of gravity safely. This area is called the *stability limit* (see Fig. 3.22).

The centre of pressure (COP) was defined as the point of application of the ground reaction force. During quiet standing the COP lies well within the BOS and the stability limit. The COP is usually located a few centimetres in front of the ankle joint and moves with an amplitude of approximately 1 cm because a person sways when standing (see Fig. 3.22).

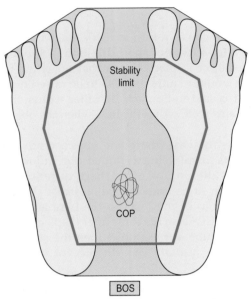

Figure 3.22   During quiet upright standing, the contact area with the floor underneath the feet and the area in between the feet is the base of support (BOS; darker area in the diagram). Because people cannot easily move their line of gravity to the outer edges of the BOS, the stability limit has been defined as the area within which people can move their line of gravity without losing balance. The centre of pressure (COP) of the ground reaction force is located well within those two areas. Because a person will always sway a bit, the COP oscillates with a certain amplitude.

WORK, ENERGY, POWER AND MOMENTUM

Work

When a force moves an object in a specified direction, the extent to which it is moved is the amount of *work* performed. The unit of work is the joule (J). Work can either be linear or rotational and can be calculated by using the following equations:

$$\text{Linear work} = \text{Force} \times \text{distance of linear displacement}$$

$$\text{Rotational work} = \text{Moment} \times \text{angular displacement}$$

Muscle work

Muscle work can be calculated in different ways using the following equations. If the muscle force and the distance between muscle origin and insertion are known:

$$\text{Work} = \text{Muscle force} \times \text{muscle length change}$$

If the net joint moment (see section on movement analysis later in this chapter) and joint rotations are known:

$$\text{Work} = \text{Net joint moment} \times \text{joint angular displacement}$$

Muscle can only actively shorten by means of a contraction. During a concentric contraction the muscle force and the muscle length change are in the same direction. The above equation will then result in a positive outcome and therefore results in positive work. During an eccentric contraction the muscle force and the muscle length change are in opposite directions. The above equation will then result in a negative outcome and therefore results in negative work. During an isometric contraction there is no length change of the muscle and therefore, in biomechanical terms, there is no work done.

Energy

The capacity of a force to do work is termed *energy*, also measured in joules (J). There are many forms that energy can take. *Metabolic* energy is the energy obtained from food by means of the metabolic process. *Heat* energy is the energy that a system can derive from a heat source. *Mechanical* energy is a measure of the state of a body at an instant in time as to its ability to do work.

Forms of mechanical energy

Potential (gravitational) energy is defined as the capacity of a body to do work due to the location of an object in a gravitational field above a certain baseline. The equation for calculating this energy is shown below:

$$E_p = \text{mass} \times \text{gravity} \times \text{height}$$

where mass is the mass of the body or object, gravity is the acceleration due to gravity and height is the position of the body above the baseline.

Kinetic energy is the capacity of an object to perform work due to its motion. It can be calculated using the equation below:

$$\text{Linear kinetic energy: } E_k = \tfrac{1}{2}\, m \times v^2$$

where m is mass and v is velocity.

$$\text{Rotational kinetic energy: } E_r = \tfrac{1}{2}\, I \times \omega^2$$

where I is moment of inertia and ω is angular velocity.

Elastic (strain) energy is the capacity a body has to do work after being deformed from its original shape. It is calculated by using the equation below.

$$E_s = k \times x$$

where k is the spring stiffness and x is the change in length.

Conservation of energy

The total sum of energy is assumed to always be constant. One form of energy can be transformed into another but the total amount of energy is never lost.

Power

The rate at which work is performed is termed the *power* of the system. Power is the product of force and distance in a specified time (velocity). This can be calculated by using the equations below.

For linear motion:

$$\text{Power} = \text{Force} \times \text{distance}/\text{time}$$

or

$$\text{Power} = \text{Force} \times \text{velocity}$$

For rotational motion:

$$\text{Power} = \text{Moment} \times \text{angular displacement}/\text{time}$$

or

$$\text{Power} = \text{Moment} \times \text{angular velocity}$$

Muscle power

The rate of doing muscle work is termed *muscle power*. Muscle power can be calculated using the following equations.

If the muscle force and the distance between muscle origin and insertion are known:

$$\text{Power} = \text{Force} \times \text{velocity of contraction}$$

If the net joint moment and joint rotations are known:

$$\text{Power} = \text{Net joint moment} \times \text{joint angular velocity}$$

During concentric contractions, power is generated (positive power) and during eccentric contractions, power is absorbed (negative power). Because there is no contraction velocity of the muscle during an isometric contraction, power will be zero, in biomechanical terms.

Momentum and impulse

Momentum can be defined as the quantity of motion possessed by an object, measured by the product of its mass and the velocity of its COM. A linear momentum is relevant when an object moves linearly and angular momentum is relevant when an object rotates.

The summation of a force over time is called the *impulse*. It is also described as the area under the force curve (Fig. 3.23) and can be interpreted as

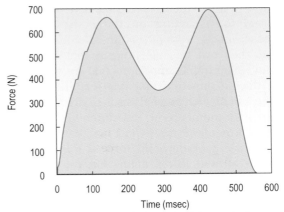

Figure 3.23 This is a typical graph of the vertical ground reaction force under one foot during gait. The double hump shape arises from the heel-strike and push-off phases. Because the foot does not move during the stance phase, this force would not result in any work. Therefore, the impulse (area under the curve) is a better indication of the impact the foot has on the ground or vice versa.

the change of momentum. Momentum and impulse have the same units, namely newton.second (N.s).

They are useful quantities when a force applied over time does not result in a change of position, as happens during gait. The ground reaction force applied to the foot during the stance phase of gait is substantial but the foot remains in the same position relative to the floor. Without a distance or velocity over which this force is applied, work or power generated by this ground reaction force would be zero. The impulse of the ground reaction force in that case is more revealing.

These quantities can also help to explain what happens during collisions (kicking a ball, rugby tackle). The sum of the colliding objects remains constant. This is also known as *conservation of momentum*.

QUANTITATIVE MOVEMENT ANALYSIS

The majority of human movements are quite complex because body segments move relative to each other and relative to the environment. This makes it difficult to predict what combination of muscle actions is required to generate a particular movement. A quantitative movement analysis can clarify which muscles should be active during a posture or movement in the context of several external forces acting on the body. For this purpose, *inverse dynamics* is an often-used technique. The word 'inverse' indicates that the causes of movement (forces and moments) are calculated from the outcome (movement as it is measured).

The aim of such an analysis is to determine the forces and moments at the different joints. In particular, net joint forces and net joint moments are calculated. A net joint force is the resultant force of all the forces acting on the different anatomical structures at the joint interface between two body segments. In equivalent terms, a net joint moment is the resultant moment. Muscles generate the main components of a net joint moment and therefore these net joint moments can be used as an indication of which muscles contribute to an activity. A limitation of the method is that it does not clearly predict the co-activation of muscles.

Once net joint forces and moments are known and given certain assumptions, it is possible to estimate what loading muscle tendons, joint surfaces and passive joint structures undergo during an activity.

Link segment model and a free body diagram (FBD)

Movement analysis by means of the inverse dynamics approach involves a number of steps. First of all, a link segment model is used to represent the body in biomechanical terms. In a two-dimensional link segment model the segments of the body can be represented by a bar or a line and the joints by a hinge. A free body diagram is a graphical representation of the whole or part of the body. To be able to do any calculations three different types of information are necessary. These are anthropometric information on the segments (for example segment mass and length), kinematic information (linear and angular segmental movement) and some information about the external forces acting on the body (for example ground reaction force). Each segment is analysed separately using a free body diagram and the equilibrium equations of force and moment. The analysis is usually started at the distal segment. The results (net joint forces and moments) from that distal segment can then be used in the analysis of the next segment in the link. The calculation therefore progresses in steps from one segment to the next.

Finding the resultant

To illustrate this process, we will use an example of the lower limb during gait. The phase of the gait cycle to be analysed is at the end of mid-stance just before the push-off phase (Fig. 3.24). At that point the foot is normally flat on the ground and not yet moving. To analyse the right leg, we need to start by constructing a link segment model of the right lower limb (Fig. 3.25). For each segment we need to know the mass, the length, the location of the centre of mass and the moment of inertia about the centre of mass. This information is available in the literature (Winter 1990). In our example information about the ground reaction force (magnitude, direction and point of application) is available from measurement.

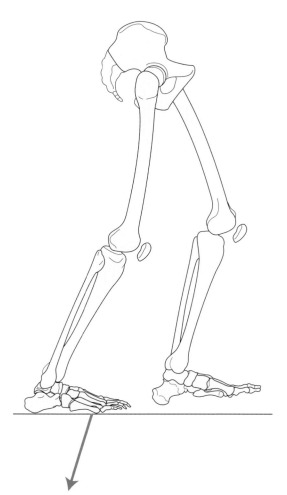

Figure 3.24 This is the phase during gait that is used in the example of movement analysis. The right foot is starting the push-off but heel-off has not yet occurred. The other limb is in terminal swing phase and heel-strike will occur soon. The vector shows the force applied by the foot on the ground (magnitude, direction and point of application).

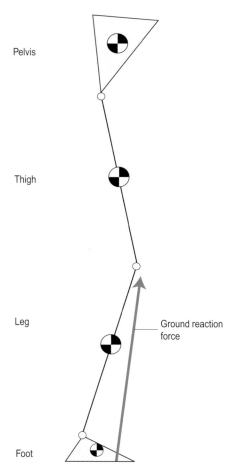

Pelvis

Thigh

Leg

Ground reaction force

Foot

Figure 3.25 A link segment model describes the relation of the body segments relative to each other in mechanical terms, using bars to represent the segments and hinges to represent the joints. The targets indicate the positions of the centre of mass of each segment. The vector shows the magnitude, direction and point of application of the ground reaction force acting on the foot.

Steps involved in quantitative movement analysis

Step 1 – creating a free body diagram

Calculations are started at the foot since sufficient information about the external forces is available. Therefore a free body diagram of the right foot is constructed (Fig. 3.26). The free body is analysed as a separate entity. The environment and neighbouring parts of the body are represented in the

FBD by arrows indicating the forces and moments that are applied by these factors to the free body.

In our example the relevant forces and moments to be included in the FBD are the ground reaction force (GRF), the effect of gravity on the centre of mass of the foot (G_{foot}), the net joint force at the ankle (F_{ankle}) and the net joint moment at the ankle (M_{ankle}). The latter two factors represent the net linear and rotational effects of the rest of the body on the foot acting at the ankle joint. These

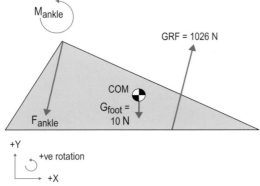

Figure 3.26 A free body diagram of the right foot. Vectors indicate forces and moments acting on the foot during the late stance phase of gait.

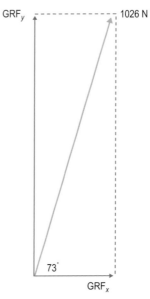

Figure 3.27 The ground reaction force (GRF) is an angled force and therefore must be resolved into its orthogonal components to be able to do further calculations.

$$\text{GRF}_x = 1026 \times \cos 73° = 300 \text{ N}$$
$$\text{GRF}_y = 1026 \times \sin 73° = 981 \text{ N}$$

influences are unknown but will be solved by calculation. These forces and moments are entered in the FBD as arrows in the locations where they act. The directions of the forces and moments are not always easy to predict. It is not essential to make an accurate prediction so long as the equilibrium equations are written on the basis of the FBD. The results of the calculations will then tell you whether the direction of the arrows was correct or not. A negative result indicates that the force or moment is pointing in the direction opposite to the one drawn.

Step 2 – type of equilibrium

The next step is to consider whether the foot is accelerating/decelerating (dynamic equilibrium) or not (static equilibrium). In our example the foot at that particular instant is not moving or starting to move. Therefore, all the forces acting on the foot should add up to zero since there is no linear acceleration/deceleration and all the moments should also add up to zero since there is no angular acceleration/deceleration (static equilibrium).

Step 3 – the equilibrium equations and finding the force

With the above information the equilibrium equations of force and moment for this free body diagram can be written and solved. The net joint force is solved first followed by the net joint moment. Before the forces can be summed they

need to be resolved into their orthogonal components. For instance, the ground reaction force can be resolved (Fig. 3.27) into a vertical component pointing upwards (positive direction) and a horizontal component pointing to the right (positive direction). The net ankle force can be resolved into a vertical component pointing down (negative direction) and a horizontal component pointing to the left (negative direction). The effect of gravity is always pointing vertically down so that it does not have to be resolved.

Step 4 – the horizontal force

The horizontal forces in this FBD are the horizontal components GRF_x and $F_{\text{ankle},x}$. These should add up to zero, as stated earlier. This results in an equation that can readily be solved.

Horizontal forces:

$$\text{GRF}_x - F_{\text{ankle},x} = 0$$
$$300 - F_{\text{ankle},x} = 0$$
$$F_{\text{ankle},x} = 300 \text{ N}$$

The result is a positive number, therefore the direction of the arrow pointing in the negative direction in the FBD was correct.

Step 5 – the vertical force

In the vertical direction there are three forces to consider: the vertical component of the GRF_y and the $F_{ankle,y}$ and the effect of gravity on the foot (G_{foot}). They should add to zero so this also results in an equation that can readily be solved.

Vertical forces:

$$GRF_y - F_{ankle,y} - G_{foot} = 0$$

$$981 - F_{ankle,y} - 10 = 0$$

$$F_{ankle,y} = 971 \text{ N}$$

The total net ankle force can now be calculated by summing the horizontal and vertical components: $F_{ankle,x}$ and $F_{ankle,y}$.

Net ankle force:

$$F_{ankle} = \sqrt{(F_{ankle,x}^2 + F_{ankle,y}^2)}$$

$$F_{ankle} = \sqrt{(300^2 + 971^2)} = 1016 \text{ N}$$

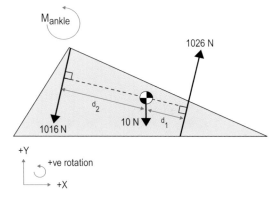

Key $d_1 = 0.02$ m
$d_2 = 0.10$ m

Figure 3.28 Once all the forces acting on the foot have been calculated, the rotatory effects of these forces also need to be considered. The same free body diagram used in Figure 3.26 is shown, but the moment arms of the GRF (d1) and ankle force (d2) are entered as well.

Step 6 – the ankle moment

Now that all the unknown forces for this FBD have been solved, the net ankle moment can also be solved. Note that the moments of force about the COM of the free body are considered and not about the ankle joint. In that case gravity does not have a moment of force about the COM. Therefore, the moment of force of the GRF and of the net ankle force and the net joint moment are to be included in the equation. The moment of force can be calculated by multiplying the force by the perpendicular distance between the axis of rotation (fulcrum) and the line of action of the force (Fig. 3.28). As mentioned before, this distance is also called the moment arm or lever arm.

Another aspect to consider is the direction in which each force would rotate the free body if acting alone. In this FBD the GRF would result in an anti-clockwise (positive) rotation around the COM if it was the only force acting on the foot. The net ankle force would result in an anti-clockwise (positive) rotation. These will therefore be entered in the moment equation as positive. The net joint moment has been drawn as an anti-clockwise moment (see Fig. 3.28) so this is also entered into the same equation as positive. All these factors should add up to zero because

the foot is not rotating, i.e. there is no angular acceleration.

Net ankle moment:

$$(GRF \times d_1) + (F_{ankle} \times d_2) + M_{ankle} = 0$$

$$(1026 \times 0.02) + (1016 \times 0.10) + M_{ankle} = 0$$

$$M_{ankle} = -122 \text{ N.m}$$

Step 7 – the internal moment

The result of this calculation of the net joint moment is negative. Therefore, the moment should be drawn as a clockwise moment, which means that it is an internal plantarflexing moment. This internal moment is mainly generated by the plantarflexors of the ankle. The triceps surae is the major contributor because of its large physiological cross-sectional area and because of its large moment arm compared to the other flexors. Therefore it is not unreasonable to assume that this muscle almost entirely generates the ankle moment calculated in our example.

This assumption that one muscle produces the net joint moment makes it possible to calculate the force that will occur within the tendo calcaneus. A muscle moment is the product of the force within the muscle and the distance between the line of

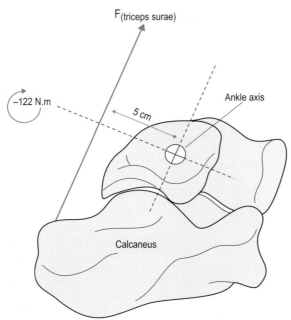

Figure 3.29   The net ankle moment calculated in the example is mainly provided by the triceps surae muscle. The moment arm of the muscle determines what muscle force is required to generate this moment. In this example the muscle moment arm is estimated to be 5 cm.

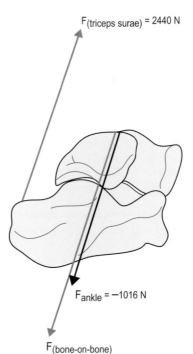

Figure 3.30   The triceps surae applies a large force in the direction opposite to the net joint force that was calculated. Therefore, there needs to be a third force that balances the force system. This would have to be the force that the bones of the leg apply to the foot. The resultant of the $F_{(triceps)}$ and the $F_{(bone-on-bone)}$ is the net ankle force (F_{ankle}).

action of the muscle and the axis of rotation of the ankle joint (Fig. 3.29). This distance or moment arm for the tendo calcaneus can be estimated at 5 cm.

Net ankle moment generated by the triceps surae:

$$M_{ankle} = Force_{(triceps)} \times distance_{(tendo\ calcaneus)}$$

$$-122\ N.m = Force_{(triceps)} \times -0.05\ m$$

$$\frac{-122\ N.m}{-0.05\ m} = Force_{(triceps)}$$

$$Force_{(triceps)} = 2440\ N$$

Step 8 – muscles, forces and their effects

The calculated force acting on the tendo calcaneus is quite high but not out of the ordinary. In fact, the tensile loading in this example is equivalent to approximately three times the body weight of an average person. In more strenuous activities, such as jumping, this loading is expected to be much higher still.

The force of the triceps muscle is much larger than the net ankle force that was calculated earlier ($F_{ankle} = -1016\ N$) and is pointing in the opposite direction. The net ankle force is the resultant force of all the different structures producing forces at the ankle joint. The muscle is just one of these structures. In this example, the other structures are therefore generating the remainder of the forces so that the resultant force equals the net ankle force that was calculated. Because all forces in this example are parallel, the force of the other structures ($F_{(bone-on-bone)}$ in Fig. 3.30) can be easily determined.

Bone-on-bone forces:

$$F_{ankle} = F_{(triceps)} - F_{(bone-on-bone)}$$

$$-1016 = 2440 - F_{(bone-on-bone)}$$

$$F_{(bone-on-bone)} = 2440 + 1016 = 3456\ N$$

It is assumed that the main structure contributing to this is the force of the tibia on the talus although the ligaments cannot be ignored.

The bone-on-bone force results in a compression of the ankle cartilage. This load is the largest of all the values calculated. It is interesting to note that the activity of the triceps muscle was the major contributor to this cartilage loading. Body weight contributed to the cartilage loading to a much lesser extent. This is mainly due to the direction of pull of the muscle, which is almost parallel to the tibia, and to the 'small' moment arm of the muscle. The tendo calcaneus has one of the largest moment arms of the muscles of the limbs. The result of this example, therefore, illustrates in general that joint loading is mostly due to muscle contractions.

Moving up the limb

The calculations so far have indicated which muscle group needs to be active to provide the appropriate moment at the ankle joint and given us an idea of the magnitude of the tissue loading at the ankle joint. The same type of calculation can be carried out for the knee joint. For this purpose, an FBD of the lower leg is required. The unknowns are the net joint force and net joint moment at the knee. The net ankle force and moment have already been solved for the FBD of the foot. These can be used for the FBD of the lower leg as well because according to Newton's Third Law of Motion, 'to every action there is an equal and opposite reaction'. In other words, the force (or moment) applied to the foot by the leg is equal but opposite to the force (or moment) applied by the foot to the leg. Once the net knee force and moment have been solved, the analysis can be progressed to the hip joint. This will not be elaborated on in this chapter.

Note that the calculation for the example provided could be done in different ways but the proposed method allows analysis of more complex situations as well. It is the process that is demonstrated and not so much the calculation of the example.

DEFORMATION OF MATERIALS

So far this chapter has considered the effects of force on an object if the object moves or has the propensity to move. There are conditions when the object to which the force is being applied does not perform linear or angular motion. If sufficient force is applied then the object will undergo deformation. The type and extent of deformation will depend on the magnitude, direction and duration of the applied force and the composition of the object itself.

Stress and strain

The application of a force to an object is termed *loading*. The standardised measurement of loading is termed *stress*. The intensity of the applied stress is a result of the applied force divided by the surface area over which the force acts. This is expressed in $N.m^{-2}$ (pascals). The equation is:

$$\sigma = \text{Force/cross sectional area}$$

Once the stress has been applied, the object will undergo a *deformation* which can be defined as the change in shape or dimensions produced by the applied force. Not all materials will deform in the same way or to the same extent. Some materials will offer greater resistance to being deformed. This resistance is known as the material's *stiffness*. The measure of deformation undergone by the object due to the stress that has been placed on it is termed the *strain*; it has no units and is denoted by the letter epsilon (ε) and expressed by the equation:

$$\varepsilon = \Delta L / L_0$$

where ΔL is change in dimension and L_0 the original dimension.

Figure 3.31 gives examples of the types of stress that can act on an object. For every stress there is a corresponding strain. The relationship between the two parameters is unique to every material.

Linear loading

There are three types of linear stress that can be applied to the object.

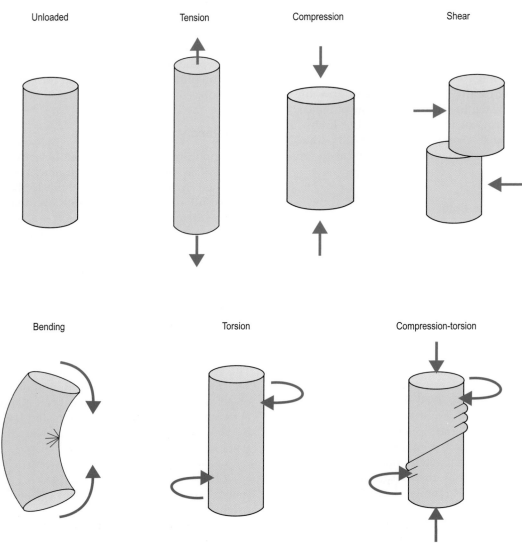

Figure 3.31   These are examples of the types of tissue loading that can occur. Included are linear and rotational types of loading.

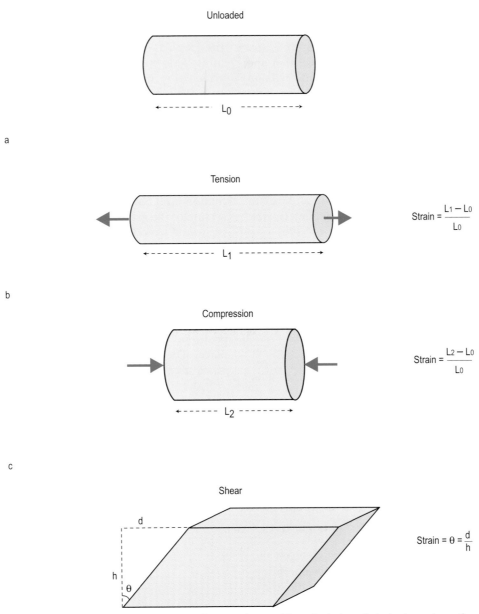

Figure 3.32   Strain occurs under the influence of stress. The calculation of strain depends on the type of stress that is active. The examples provided are for the linear stresses of tension, compression and shear.

Linear tension occurs when two equal loads are applied to an object in such a way that they act along the same action line but in opposite directions. The resultant deformation is a lengthening and some narrowing. This is shown in Figure 3.32a.

Linear compression occurs when two equal loads are applied to an object such that they act along the same action line towards each other, i.e. squeezing. The resultant deformation will therefore be shortening with some widening, as shown in Figure 3.32b.

Shear occurs when two parallel and equal loads are applied in opposite directions but not on the same line of action. This is shown in Figure 3.32c.

It can also be seen from Figure 3.32 that the calculation of the linear compression and tension strain is relatively straightforward. When considering the shear stress and strain there is no change in length but there is an angular deformation. If, as illustrated in Figure 3.32c, the block is acted upon by a stress and the top of the block moves a distance d relative from the bottom of the block, then there is an angle Θ produced, as shown. This is the angle of shear strain and can be calculated by dividing the displacement by the height.

Young's modulus

The relationship of the changing stress and strain results in a constant of proportionality for each individual material. This constant is called *Young's modulus* and is represented by the equation:

$$\text{Young's modulus} = \Delta\sigma/\Delta\varepsilon$$

where $\Delta\sigma$ is the change in linear stress and $\Delta\varepsilon$ is the change in linear strain.

The constant of proportionality for shear stress is the *shear modulus* and is represented by the equation:

$$\text{Shear modulus} = \Delta\sigma/\Theta$$

where $\Delta\sigma$ is the change in shear stress and Θ is the change in shear strain.

Stress/strain curves

One of the more useful relationships between the stress placed on an object and the corresponding strain is seen when a graph is plotted with strain on the *x*-axis and stress on the *y*-axis. A general stress/strain curve is illustrated in Figure 3.33. The relationship found for any material is dependent only on the type of loading and the mechanical properties of the material. It is interesting to note that the relationship will stay the same for any object made from the same material irrespective of its size or shape. By experimentation, the relationships between stress and strain for different materials have been found and each displays variations of a basic pattern.

As can be seen from the diagram, there are two distinct regions. The first is the linear section of the graph as seen between the start and the elastic limit. This is referred to as the elastic region, in which the material under stress obeys Hooke's Law. This means that for every incremental unit of stress, there is a corresponding incremental increase in strain, i.e. there is a linear relationship between the two. If the stress is released before the elastic limit is reached, the material will return to its original position. Therefore, there is no permanent deformation occurring and the deformation (and material) is referred to as *elastic*. This section of the graph is represented mathematically by Young's modulus.

Once the stress has increased past the elastic limit, the graphical representation is seen to occur in the plastic region (up to the *yield point*). If the stress does not exceed the yield point then the material will still exhibit some elastic properties but the material will not return to its original position. Some permanent deformation has taken place. The material is said to have undergone *plastic change*.

If the stress is maintained at the yield point the material will undergo *plastic flow* where the strain continues with no increase in stress until *failure* occurs and the material will fracture. The amount of stress that a material can absorb prior to failure

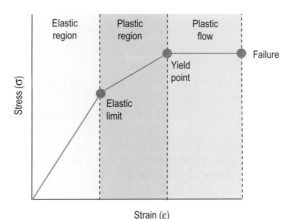

Figure 3.33   A typical stress-strain curve that applies to many types of materials. Generally, materials have an elastic region and a plastic region until failure. The elastic limit and the yield point are shown in the graph marking the transition from one region to the next.

is called its *ductility* and will vary for different materials.

MECHANICAL PRINCIPLES OF FLUIDS

Hydrostatics and hydrodynamics

Hydrostatics is the study of the effects of force and pressure on a fluid at rest whereas hydrodynamics is the study of fluid in motion (flow). To understand hydrostatics we must look first at some of the physical properties of liquids. In this section only water will be described, as it is water that is generally used in the treatment of patients. Water itself can take the form of any of the three states of matter, being solid below temperatures of 0°C and gaseous above 100°C. Hydrotherapy pools are normally heated to temperatures of between 33°C and 38°C and thus the water is always a liquid.

The structure of a liquid is such that its properties are different from those of solid objects. At a basic level the atomic structure of a liquid can be said to have weaker cohesive bonds (attractive forces between the same type of molecules) than a solid. This means that the motion of these molecules is much greater than in solids, so much so that a liquid is unable to maintain its own shape and therefore has to take the shape of the receptacle in which it is placed. A liquid also has the property of retaining its volume, showing a molecular repulsive force when it is being compressed. It is this repulsive force that produces the almost continuous flow of the liquid when an outside force is applied to it, hence the term 'fluid'.

The cohesive force is responsible for giving water its property of *surface tension*. This is the 'film-like' covering on the surface of the water which is caused by the cohesive forces of the water-to-water molecules which are stronger than the adhesive forces (the attractive forces between different molecules) of the water-to-air molecules. The force of surface tension for a hydrotherapy pool is so weak that it can be ignored. The adhesive forces between the water and whatever is placed in it, part of the body or an oar for example, are also very weak, being greater than moving through the air but insignificant when compared to the frictional forces experienced on land.

Pressure

When a force is applied to a fluid in a confined container, the fluid experiences pressure. Earlier in the chapter pressure was described as the force per unit area and this was the pressure on a plane surface. In fluids, however, the pressure is said to be acting at a point and this point can be thought of as a small plane surface (Bell 1998). Even without an additional force, hydrostatic pressure is felt within the fluid in all directions as the randomly moving molecules collide into each other, the container and any object immersed in it. Pascal's Law states that this force is equal in all directions and is independent of gravity. Pressure within the fluid is also the result of the weight of the fluid above a given point and it is equal to the vertical distance from the point to the surface, multiplied by the weight density of the fluid. So it can be seen that the deeper an object is in the fluid, the greater the pressure it will experience. Hydrostatic pressure is usually measured in pascals (one pascal equals $1 \ N.m^{-2}$).

Density

Along with depth, pressure in a fluid will change when the density of the fluid changes. Density is defined as the mass of the fluid divided by its volume. This then gives us the fluid's mass density (ρ) expressed in $kg.m^{-3}$. If we multiply the fluid's mass by the acceleration due to gravity and divide it by its volume then we have the fluid's weight density.

Relative density/specific gravity

This is the density of a material (solid or liquid) relative to that of pure water at 4°C. As the relative density of water is, by definition, 1 then the relative densities of other materials will determine whether they will float or sink in water. A relative density less than 1 will mean that the material will float and with a relative density greater than 1 it will sink. The relative density of the human body is in the region of 0.86–0.97 (Bell 1998). This number will vary depending on the proportion of the different body tissues and the amount of air within the lungs.

Buoyancy

It has already been said that the pressure on a body within the water is equal on all aspects of that body and this pressure increases with the depth of the water. The point forces will be greater on the deeper aspects of the object, thus there will be a resultant upward force on that body. This resultant upward force is the upthrust experienced in the water and is termed the force of *buoyancy*.

The amount of force a body will experience is governed by Archimedes' principle which states that any body which is wholly or partially immersed in a fluid will experience an upward thrust equal to the weight of fluid displaced. The force of buoyancy can be said to be acting through the *centre of buoyancy*, which is the centre of gravity of the displaced fluid. Therefore, the centre of buoyancy does not have to coincide with the centre of gravity of the body in the water.

Stability

The stability of a body on dry land is subject to the relationship of the centre of gravity to the base on which it rests. In fluids, however, the relationship of the centre of gravity to the centre of buoyancy is the predominant factor controlling stability. If a body is placed in water it will rotate until the centre of buoyancy and the centre of gravity are coincident. This point is referred to as the *meta-centre*. This is illustrated in Figure 3.34.

Moment of buoyancy

If the centres of buoyancy and gravity do not lie in the same vertical line then the body, as explained above, will not be in equilibrium and will rotate. The cause of this rotation is the *moment of buoyancy*. The moment of buoyancy is the same as any turning effect of a force on dry land in that it causes the body to rotate until it is compelled to stop by another force or, in this example, because the forces of buoyancy and gravity are co-linear.

The moment of buoyancy is calculated, as on dry land, by multiplying the force (buoyancy) by the perpendicular distance from the fulcrum. As can be seen from Figure 3.35, the nearer the body

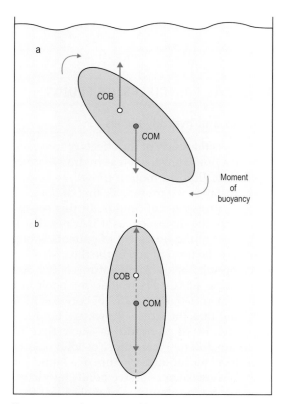

Figure 3.34   A moment of buoyancy occurs when the forces due to gravity and buoyancy are not co-linear (a). The object will rotate until co-linearity has been achieved (b). In this example the centre of buoyancy and the centre of mass never coincide.

segment is to the water's surface, the greater the perpendicular distance from the knee axis of rotation and hence the greater the moment of buoyancy, thus facilitating knee extension.

Types of flow

When a fluid flows from a point of higher to a point of lower pressure, the fluid molecules form themselves into layers or *laminae*. The layers at the centre of the flow move faster than those nearer the edge of the fluid, whilst those at the very edge may even be stationary. If these layers run smoothly along without any disturbance then the flow is said to be *laminar* or *streamlined*.

The fluid will flow in a streamlined way until it reaches a critical velocity. At this velocity the

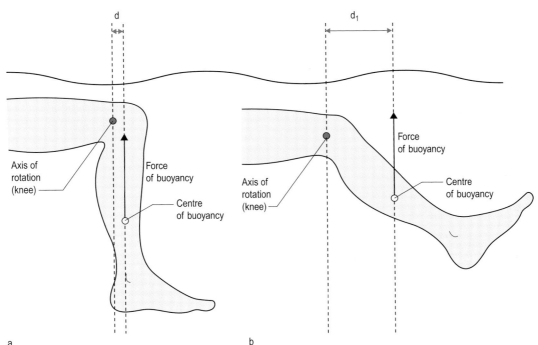

a   b

Figure 3.35 The moment of buoyancy depends on the perpendicular distance between the line of action of the force of buoyancy and the knee axis of rotation. In (a) the moment of buoyancy will be smaller than in (b) because of the greater distance (moment arm).

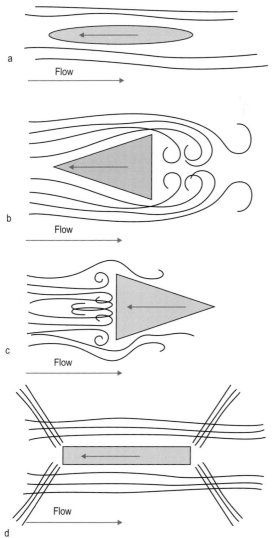

velocity in the direction of flow and perpendicular to the flow. Thus, with the increase in the flow rate, the laminar pattern will break up and the molecules will no longer travel in layers but take on an irregular pattern of motion. Once turbulent flow has been established, the back current or *eddy currents* may become exaggerated and cause areas of reduced pressure downstream (in the wake) of these eddy currents.

Movement through a fluid

If a streamlined object moves through a fluid then the fluid offers little resistance to its flow. Very little turbulence is caused by the movement of the object and thus the frictional resistance is low. If the object is not streamlined then there will be a much greater resistance to its progress. The type of resistance it will meet will depend on the shape of the object. As can be seen from Figure 3.36a, a streamlined object produces little disturbance in the fluid. Figure 3.36b shows the formation of eddy currents and an area of reduced pressure, which together form a *wake*. Figure 3.36c shows the formation of eddy currents with the turbulent flow in front of the object, which provides a much greater resistance to movement. As seen from Figure 3.36d, there is also the formation of waves, one travelling out in front of the object and one travelling out from behind. Both these waves will require energy to overcome their resistance. The resistance to movement is increased even further if the fluid in which the movement is taking place is already turbulent.

Figure 3.36 Four examples of the flow of fluid around objects of different shapes. The arrows inside the objects indicate movement of the objects from right to left. The fluid is moving in the opposite direction as indicated. In (a) there is a streamlined object that does not disturb the flow in laminae. In (b) the shape of the object results in turbulence with an area of reduced pressure and eddy currents in its wake. In (c) there are turbulence and eddy currents in front of the object. In (d) waves form at the front and the back of the object.

laminae break up and the flow is said to be *turbulent*. Turbulence is created because shear stress between the different laminae depends on the viscosity of the fluid and the rate of change of

---

Task 3.3

With a group of colleagues walk around in a circle in single file in a swimming pool. After a few seconds change the direction you are all walking (from clockwise to anti-clockwise). What happens? Try this again but this time vary the depth and speed of your walk and the frequency of your direction change. What differences do you find?

REFERENCES

Bell F 1998 Principles of mechanics and biomechanics. Stanley Thornes, Cheltenham, UK

Winter D 1990 Biomechanics and motor control of human movement. John Wiley, New York

FURTHER READING

Craik RL, Oatis CA (eds) 1995 Gait analysis: theory and application. Mosby-Year Book, St Louis

Enoka RM 1994 Neuromechanical basis of kinesiology. Human Kinetics, Champaign, Illinois

Hollis M 1989 Practical exercise therapy. Blackwell Scientific Publications, Oxford.

Zatsiorsky VM 1998 Kinematics of human motion. Human Kinetics, Champaign, Illinois

Chapter 4

The neural control of human movement

Bernhard Haas

LEARNING OUTCOMES

When you have completed this chapter you should
be able to:

1. Outline the roles of the various nervous system
   centres in the control of movement

2. Explain how movements are generated and
   controlled

3. Explain how posture and balance are controlled
   by the nervous system

4. Explain how the nervous system controls gait

5. Demonstrate knowledge of information
   transmission within the nervous system.

INTRODUCTION

The purpose of this chapter is to help you
understand the human nervous system and how
it participates in the control of movement.
Traditionally, this has been done by reducing the
function of this complex system to the properties
of its individual elements, the neurones and
control centres. Although it is essential to understand the language used to describe the system
and to have a basic knowledge of which elements
contribute to the complex affair of human movement, this reductionist view is not sufficient and
sometimes you will have to 'ignore' the individual

elements in order to better understand the system as a whole.

One of the traditional views of the nervous system has been that it is purely hierarchical with a 'top-down' approach of control. According to this view, the cortical areas of the brain would exert a higher level of control and organise voluntary skilled movement. At the other end, the spinal cord would be fairly low down in the control stakes and mainly execute plans designed and refined above. A number of textbooks, such as Tortora and Grabowski (2003), Ganong (1995), Kiernan (1998) and Martini (1998) will provide you with further details. The section in this chapter on 'The structures of the nervous system for controlling movement' will also give you an overview of the individual parts of the movement control system. In reality there is, however, no real separation between voluntary movements and the background of postural control that maintains the body in an upright position with the aid of automatic reflexes and responses. (See also Chapter 13 for more information on posture and balance.)

Therefore, parallel systems of control, with integration of all levels rather than just a serial hierarchy, may be a more appropriate description. All levels of control, from the spinal cord up to the cerebral cortex, are necessary and integrate to provide the base of axial stability for more normal distal mobility and skilled or refined coordinated limb movements (Kandel et al 2000). In addition, the environmental context and the movement task itself will influence how the nervous system organises movement.

INFORMATION TRANSMISSION

The vast numbers of neurones in the human nervous system need to communicate with each other, often very rapidly. Information is carried within neurones and between neurones by electrical and chemical signals. The rapid transmission of signals, which is vital for human movement, is a function of the 'action potential'. This action potential is achieved by temporary changes of current flow in and out of cells which then propagates a signal along the nerve axon. A necessary

precondition for action potentials is the creation of a membrane potential, the 'resting potential' (Tortora & Grabowski 2003). Please note that no movement is possible if the action potential is completely interrupted and that movement will be impaired if the signal propagation is abnormal. This may be the case if the myelin sheath that surrounds nerve axons is damaged, such as in multiple sclerosis. Figure 4.1 shows the concentrations of ions inside and outside the cell during the resting potential. Figure 4.2 shows the changes in membrane potential during the action potential. Box 4.1 summarises the key facts about the action potential.

Information transmission from one cell to another occurs at the synapse. The most important components of a synapse are the presynaptic membrane, the synaptic cleft and the postsynaptic membrane (Latash 1998). An action potential arrives at the presynaptic membrane. This leads to the influx of calcium ions which in turn facilitates the fusion of neurotransmitter vesicles to the membrane for the release of the neurotransmitter into the synaptic cleft. Neurotransmitter molecules diffuse across the synaptic cleft and bind at specialist receptor sites in the postsynaptic neurone. This changes the potential in the postsynaptic neurone as ion channels are opened and the voltage across the cell membrane changes. Depending on the particular type of channel that is being activated, either depolarisation or hyperpolarisation may occur. This explains how an action potential in the presynaptic neurone can cause either excitation or inhibition of the postsynaptic membrane. Opening of Na^+ channels would lead to depolarisation and therefore excitation, whereas opening of the Cl^- channels would hyperpolarise the postsynaptic neurone and lead to inhibition. Figure 4.3 summarises the events that occur at a synapse.

Receptors

The central nervous system (CNS) needs to receive continuous feedback about movement. It receives this information in the form of the status of muscles, i.e. length, instantaneous tension and rate of change of length and tension (Guyton 1992). Muscle spindles detect the rate of change

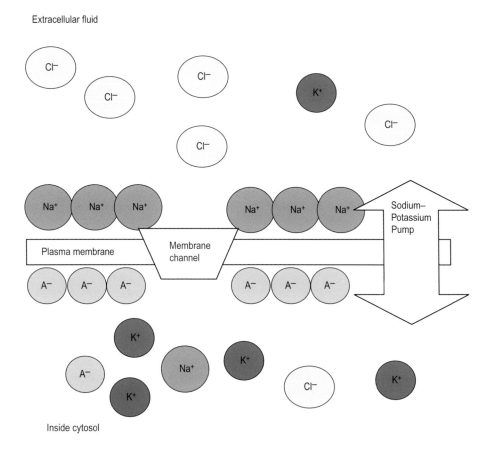

Extracellular fluid

Inside cytosol

Ion	Concentration inside cytosol	Concentration in extracellular fluid
K^+ – Potassium	150 mmol/l	5 mmol/l
Na^+ – Sodium	12 mmol/l	150 mmol/l
Cl^- – Clorine	5 mmol/l	125 mmol/l
A^+ – Organic anions	150 mmol/l	–

Figure 4.1   Distribution of ions across the cell membrane during the resting potential.

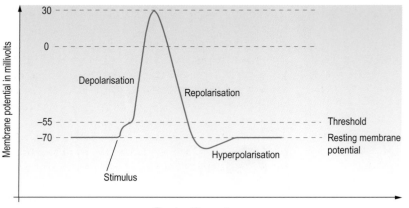

Figure 4.2   The action potential.

Box 4.1 Summary of important facts associated with the action potential.

- A necessary precondition for the creation of an action potential is the resting potential.
- The resting potential creates the excitability of the cell.
- The resting potential is the unequal distribution of ions across the cell membrane with a negative charge of –70 mV inside the cytosol.
- The action potential emerges if a stimulus is large enough to take the membrane potential above the threshold (–55 mV).
- When the threshold level is reached, voltage-gated Na^+ channels open and Na^+ rushes into the cell which produces the 'depolarisation' period.
- Voltage-gated K^+ channels open to allow K^+ to flow out of the cell and produce the 'repolarisation' period.

- Another action potential cannot be generated during the depolarisation period and during most of the repolarisation period.
- The action potential propagates along the axon segment by segment until it reaches the synaptic end bulb at the end of the axon.
- Propagation is more rapid in myelinated axons where the signal 'leaps' from node to node. Large-diameter axons also propagate signals faster than small-diameter axons.
- Axons of sensory neurones transmitting information about touch, pressure and movement as well as the axons of motor neurones transmitting movement instructions to the skeletal muscles are all large and myelinated.

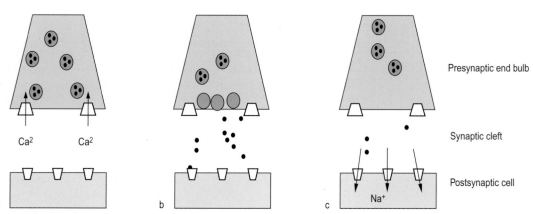

Figure 4.3   Synaptic events associated with the action potential.

and changes in the length of a muscle whereas Golgi tendon organs detect degree and rate of change of tension. Signals from these sensory receptors operate at an almost subconscious level, transmitting information into the spinal cord, cerebellum and cerebral cortex which assists in the control of muscle contraction.

The muscle spindle has both a static and a dynamic response. The primary and secondary endings respond to the length of the receptor, so impulses transmitted are proportional to the degree of stretch and continue to be transmitted as long as the receptor remains stretched. If the spindle receptors shorten, the firing rate decreases. Only the primary endings respond to sudden changes of length by increasing their firing rate, and then only whilst the length is actually increasing. Once the length stops increasing, the discharge returns to its original level, though the static response may still be active. If the spindle receptors shorten, then the firing rate decreases.

The static and dynamic response is controlled by the gamma motor neurone. Normally, the muscle spindle emits sensory nerve impulses continuously, with the rate increasing as the spindle is stretched (lengthened) or decreasing as the spindle shortens.

The spinal reflexes associated with the muscle spindle and Golgi tendon organ are the stretch reflex and tendon reflex respectively. Stimulation of the stretch reflex leads to a reflex contraction of the muscle that has been stretched whereas the tendon reflex will lead to a reflex relaxation of the muscle if there is tension build-up. Both reflexes have a protective function.

The stretch reflex also has the ability to prevent some types of oscillation and jerkiness of body movements even if the input is jerky, i.e. a damping function (Guyton 1992).

When the motor cortex or other areas of the brain transmit signals to the alpha motor neurones, the gamma motor neurones are nearly always stimulated simultaneously, i.e. a co-activation of the alpha and gamma systems so that intra- and extrafusal muscle fibres (usually) contract at the same time. This stops the muscle spindle opposing the muscle contraction and maintains a proper damping and load responsiveness of the spindle regardless of change in muscle length. If the alpha and gamma systems are stimulated simultaneously

and the intra- and extrafusal fibres contract equally, then the degree of stimulation of the muscle spindle will not change. If the extrafusal fibres contract less because they are working against a great load, the mismatch will cause a stretch on the spindle and the resultant stretch reflex will provide extra excitation of the extrafusal fibres to overcome the load (Cohen 1999).

The gamma efferent system is excited/controlled by areas in the brain stem with impulses transmitted to that region from the cerebellum, basal ganglia and cerebral cortex.

The Golgi tendon organ, as a sensory receptor in the muscle tendon, detects relative muscle tension. Therefore, it is able to provide the CNS with instantaneous information about the degree of tension on each small segment of each muscle. The Golgi tendon organ is stimulated by increased tension. When the increase in tension is too great, the tendon reflex response is evoked in the same muscle and this response is entirely inhibitory. The brain dictates a set point of tension beyond which automatic inhibition of muscle contraction prevents additional tension. Alternatively, if the tension decrease is too low, then the Golgi tendon organ reacts to return the tension to a more normal level. This leads to a loss of inhibition, so allowing the A-alpha motor neurone to be more active and increase the muscle tension.

The key facts about receptors and reflexes are summarised in Box 4.2.

MOVEMENT CONTROL

Controlling 'simple' movements

Human movement is anything but simple. There is infinite variability and any attempt to describe a complex system in simple terms is likely to tell you only part of the 'story'. However, if you understand the 'simple' then you are more likely to grasp the more complex.

Most human voluntary movements require the design and planning of movement by a control centre. This control centre will use previous experiences in the planning of movements. Once a movement plan has been designed, it will be supplied as a signal by the control centre in a feedforward manner to an execution centre, responsible

Box 4.2 Summary of important facts associated with receptors and reflexes.

- Sensory feedback for movement control is mainly provided by receptors inside the muscle and between the muscle and tendon.
- The receptors are the muscle spindle and the Golgi tendon organ.
- The muscle spindle provides information about muscle length changes.
- The Golgi tendon organ provides information about tension changes.
- Both of these receptors are also closely linked to spinal reflexes.
- The stretch reflex relies on muscle spindle information and is triggered when a muscle is lengthened. It is designed to prevent overstretching of a muscle by causing a reflex contraction of the lengthened muscle.
- The tendon reflex relies on Golgi tendon information and is triggered when tension is building up at the interchange of muscle and tendon. It is designed to prevent tearing of a muscle by causing a reflex relaxation of the muscle.
- Stretch reflex and tension reflex therefore have opposite effects on a muscle.

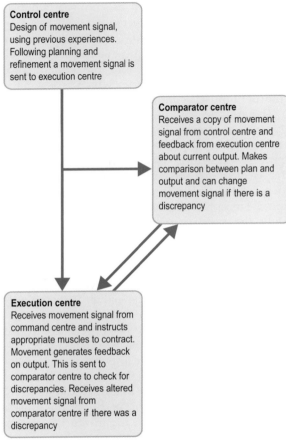

Figure 4.4 Feed-forward and feedback system of a 'simple' voluntary movement.

for activating muscles to produce the movement. Feed-forward implies that the signal is independent of the output or any other variable (Latash 1998). The feed-forward signal uses knowledge of the dynamics of the musculoskeletal system and the environment it is in (Stroeve 1999). Once the movement has started, receptors will be able to provide feedback about the movement. The controller may then be able to alter the signal according to this feedback. The addition of a 'comparator centre' provides a mechanism to speed up the refinement of movement according to its feedback. Over a period of time the feedback will in turn influence the feed-forward signal designed by the control centre and motor learning will have taken place (Houk et al 1997). It may be worth visiting Chapter 7 on 'Motor Learning' before you move on. Figure 4.4 shows such a 'simple' movement control system using feed-forward and feedback mechanisms.

Postural control and balance

Postural control and balance involve controlling the body's position in space for stability and orientation (Shumway-Cook & Woollacott 2001). The nervous system participates in postural control by designing command signals and by providing feedback through a number of receptors. The interpretation and integration of all the feedback signals would also be undertaken by the nervous system.

The postural control requirements vary with the task. For example, sitting in a chair and watching television requires minimal stability control, whereas standing on one leg and watching television is a lot more demanding on the postural

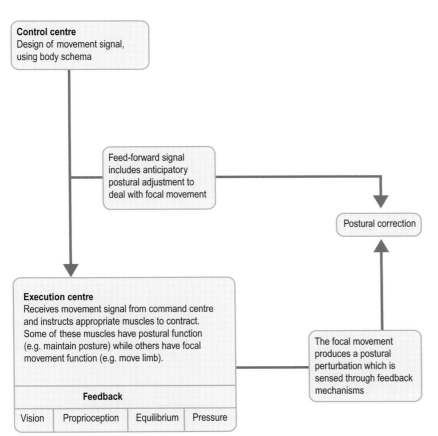

Figure 4.5 Feed-forward and feedback system for postural control.

control system. Therefore, we need to have a flexible control system that can adapt to these varying demands. Postural control requires the production of movements or muscular contractions that help keep the body upright in space. Like the simple movement system above, postural control is also achieved by a combination of feed-forward and feedback mechanisms. The control centre for posture will utilise previous experiences which contribute to an internal representation of the body or body schema (Massion 1994). This body schema provides reference points for body alignment, movement and orientation in space. The aim of the nervous system is then to maintain this body schema during changes in the environment or during movement.

The feedback mechanisms for posture and balance involve more than just the receptors for movement in the muscles. In addition, there will be feedback about movements of the head through the vestibular system in the inner ear, visual feedback and feedback about pressure changes through the support surfaces of the body (Kandel et al 2000). The feed-forward mechanisms will have to include signals that are able to anticipate disturbances to the postural control system that will arise as a consequence of movement (Aruin et al 2001). Figure 4.5 shows the system of feed-forward and feedback for the control of posture and balance. It may be worth also visiting Chapter 13 in this book.

Gait

Walking requires the cooperation of large numbers of muscles and joints. Research on animals has shown that a neural network in the spinal cord is responsible for regulating the stepping motions

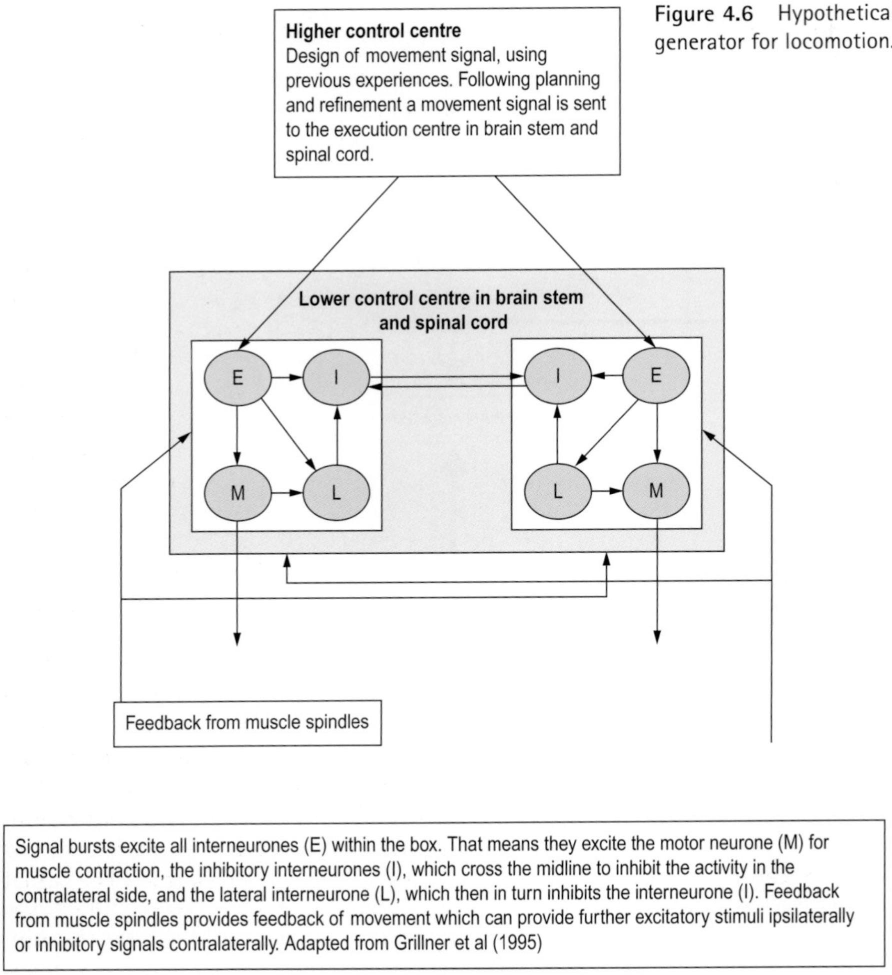

Higher control centre
Design of movement signal, using previous experiences. Following planning and refinement a movement signal is sent to the execution centre in brain stem and spinal cord.
Lower control centre in brain stem and spinal cord
E
I
M
L
I
E
L
M
Feedback from muscle spindles
Signal bursts excite all interneurones (E) within the box. That means they excite the motor neurone (M) for muscle contraction, the inhibitory interneurones (I), which cross the midline to inhibit the activity in the contralateral side, and the lateral interneurone (L), which then in turn inhibits the interneurone (I). Feedback from muscle spindles provides feedback of movement which can provide further excitatory stimuli ipsilaterally or inhibitory signals contralaterally. Adapted from Grillner et al (1995)

Figure 4.6 Hypothetical model of a central pattern generator for locomotion.

during gait. There is controversy over whether such a network also exists in humans (Guadagnoli et al 2000, Vilensky & O'Connor 1997). The brain stem together with the spinal cord could provide such a network, or 'central pattern generator', to co-ordinate locomotion. The impulse for walking may come from higher cortical centres but these central pattern generators could provide the motor pattern. Figure 4.6 provides a proposed diagram of a central pattern generator for movement in the lamprey fish (Grillner et al 1995). A similar neural network may also exist in humans. You may find it helpful to visit Chapter 10 on 'Function of the Lower Limb'.

The structures of the nervous system for controlling movement

This chapter has so far given you an overview of how the nervous system controls all types of movements (summarised in Box 4.3) and how the necessary signals for this control are generated and propagated. This has been the difficult part of the chapter and once you have understood it, you should move on to the next section, which will add more detail about the individual parts of the nervous system, which have been described only in very broad terms until now. For example, you will find that the 'comparator centre' described in Figure 4.4 is in reality called the cerebellum.

- The nervous system as a WHOLE controls all types of movements.
- These movements can differ in complexity and characteristics. They can range from a relatively simple contraction of a muscle over one joint to multi-joint and whole-body movements such as those used during walking.
- Voluntary movements are designed utilising previous experiences and use feed-forward signals towards the muscles.
- In addition to the feed-forward signals, there will also be feedback about movement and the body in relation to the environment.
- All voluntary movements, including posture, balance and gait, are based on these feed-forward and feedback principles.
- The feedback generated through movement experience also provides for the possibility of motor learning.

Cerebral cortex

The cerebral cortex is the main centre for the control of voluntary movement. It uses the information it receives from the cerebellum, basal ganglia and other centres in the CNS, as well as the feedback from the periphery, to bring movements under voluntary control.

The cerebral cortex or, more specifically, the association areas of the cerebral cortex, provide the advanced intellectual functions of humans, having a memory store and recall abilities along with other higher cognitive functions. The cerebral cortex is, therefore, able to perceive, understand and integrate all the various sensations. This provides the transition from perception to action (Shumway-Cook & Woollacott 2001). Its primary movement function is in the planning and execution of many complex motor activities, especially the highly skilled manipulative movements of the hand. This fact becomes clear when one considers the size of a cortical area for a particular part of the body.

The motor cortex occupies the posterior half of the frontal lobes. It is a broad area of the cerebral cortex concerned with integrating the sensations from the association areas with the control of movements and posture. It is closely related to other motor areas including the primary motor area and the premotor or motor association area. The primary motor area contains very large pyramidal cells which send fibres directly to the spinal cord and anterior horn cells via the corticospinal pathways. In contrast, the premotor area has a few fibres connecting directly with the spinal cord but it mainly sends signals into the primary motor cortex to activate multiple groups of muscles, i.e. signals generated here cause more complex muscle actions, usually involving groups of muscles which perform specific tasks rather than individual muscles. This area connects to the cerebellum and basal ganglia which both transmit signals back, via the thalamus, to the motor cortex. Projection fibres from the visual and auditory areas of the brain allow visual and auditory information to be integrated at cortical level to influence the activity of the primary motor area.

Each time the corticospinal pathway transmits information to the spinal cord, the same information is received by the basal ganglia, brain stem and cerebellum. Nerve signals from the motor cortex cause a muscle group to contract. The signal then returns from the activated region of the body to the same neurones that caused the contraction, providing a general positive feedback enhancement if the movement was successful and recording it for future use. The role of the cerebral cortex and its subdivisions is described in Figure 4.7.

Basal ganglia

The basal ganglia consist of five nuclei deep inside the brain (putamen, caudate nucleus, globus pallidus, subthalamic nucleus and substantia nigra). They serve as side loops to the cerebral cortex since they receive their input from the cerebral cortex and project exclusively back to the cerebral cortex. The basal ganglia are involved in all types of movements but have a predominant role in the provision of internal cues for the smooth running of learned movements (Morris & Iansek 1996).

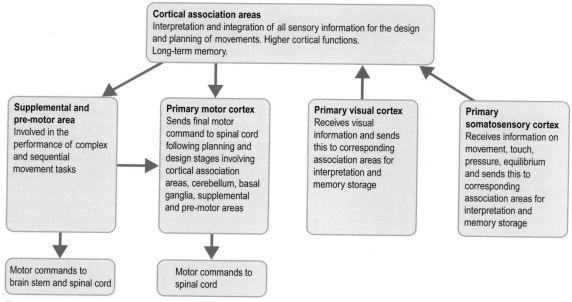

Figure 4.7   The cerebral cortex in movement control.

It is believed that the basal ganglia play an essential role in the selective initiation of most activities of the body as well as the selective suppression of unwanted movements. A number of distinct loops have been described and the interconnections of inhibitory or excitatory neurotransmitters explain the variety of symptoms that emerge in disorders of the basal ganglia. The direct pathway is responsible for the facilitation of movement, whereas the indirect pathway is more involved in the inhibition of unwanted movements (Rothwell 1994). Figure 4.8 shows the direct loop through the basal ganglia.

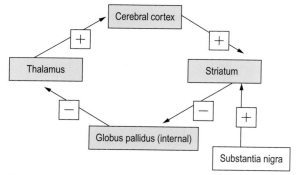

Figure 4.8   Hypothetical model of the direct loop in the basal ganglia.

Cerebellum

The cerebellum is vital for the control of very rapid muscular activities such as running, talking, typing, playing sport or playing a musical instrument. Loss of the cerebellum leads to incoordination of these movements such that the actions are still available but no longer rapid or coordinated. This is due to the loss of the planning function.

The cerebellum makes comparisons between the movement plan and the output and can change the movement signal if there is a discrepancy.

Extensive input and output systems operate to and from the cerebellum. Input pathways to the cerebellum from the cerebral cortex, carrying both motor and sensory information, pass through various brain stem nuclei before reaching the deep nuclei of the cerebellum. Likewise, output from the cerebellum exits via the deep nuclei to the cerebral cortex to help coordinate voluntary motor activity initiated there.

The cerebellum does not initiate motor activities but plays an important role in planning, mediating, correcting, coordinating and predicting motor activities, especially for rapid movements. It is vitally important for the control of posture and equilibrium where it works in close relationship with the brain stem. Working with the basal ganglia and thalamus, the cerebellum helps to control voluntary movement by utilising feedback circuits from the periphery and the brain. The distal parts of the limbs are controlled by information from the motor cortex and from the periphery and this information is integrated in the cerebellum. This provides smooth, coordinated movements of agonist and antagonistic muscle groups, allowing the performance of accurate, purposeful intricate movements, which are especially required in the distal part of the limbs. This is achieved by comparing the intentions of the higher centres of the motor cortex with the performance of respective parts of the body. Overall, the cerebellum serves as an error-correcting device for goal-directed movements. It receives information on body position and movements in progress and then computes and delivers appropriate signals to the brain stem effector centres to correct posture and smooth out movements. The cerebellum is also important in the process of learning and acquisition of motor skills (Houk et al 1997). Figure 4.4 showed the position of the comparator centre in the control of movement.

Brain stem

The principal role of the brain stem in control of motor function is to initiate background contractions of the postural muscles of the trunk, neck and proximal parts of limb musculature and so provide support for the body against gravity. The relative degree of contraction of these individual antigravity muscles is determined by equilibrium mechanisms, with reactions being controlled by the vestibular apparatus, which is directly related to the brain stem region.

The brain stem connects the spinal cord to the cerebral cortex. It is composed of the midbrain, pons and medulla oblongata. The central core of this region is often referred to as the reticular formation. This region of the central nervous system comprises all the major pathways connecting the brain to the spinal cord in a very compact, restricted space. It is also the exit point of the cranial nerves from the central nervous system.

It is through the integration of the information reaching the reticular formation that axial postural control and gross movements are controlled. Input to the reticular formation is from many sources, including the spinoreticular pathways, collaterals from spinothalamic pathways, vestibular nuclei, cerebellum, basal ganglia, cerebral cortex and hypothalamus. The smaller neurones make multiple connections within the area whereas the larger neurones are passing through, being mainly motor in function.

The vestibular nuclei are very important for the functional control of eye movements, equilibrium and support of the body against gravity and the gross stereotyped movements of the body. The direct connections to the vestibular apparatus of the inner ear and cerebellum, as well as the cerebral cortex, enable the use of preprogrammed, background attitudinal reactions to maintain equilibrium and posture. Working with the pontine portion of the reticular formation, the vestibular nuclei are intrinsically excitable; however, this is held in check by inhibitory signals from the basal ganglia (Guyton 1992). Overall, the motor-related functions of the brain stem are to support the body against gravity, generate gross, stereotyped movements of the body and maintain equilibrium. This is achieved in association with the cerebellum, basal ganglia and cortical regions.

Spinal cord

The grey matter of the spinal cord is the integrative area for the spinal reflexes and other automatic motor functions. As the region for the peripheral execution of movements, it also contains the circuitry necessary for more sophisticated movements and postural adjustments.

Sensory signals enter the cord through the sensory nerve roots and then travel to two separate destinations:

• same or nearby segments of the cord where they terminate in the grey matter and elicit local segmental responses (excitatory, inhibitory, reflexes, etc.)

• higher centres of the CNS, i.e. higher in the cord, and brain stem cortices where they provide

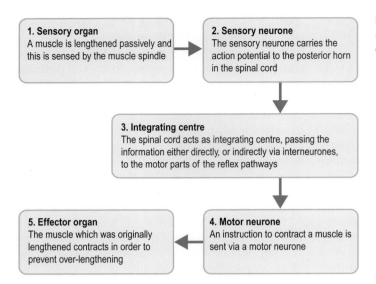

1. Sensory organ
A muscle is lengthened passively and this is sensed by the muscle spindle

2. Sensory neurone
The sensory neurone carries the action potential to the posterior horn in the spinal cord

3. Integrating centre
The spinal cord acts as integrating centre, passing the information either directly, or indirectly via interneurones, to the motor parts of the reflex pathways

5. Effector organ
The muscle which was originally lengthened contracts in order to prevent over-lengthening

4. Motor neurone
An instruction to contract a muscle is sent via a motor neurone

Figure 4.9   The components of a basic spinal reflex pathway using the stretch reflex as an example.

conscious (and unconscious, i.e. cerebellum) sensory information and experiences.

Each segment of the cord has several million neurones in the grey matter which include sensory relay neurones, anterior motor neurones and interneurones.

Interneurones are small and highly excitable with many interconnections, either with each other or with the anterior motor neurones. They have an integrative/processing function within the spinal cord as few incoming sensory signals to the spinal cord or signals from the brain terminate directly on an anterior motor neurone. This is essential for the control of motor function. One specific type of interneurone is called the Renshaw cell, located in the anterior horn of the spinal cord. Collaterals from one motor neurone can pass to adjacent Renshaw cells which then transmit inhibitory signals to nearby motor neurones. So stimulation of one motor neurone can also inhibit the surrounding motor neurones. Termed recurrent or lateral inhibition, this helps the motor system to focus or sharpen its signal by allowing good transmission of the primary signal and suppressing the tendency for the signal to spread to other neurones (Rothwell 1994). Together with the brain stem, the spinal cord contains a network of neurones which control walking. Figure 4.9 shows the basic components of a spinal reflex pathway.

Control processes of voluntary movement

Figure 4.10 summarises in a 'simplistic' diagram the control processes for voluntary movement. Follow the arrows and boxes from the design to the execution and then the return of feedback which is finally stored as memory traces.

1. The cortical association areas play the key role in the design and planning of voluntary movements. Action potentials from the cortical association areas project to the basal ganglia for refinement and selective activation of movements and/or inhibition of unwanted movements.

2/3. The thalamus here is part of the basal ganglia loops and sends impulses to the motor cortex, which is seen as the final common pathway.

4. Impulses from the motor cortex are almost simultaneously sent to the cerebellum, the brain stem and the spinal cord. The cerebellum will compare this information with the movement sensory information received from the periphery (6). The brain stem will play a role in maintaining background postural control, whilst impulses to the spinal cord are more of a focal nature for the activation of individual muscles or groups of muscles.

5. Alpha motor neurones cause muscle contraction.

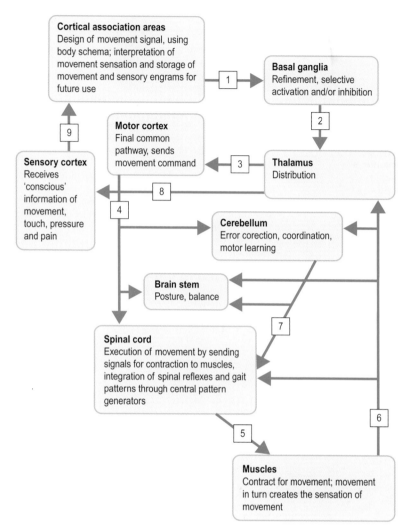

Figure 4.10   Control processes for voluntary movement.

6.   The sensation of movement, together with other relevant feedback information, is sent towards the central nervous system. This sensory information is needed by various centres. The spinal cord will use it in its integration of spinal reflexes and the control of walking patterns. The brain stem utilises sensory feedback mostly for postural control and balance. Sensory feedback is also sent to the thalamus. The cerebellum compares the movement as it occurs with the original movement instruction sent by the motor cortex.

7.   If there is a discrepancy between the intended movement and the actual movement, cor-recting signals can be sent directly to the execution centres.

8.   The thalamus distributes sensory feedback to its appropriate location on the sensory cortex.

9.   Sensory experiences are interpreted by the cortical association areas and memorised movements are stored for future use in the design and planning of movements.

Acknowledgement

This chapter has been substantially rewritten for the fifth edition. However, it would not have been possible without the inspiration and hard work of the previous co-author, J. Lesley Crow.

REFERENCES

Aruin A, Ota T, Latash ML 2001 Anticipatory postural adjustments associated with lateral and rotational perturbations during standing. Journal of Electromyography and Kinesiology 11:39–51

Cohen H 1999 Neuroscience for rehabilitation. J B Lippincott, Philadelphia

Ganong WF 1995 Review of medical physiology. Prentice-Hall, London

Grillner S, Deliagina T, Ekeberg O 1995 Neural networks that co-ordinate locomotion and body orientation in lamprey. Trends in Neurosciences 18(6):270–279

Guadagnoli MA, Etnyre B, Rodrigue ML 2000 A test of a dual central pattern generator hypothesis for subcortical control of locomotion. Journal of Electromyography and Kinesiology 10:241–247

Guyton AC 1992 Basic neuroscience: anatomy and physiology. WB Saunders, Philadelphia

Houk JC, Buckingham JT, Barto AG 1997 Models of the cerebellum and motor learning. In: Cordo PJ, Bell CC Harnad S (eds) Motor learning and synaptic plasticity in the cerebellum. Cambridge University Press, Cambridge

Kandel ER, Schwartz JH, Jessell TM 2000 Principles of neural science. McGraw-Hill, New York

Kiernan JA 1998 The human nervous system. Lippincott-Raven, Philadelphia

Latash ML 1998 Neurophysiological basis of movement. Human Kinetics, Champaign, Illinois

Martini FH 1998 Fundamentals of anatomy and physiology. Prentice-Hall International, London

Massion J 1994 Postural control system. Current Opinion in Neurobiology 4:877–887

Morris ME, Iansek R 1996 Characteristics of motor disturbance in Parkinson's disease and strategies for movement rehabilitation. Human Movement Science 15:649–669

Rothwell JC 1994 Control of human voluntary movement. Chapman and Hall, London

Shumway-Cook A, Woollacott MH 2001 Motor control – theory and practical applications, 2. Lippincott Williams and Wilkins, Philadelphia

Stroeve S 1999 Analysis of the role of proprioceptive information during arm movements using a model of the human arm. Motor Control 3(2):158–185

Tortora GJ, Grabowski SR 2003 Principles of anatomy and physiology. John Wiley, New York

Vilensky JA, O'Connor BL 1997 Stepping in humans with complete spinal cord transection: a phylogenetic evaluation. Motor Control 1:284–292

Chapter **5**

Joint mobility

Tony Everett

LEARNING OUTCOMES

At the end of this chapter you should be able to:

1. Describe the structure and function of joints

2. Discuss ranges of joint movement

3. Describe how movement is produced at joints

4. Discuss factors that influence normal facilitation and restriction of joint range

5. Discuss the causes of abnormal restriction of joint range

6. Classify joint movement

7. Discuss the rationale of the use of movement to increase joint mobility.

INTRODUCTION

Biomechanically the body can be considered as composed of segments divided between the axial and appendicular skeleton. There are many models which describe this segmental arrangement; the one that is used in this book divides the body into eight segments. The head and neck, and trunk, make up the two segments of the axial skeleton. The other six segments comprise the appendicular skeleton and are equally divided between the upper and lower limbs; the upper limb consists of arm, forearm, and wrist and hand, whilst the lower limb consists of the thigh, leg, and foot and ankle. All movements, including locomotion, involve the motion of these bony segments, be they in the appendicular or axial skeleton.

Junctions between these segments are provided by the joints (juncture, articulations or arthroses) which are themselves classified into three groups: fibrous or fixed (synarthroses), cartilaginous (amphiarthroses) or synovial (diarthroses), the last being the only freely moveable joints (Williams 1995). It is at these joints that the motion actually takes place. Movements of the segments are produced by forces, mainly the internal forces provided by muscles but also the force of gravity, which is modified by the internal muscle forces acting in opposition.

This combination of the bones that form the core of the segments and the muscles that produce the force that provides movement is described as the musculoskeletal system. It is vital that this musculoskeletal system is intact for functional movement to occur. The role of the muscles producing the movement is covered in Chapters 2 and 6 of this text but the vital components of this system, the synovial joints, will be described below.

The major characteristics of a synovial joint include the surface of opposing bones being in contact, but not in continuity, and covered in hyaline cartilage. These bony ends are joined together via ligaments and the whole joint complex, which may or may not include the ligaments, is surrounded by an extensive synovium-lined fibrous joint capsule. The viscous synovial fluid secreted by this synovial membrane not only provides the articular cartilage with nutrition but acts with it to decrease the coefficient of friction within the joint to a level that is low enough to reduce the possibility of joint surface destruction. Intracapsular structures are usually covered by synovium. Intra-articular discs or menisci may be found within the synovial joint, helping congruity and acting as shock absorbers. Labra and fat pads may also be found within the joints, having the function of increasing joint surface area (and possibly stability) and shock absorption respectively.

There are a large number of different types of synovial joints, classified according to their shape,

for example plane, saddle, hinge, pivot, ball and socket, condylar or ellipsoid (Palastanga et al 1998), but movement at all of these joints can be considered as either physiological or accessory. A *physiological* movement is the movement that the joint performs under voluntary control of the muscles or is performed passively by an external force but still within the available range of the joint. Maitland (1986) defines *accessory* movements as those movements of the joints that a person cannot perform actively but that can be performed on that person by an external force. They are an integral part of the physiological movement that cannot be isolated and performed actively by muscular effort.

Although there may seem to be a large number of directions in which joints may move, a system of description has been devised to make the visual analysis of movement more simple. From the anatomical position (standing upright with the upper limbs at the sides and palms and head facing forward), movements can be described as occurring in three planes and around three axes (Fig. 5.1).

The frontal plane splits the body into front and back halves, the sagittal plane splits the body into right and left halves and the transverse plane splits the body into top and bottom halves.

Movements within these planes take place around three axes. The axes can be described as being perpendicular to the plane of movement. Therefore, there are two horizontal axes and one vertical axis. The sagittal axis is at 90° to the frontal plane and therefore allows movements within that frontal plane. These movements consist of abduction, adduction, deviation and lateral flexion. The frontal axis allows movements of the segments within the sagittal plane and consists of the movements of flexion and extension. Both frontal and sagittal are horizontal axes. The vertical axis is at 90° to the horizontal plane and movements around this axis give rotatory motion.

The actual movements performed can be described in terms of the degrees of freedom the joint allows. A uniaxial joint will possess only one degree of freedom, i.e. rotation about only one axis. An example of this is flexion and extension at the elbow. A biaxial joint has two degrees of freedom, such as the radiocarpal joint which has

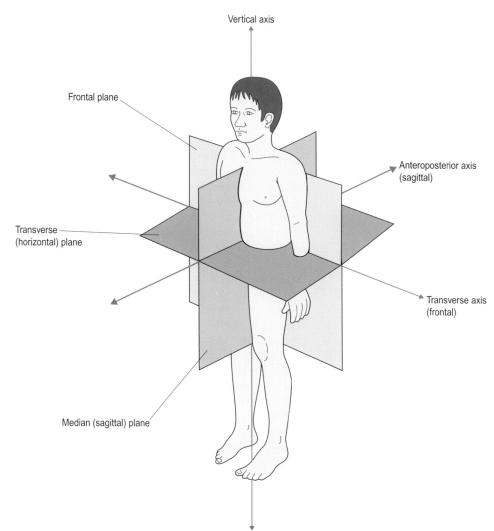

Vertical axis

Frontal plane

Anteroposterior axis
(sagittal)

Transverse
(horizontal) plane

Transverse axis
(frontal)

Median (sagittal) plane

Figure 5.1   Planes
and axes.

Task 5.1

Movements of the body segments are described in terms of their planes and axes. For each of the major joints of the body, describe the planes in which the segments move followed by the axes that they move around.

flexion and extension at the wrist about one axis and ulnar and radial deviation about the other axis. The movement available at a multiaxial joint can be described as having three degrees of freedom. This type of movement can be described at the shoulder where flexion, extension, abduction, adduction and internal and external rotation all take place.

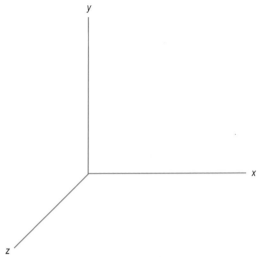

Figure 5.2   The Cartesian coordinate system.

The above system of movement analysis is only truly applicable if the movement takes place within the anatomical position and does not cross planes and axes. This, however, is not really the case. The shape of most joints is rather complex and they have axes that permit movement in more than one direction. Most movements are also functional in nature and therefore do not take place from the anatomical position. This makes the analysis system rather artificial.

An alternative system for describing movement is the Cartesian coordinate system which allows any permutation of movement to be described in the three planes. It has, as shown in Figure 5.2, three coordinates in the directions of:

- anteroposterior: the x coordinate
- mediolateral: the z coordinate
- superior-inferior: the y coordinate.

RANGE OF MOVEMENT

With the combination of uniaxial, biaxial and multiaxial joints, the body may adopt a multitude of functional positions. When these positions or movements are analysed, the components are broken down to each individual joint with the range of movement (ROM) of that joint being

described. This movement may not be the maximum movement that the joint is capable of achieving, i.e. its full range of movement (FROM), but only a functional component of it.

Movements of the joints are dependent on many factors and the description of these factors is largely dependent on the discipline by which the movement is being studied. One such discipline is arthrokinematics. This is the intimate mechanics of the joints and is dependent, for its description, largely on the shape of the joint surfaces. Most of the synovial joints are complex in their formation, having more than one axis within the joint. These joints, being ovoid in different axes of the same joint, have the ability to bring about these different movements. This means that, although joints have roughly reciprocally shaped surfaces, the maximum congruity of the articular surfaces occurs at specific positions within the range of movement and does not necessarily equate with the end of range of the physiological movement. This position of maximum congruity is called the *close packed* position and is the position of greatest joint stability. At this close packed position, not only is there most joint surface contact but the ligaments are often taut. The *loose packed* position, conversely, is where the apposition of the joint surface is the least; muscle, ligaments and capsule are usually lax and the joint is in its least stable position (Hall 1995).

Physiological movements always contain different combinations of physiological or accessory movements. These may be a combination of physiological movements, such as side flexion of the cervical spine which, if examined closely, will be seen to involve both side flexion and rotation in combination. By studying the arthrokinematics of the joint it can be shown that there is a combination of accessory type movements occurring during the physiological joint movement. These accessory movements are considered to be of three types: spin, roll and glide. A roll refers to one surface rolling over another, like a ball rolling over a surface. An example of roll is seen when the femoral condyle rolls over a fixed tibial plateau during knee extension. Gliding is a pure translatory movement, one fixed point sliding over the other joint surface. A glide usually takes place in an anteroposterior or mediolateral direction and

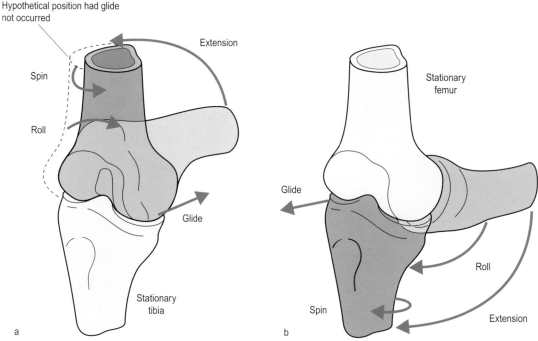

Figure 5.3 Diagrammatic representation of roll, spin and glide at the knee. (a) With stationary tibia; (b) with stationary femur.

this type of movement is again seen when the femur slides forward on a fixed tibia at the knee joint. Spin is like a top spinning, a pure rotatory motion. These movements are illustrated in Figure 5.3. Accessory movements enable the range of movement to be increased at the joint and also maximise the congruency of the joint surfaces to improve stability (Norkin & Levangie 1992). Descriptions of these movements and their combinations for specific joints can be found in many anatomical texts.

So it can be seen that movement at joints is not the straightforward unidimensional process that it may at first appear. Movement is caused by a force acting on the bony segment, which in turn produces the movement at the joint. This force may be an internal force, the concentric or eccentric work of the muscle, or an external force, the force of gravity for example.

When the joint is moved by the force of muscle contraction, either concentrically or eccentrically, the range of joint movement may be described in terms of the excursion of the muscle. This excursion consists of the full range of the muscle, i.e. the inner, middle and outer range, each being roughly a third of the full range of movement. The inner range is where the muscle is at its shortest, middle range is the middle third of the muscle excursion and the outer range is where the muscle is at its longest. This is graphically illustrated in Figure 5.4.

The actual range through which the joint moves, either actively or passively, is measured in degrees of a circle. Range of movement is usually measured by goniometry. This gives an accepted objective measurement that may be used when analysing joint motion as a part of movement analysis or used as an objective marker when assessing patients.

FACILITATION AND RESTRICTION/LIMITATION OF MOVEMENT

Anatomical, physiological and arthrokinaesiological factors combine to give normal facilitation to, and restriction of, movement within a joint.

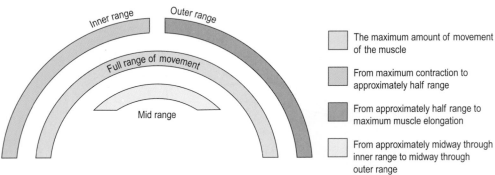

Figure 5.4   Diagrammatic representation of ranges of movement.

Task 5.2

Work in small groups and choose some simple activities. One person performs the activity whilst the others observe the movement very closely. Try to estimate the range of movement of each joint and identify the muscles that are working to produce the movement. Describe the range of movement of the muscle and the type of muscle contraction throughout the activity.

Normal facilitation

ROM is facilitated by the following:

- bony shape
- hyaline cartilage
- capsule supporting synovial membrane
- additional structures
- elastic ligaments
- intact neuromuscular and musculoskeletal system
- muscle strength.

The reciprocal convex and concave shapes of the joint surfaces combined with the accessory movements of roll, spin and glide provide a greater surface area over which the two bone ends can move. Hyaline cartilage, present on the articulating surfaces of the bone ends, has the dual function of providing a smooth surface over which the bone ends can glide and affording the joint protection from wear and tear. Both the functions of the hyaline cartilage are enhanced by the presence of synovial fluid within the joint. The fluid layer over the two joint surfaces will reduce the amount of friction between the bone ends when movements occur and act as a form of shock absorber to reduce the trauma of constant impact, particularly in weight-bearing joints. Synovial fluid produced by the synovial membrane also provides the joint with some of its nutrition. Most of the capsule surrounding joints is lax, thus permitting a large range of movement by the joint.

Many joints have additional structures within them; examples of these are the menisci in the knee or the glenoidal labrum within the shoulder. Both these structures, and others like them, can act as a mechanism for increasing joint surfaces, increasing congruity or affecting stability within the joint. Occasionally, the ligaments surrounding the joints contain yellow elastic fibres in addition to the usual collagen, enabling the ligament to allow the joint an increase in range by providing more flexibility. An example of this is the ligamentum flavum which connects adjacent laminae of the spine. It permits separation of these laminae in flexion and ensures that the end range is not reached abruptly. It also assists in returning the spine to the erect position after flexion has occurred (Williams 1995).

Normal limitation/restriction of an intact system

Normal limitation of range of movement is brought about by:

- articular surface contact
- limit of ligament extensibility
- limit of tendon and muscle extensibility
- apposition of soft tissue.

The two main factors that limit joint mobility are the shape of the joints and the type of structures that run over them. Articular surface contact could mean that the joint is in the close packed position, as in the elbow, where the joint is actually prevented from extending beyond approximately 180° by the olecranon of the ulna impinging onto the humerus. Flexion of the elbow, on the other hand, is limited by the bulk of the biceps brachii pressing against the forearm, this being an example of soft tissue apposition.

Most ligaments and all tendons are primarily composed of white fibrous collagen. One of the properties of collagen is that it is fairly inelastic and stretching achieved by deformation requires strong forces. Therefore, within normal activities, if the ligaments or tendons are at their maximum length, no more movement is possible at that joint. This is illustrated by McMahon et al (1998) who point out that the inferior band of the inferior glenohumeral ligament is the primary restraint to anterior stability post shoulder dislocation. When considering normal movement, Branch et al (1995) point out that the anterior and posterior components of the glenohumeral capsuloligamentous complex limit the external and internal rotation of the glenohumeral joint respectively.

It must be remembered, as O'Brien et al (1995) describe, that differing positions of joints enable different structures to limit movement. This point is taken a stage further by Warner et al (1999) who show that glenohumeral compression through muscle contraction provides stability against inferior translation of the humeral head and this effect is more important than intercapsular pressure or ligament tension. This agrees with Wuelker et al (1998) who found that the rotator cuff force significantly contributes to stabilisation of the glenohumeral joint during arm motion.

The structure of muscle, on the other hand, offers the opportunity of more stretch as it crosses the joint and thus affords greater mobility but it still has a limit of extensibility. The limitation that muscle offers to joint mobility is seen particularly when the muscle stretches over two joints, such as the hamstrings stretching over the hip and knee. If the hip is flexed then the amount of knee extension is limited as the muscle is already near its maximum possible length. If the hip is

---

Task 5.3

Work with a partner and move the major joints of the body passively to their physiological limits. Identify (by end-feel if possible) what is preventing further movement and remember what the end-range feels like. Move to a different partner and perform the same passive movements. See if you can detect any differences and similarities. Discuss your findings with your colleagues.

---

extended then the hamstrings are no longer near the limit of their potential length and will therefore allow for a greater range of knee extension.

It is important that the therapist becomes aware of the normal limitations and can recognise these both by visual analysis and recognising how the joint feels at the end of passive range. This is referred to as the 'end-feel' of the joint and will be different according to the circumstance of the particular joint. For example, the feel of a bony end block, as in the elbow extension, is quite different from that of soft tissue apposition, as in full flexion of the elbow. There is also the 'springy' end-feel of normal tendon, ligamentous and other joint structures. It is only by recognising the normal end-feel of joints that the therapist will become skilled at recognising pathological joint changes.

Abnormal limitation

Although both normal facilitation and limitation are important factors to consider when discussing joint range, joint range becomes an issue when there is an abnormal limitation in that range. Abnormal limitation of joint range is usually brought about by either injury or disease to its structure, surface or surrounding soft tissue, i.e. the muscles producing the movement or their functioning.

The above factors can be summarised as:

- destruction of bone and cartilage
- bone fracture
- foreign body in joint
- tearing or displacement of intracapsular structures

- adhesions/scar tissue
- muscle atrophy or hypertrophy
- muscle tear, rupture or denervation
- pain
- psychological factors
- oedema
- neurological impairment.

Destruction of bone and cartilage

Any disease that destroys the articular cartilage, such as osteo-arthritis or rheumatoid arthritis, will impair the functioning of the joint and thus the movement will be limited. This may be for two reasons. Either the destroyed surface will physically prevent the movement or the pain produced when the two exposed surfaces grind together may lead to a reduction in range or a deterioration in the quality of the movement. Either singly or in combination, these factors may actually prevent movement altogether.

Fracture

A fracture near to or within the joint will also prevent movement via mechanical obstruction or pain. The same applies to a foreign body within the joint complex.

Tearing or displacement of intracapsular structures

Field et al (1997) demonstrate that recurrent anterior unidirectional shoulder instability is most commonly associated with an avulsion of the glenoidal attachment of the labroligamentous complex (Bankart lesion). This would limit the range of movement available. Tearing of the meniscus of the knee is a common example of this.

Soft tissue lesions

If there has been an injury to the soft tissue surrounding or within the joint, then repair to that tissue usually takes place by the formation of fibrous or scar tissue which does not have the same extensibility as the tissue it is replacing. Fibrous adhesions may also form and these would bind structures together and hence movement would be restricted.

Injury or immobilisation

If immobilisation of soft tissue occurs there are biomechanical, biochemical and physiological changes that take place within 1 week. These changes are magnified in the presence of trauma or oedema (Cyr & Ross 1998). These structural changes are a result of stress deprivation which causes the matrix of the tissue to be remodelled to its new resting length while being held immobile (Hardy & Woodall 1998). The net result of this will be a decrease in the range of movement. If muscle tissue is held in a shortened position there appears to be absorption of the sarcomeres, causing a change in length. This shortening in length is termed 'adaptive shortening' and will limit joint movement.

Muscular changes and pathology

The joint itself may be intact but if the muscles that produce the movement have a dysfunction then the net result is a decrease in ROM. If the muscle is atrophied to a large degree then it would not create sufficient force to move the joint through its full range. Conversely, if there was a large amount of muscle hypertrophy, ROM would also be decreased due to the increased amount of soft tissue apposition.

Neurological impairment

The muscle itself may be intact but its neural control may be impaired. This could range from total denervation, causing flaccidity of the muscle, to lack of higher centre control, which may cause spasticity. Local spinal reflexes may also have the effect of limiting movement by causing the muscle to be in spasm.

Pain

The body's response to pain is usually to keep the part still and avoid movement. This may be only short term but if the pain becomes chronic then adaptive shortening may occur. The pain may disappear but the pattern that the brain adopted due to the memory of pain that occurred on movement may continue. Other psychological problems such as depression or lack of motivation or self-confidence may also be responsible for the subject not moving. This may also be transient and cause no physical limitation of movement but if the condition persists then adaptive shortening may occur.

Hypertrophy

When a muscle is overdeveloped, as in a body builder or sportsperson for example, soft tissue apposition may cause a decrease in range of movement.

Hypermobility

It is important to remember that what has so far been discussed describes a decrease in movement (hypomobility) but the opposite may also occur. This is termed 'hypermobility' where the range of movement exceeds that of the expected physiological range. This could be due to pathological change either at the joint or elsewhere within the musculoskeletal or neuromuscular systems. It may, however, be a natural phenomenon caused mainly by laxity of ligaments or a congenital joint deformity but it can also result from a deliberate attempt to stretch the joint range well beyond that which is functionally acceptable, as in a gymnast or ballet dancer for example. As Lewit (1993) states, this may be an advantage to these sportspeople but with increased mobility there may be a decrease in stability, with the disadvantage of possible problems in the future. There is also the possibility of subluxation of the joint occurring during movement, which could result in neurological damage. If the joint is hypermobile there is also the possibility that the joint will articulate on bone that is not designed for this function and therefore there is a great risk of degenerative changes occurring at the joint surfaces.

Task 5.4

In groups, look at the major joints of the body and assess visually the differences in the range of movement between each person. Can you discover what is limiting the movement for each joint? Can you find anyone with hypermobility? Are there any differences between males and females in ROM or hypermobility?

Effects of decreased range of movement

The effects of a decreased range of joint movement will obviously depend on how much the range is decreased and the importance that joint plays in functional activity. Limited flexion at the knee, for example, will have a major effect on essential functional activities like toileting and walking. Limitation of range of movement at one of the metatarsals, however, may have little obvious major effect on any functional activity, even gait. The human body is very adaptable and decrease in range of one joint is sometimes compensated by hypermobility at another joint.

Treatment

Before treatment can be given for any decrease in ROM, it is obvious from the above that the cause of the decrease will have to be known. It has been shown that the cause may be in the joint structure (surface or intracapsular), the structures surrounding or running over the joint (ligaments or tendons) or the neuromuscular system that produces the movements. So, to establish the pathological changes that have occurred, it is vital that the therapist performs a full and detailed assessment. Once the pathology is known, the therapist can choose a method of treatment whose physiological effects alter the pathological changes that have occurred to limit joint movement.

Once the assessment has been made it is important to know the physiological effects of the possible treatment options and match them with the effects they will have on the pathological changes. This is the rationale of the treatment.

Limitation of movement, from whatever cause, impairs function of the joint and the muscles producing the movement. Measures that increase the range of movement must also include methods that strengthen the muscles in their new, lengthened position. The degree of ROM gained must be able to be controlled, and the stability of the joint maintained, or further injury may result.

It is important that details of the anatomy and arthrokinaesiology are understood as well as the pathology of the joint, as these have an effect on the rationale of treatment choice when there is a pathological reduction in joint range.

Many studies have looked at actual joint ranges of physiological ROM and presented tables of values (Norkin & White 1995). It is accepted, however, that each ROM is specific to each individual and discrepancies may even exist when comparing both sides of an individual. Two of the factors that have an effect on the ROM are age and gender. Younger children appear to have a greater amount of hip flexion, abduction and lateral rotation, and ankle dorsiflexion than an adult. Elbow movements are also greater than those of an adult, whilst there is less hip extension, knee extension and ankle plantarflexion. Older age groups seem to have a generalised appendicular and axial joint decrease. Gender appears to have different effects on different joints depending on what movement that joint is performing (Norkin & White 1995).

There are many physiotherapy modalities to increase the ROM. The most obvious is the use of movement itself. The main classifications of the therapeutic movements are described below.

TYPES OF JOINT MOVEMENT

Movement is one of the main methods that therapists use to increase joint range. The therapist will use the different ways in which the joint moves as a basis for these different methods. There are two main types of movement:

- passive movement
- active movement.

Passive movement is defined as those movements produced entirely by an external force, i.e. no voluntary muscle work. These can be subdivided into:

- relaxed passive movements
- stretching
- accessory movements
- manipulations.

Active movements are those movements within the unrestricted range of a joint produced by an active contraction of the muscles crossing the joint. These can be subdivided into:

- active assisted exercise
- free active exercise.

Passive movement

Relaxed passive movements

These are movements performed within the unrestricted range by an external force and involve no muscle work of the particular joint, or joints, at which the movement takes place. These movements can be performed in three ways:

- *Manual relaxed passive movements* are movements performed by another person, usually the physiotherapist, within the unrestricted range.
- *Auto-relaxed passive movements* are performed within the unrestricted range by the patients themselves, i.e. with their unaffected limbs.
- *Mechanical relaxed passive movements* are performed by a machine but still occur within the unrestricted range.

Manual relaxed passive movements Relaxed passive movement has been a core skill of the physiotherapist for many years and is still widely used today. As with many of the traditional skills, little evidence of its clinical effectiveness has been published (Basmajian & Wolf 1990) but the following is the accepted rationale for its use.

Indications These movements are indicated when the patient is unable to perform an active full range movement. The reasons for this inability may include unconsciousness, weak or denervated muscle, spinal injury, pain, neurological disease or enforced rest.

Effects

- Maintain ROM
- Prevent contractures
- Maintain integrity of soft tissue and muscle elasticity
- Increase venous circulation
- Increase synovial fluid production and therefore joint cartilage nutrition
- Increase kinaesthetic awareness
- Maintain functional movement patterns
- Reduce pain.

Maintaining ROM and preventing contractures If muscle is not moved through its full range then it will adapt to the demands being placed upon it. The actin and myosin protein filaments (the contractile element) will be reabsorbed and thus the area for crossbridge formation will be decreased. This will cause muscle weakness and the inability to perform the movement. The muscles will adopt the new position and will be shortened, i.e. they will have adaptive shortening. The non-contractile elements within the muscle, the connective tissue, will add to this effect by altering the collagen turnover rate, which is the balance of collagen production and destruction (Basmajian & Wolf 1990). If more collagen is produced, as in immobilisation, it increases the stiffness of the muscle and decreases its propensity to stretch. If no movement takes place then the muscle will adapt to the new position and thus contractures will occur.

Other soft tissues, such as ligaments and tendons, will also be similarly affected. As they have a greater proportion of collagen, the increase and change in consistency will also lead to stiffness and eventually to contractures.

Maintaining integrity of soft tissue and muscle elasticity   By placing stresses on these tissues the collagen turnover rate is normalised and the elasticity of the tissues is maintained. As Cyr and Ross (1998) conclude, early controlled motion is vital to prevent the negative effects of immobilisation and maintain normal viscoelasticity and homeostasis of connective tissue. Passive movements will not, however, increase the strength of the muscle as this requires the greater physiological demand of active and resisted work.

Increase venous circulation   If a limb, particularly the lower limb, is not moved, venous congestion may occur. This is because the muscle pump does not work to aid venous return. Pooling occurs and is increased through dilation of the vessels caused by the physical pressure of the blood on the veins and the possible lack of sympathetic tone. This decrease in flow can lead to an increased risk of deep vein thrombosis. Passive movements will act as a prophylaxis to prevent stagnation. This is achieved by physically compressing the veins and one-way flow is achieved via the valves within the veins themselves. Lymph is also encouraged to move. Compression of the tissues increases the hydrostatic pressure and thus encourages tissue perfusion and fluid reabsorption. This may be useful in reducing oedema.

Joint cartilage nutrition   If the synovial fluid is swept over the articular cartilage it will provide nutrition and help prevent deterioration of the surface. Production and absorption of the synovial fluid by the synovial membrane are stimulated by movement of the joint. This is quite an important effect and is lost if the joint is immobile for any length of time. If the immobility is due to injury then movement is of greater importance as one of the consequences of injury is inflammation and repair by fibrosis, which in itself will increase the risk of adhesions forming within the joint. Thus, with passive movement, this risk will be decreased.

Kinaesthetic awareness   To perform coordinated, energy-efficient and safe movement, it is important for the central nervous system to receive information about the position and movement of the joints and soft tissue. This information is supplied by sensory nerve endings in the many structures in and surrounding the joints. This kinaesthetic awareness may be lost if there is a long period of immobilisation. The kinaesthetic pathways may be maintained when performing passive movements by stimulating the nerve endings within the joint complex.

Maintain functional patterns   The brain is said to recognise gross movement patterns, so if these patterns cannot occur then the memory of the pattern may be lost. Passive movement in these patterns will decrease this risk.

Reduce pain   Rhythmical movements are said to reduce pain by causing a relaxation effect within the muscles (Gardiner 1981). This may partly be achieved by removing waste products and chemical irritants from the area through increased circulation. Stimulation of the joint mechanoreceptors may also subserve the sensations from the pain nerve endings and thus decrease their effect (see section on accessory movements below, for further explanation).

Contraindications
- Immediately post injury as this may increase the inflammatory process.
- Early fractures where movement may cause disruption of the fracture site.
- Where pain may be beyond the patient's tolerance.

- Muscle or ligament incomplete tears where further damage may occur.
- Where the circulation may be compromised.

Principles of application Passive movements may either be performed in the anatomical planes or in functional patterns. The choice and type of movement will depend on the findings of the assessment and the aims of the treatment. The same basic principles of application need to be considered whichever movement is chosen, as follows:

- The segment should be comfortable, supported and localised to the specific joints.
- The patient should be comfortable, warm and supported.
- Handholds should support the segment and protect the joint.
- The motion should be smooth and rhythmical.
- Speed and duration should be appropriate for the desired effects.
- Range should be the maximum available without stretching or causing pain.
- Segments should be positioned so that muscles that stretch over two or more joints are not restricting joint range (after Hollis 1989).

Auto–relaxed passive movements Although the rationale is the same, the method of application must be modified. Patients who have to perform their own passive movements are usually those with a long-term problem. People with spinal injuries, for example, must retain their joint range and muscle length if they are to perform the functions necessary for daily living (Bromley 1998).

Mechanical relaxed passive movements Unlike manual or auto-passive movements which, by their nature, have to be carried out intermittently, mechanical passive movements may be carried out continuously. Mechanical devices for producing continuous passive movement (CPM) were first used by Salter in 1970 (McCarthy et al 1993). Although their designs and protocols of use may differ, they all have essentially the same function.

The rationale is the same as for any relaxed passive movement but the benefits of continuous movement are particularly evident following surgery (Kisner & Colby 1990). Basso and Knapp (1987) found that CPM decreased joint effusions and wound oedema whilst increasing range of movement and decreasing pain in postoperative knee patients.

Stretching

Stretching differs from relaxed passive movement in that it takes the movement beyond the available range. This available range may be limited due to disease or injury. Stretching may also take the joint beyond the normal physiological range. Whereas relaxed passive movements are designed to maintain length of soft tissue and hence joint range, stretching should result in a change in length of the soft tissue structures crossing over the joint, with the consequent increase in joint range. Passive stretching is not the only method of increasing joint range via the soft tissues. This can also be attained via active stretching which will be discussed later.

Stretching of biological material Most biological materials are viscoelastic. This means that they exhibit both viscous and elastic properties. Viscosity is the property of a fluid that is a measure of the resistance to flow. Elasticity is the property of a solid. Therefore, viscoelastic materials possess both solid and liquid properties, which means that stress is not the only function of strain. There is also a strain rate. This differs from most of the purely elastic materials discussed in Chapter 3 where there was no time dependency, i.e. how quickly the stress was applied to the material. This time dependency is described in the equation below:

$$E = de/dt$$

where E is the strain rate and t is the time.

As was discussed in Chapter 3, a useful way of describing the relationship between stress and strain is to plot a graph of the stress versus strain and discuss the resulting curves.

Loading and unloading paths For elastic materials, strain energy is stored within the substance as potential energy. When the load is released it is this energy that returns the material to its original stress. This is represented graphically in Figure 5.5.

For viscoelastic materials some of the strain energy is stored as potential and some is dissipated as heat. Therefore, once the applied load is removed there is not enough stored energy to regain the normal configuration. This is shown in Figure 5.6.

Within the enclosed area shown in the graph is the hysteresis loop which represents the energy dissipated as heat when the material is stretched and the stress released, allowing a return to the non-stressed condition. Therefore continual loading and unloading will produce heat. The amount of hysteresis (heat produced) is dependent on the strain rate. This loss of energy does not allow the material to return to its original state; hence permanent deformation has taken place.

When considering biological tissue, it is important to know the micro- and macrostructure of the tissue concerned. Not many biological tissues are pure, as most are a composite of materials. This may mean that they have fibres in an aqueous matrix (which therefore makes them viscoelastic) or that they have a combination of different fibres or both. Orientation of the composite fibres is also of importance. If the fibres are arranged in parallel and the stress is applied in the direction of the fibres then the material will be strong and possibly *stiff* (a measure of the resistance to stress). If there is irregular orientation of the fibres then there will be less strength but what strength there is will be multidirectional.

The stress/strain curve for a 'general' biological tissue can be seen in Figure 5.7. Although not presenting the graph of any particular tissue, it shows the characteristics that are common to most biological tissues.

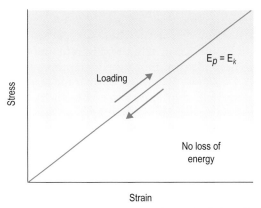

Figure 5.5   Loading and unloading paths (where $E_k = E_p$).

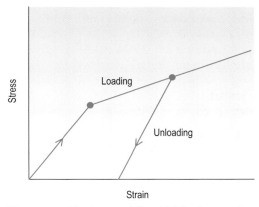

Figure 5.6   Elastic materials exhibiting hysteresis.

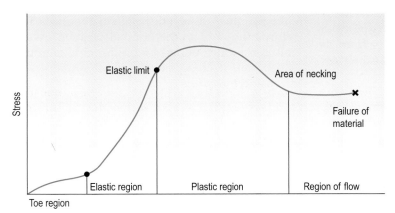

Figure 5.7   Typical stress/strain curve for biological material.

The *toe region* of the graph represents the straightening of the wavy collagen (see p. 100). It represents no change in the structure of the tissue under stress. The *elastic range* is the area under the graph that obeys Hooke's Law in that the tissue will return to its original length once the tension is released (between elastic region and elastic limit). The *elastic limit* is that point beyond which the tissue does not return to its original length when the stress is removed. *Plastic range* refers to that area in which the tissue will undergo permanent deformation and will not return to its original position. The strength of the tissue at this point is referred to as its *yield strength*, whereas the *ultimate strength* is the greatest load the tissue can sustain before strain occurs without further stress. There is a point, which is usually greater than the ultimate strength, where *necking* occurs. Necking is where considerable weakening occurs and strain continues to increase even if the stress or loading is greatly reduced or even removed. At the point of *failure* of the tissue, it has reached its *breaking strength*, i.e. the load at the time the tissue fails and rupture occurs.

Another property of tissue that is important when considering stretching is its *stiffness* which is a measure of the resistance offered by the tissue to deformation. The stiffness of a tissue is often rate and speed dependent. The *ductility* of the tissue is its capacity to absorb plastic deformation before failure occurs. If the tissue has an increase in strain with a constant stress then this increase in length is referred to as *creep*. This phenomenon is often used in serial splinting where the tissue is held in a cast under constant load and over time the tissue undergoes further lengthening. The *resilience* of material is its ability to recover quickly from its deformation whereas *damping* refers to the slow return to shape (Soderberg 1997).

Bone   Bone is non-homogenous, thus it will vary in its response to stress. It is a composite of compact and cancellous material and during loading compact bone is seen to be stiff, with a high ultimate strength and a large modulus of elasticity (see p. 65 on deformation of materials). It can resist rapidly applied loads better than loads that are applied slowly. Cancellous bone, on the other hand, is more compliant, hence it has greater

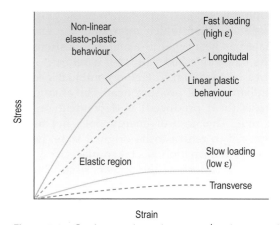

Figure 5.8   Strain rate-dependent stress/strain curves for cortical bone under longitudinal stress (continuous line) and direction-dependent stress (dotted line).

shock-absorbing capacity. These properties are shown in Figure 5.8, where the different amounts of stress needed to produce the same amount of strain and ultimate failure are shown for loads in the longitudinal and transverse directions. The graphs of fast and slow loading also illustrate the time-dependent response of the bone to stress (Fig. 5.8).

Soft tissue   Most soft tissue found in the musculoskeletal system is a composite material of mainly collagen, elastin and the aqueous ground substance. The collagen is composed of crimped fibrils which are aggregated into fibres and its prime function is to withstand axial tension.

On stretching, the crimps straighten out and the collagen then stores the potential energy that returns the fibril to the original position. As the collagen is surrounded by fluid (gel-like ground substance), it also possesses fluid properties of creep and hysteresis.

Elastin is highly elastic even at high stress strains, i.e. it possesses a low modulus of elasticity, whereas that for collagen is high. The importance of these properties is illustrated in Figure 5.9 which shows the stress/strain curves for the ligamentum flavum (70% elastin) and the anterior cruciate ligament (90% collagen).

Tendons   Fibrous connective tissue is mainly composed of collagen and ground substance,

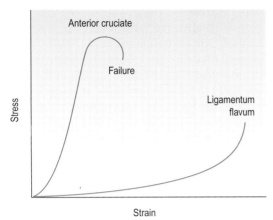

Figure 5.9   Stress/strain curves for anterior cruciate ligament and ligamentum flavum.

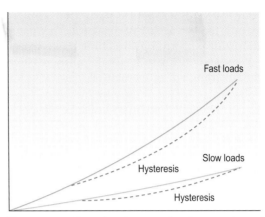

Figure 5.11   Stress/strain curve showing rate dependency and hysteresis for the tendon.

functioning primarily as a passive transmitter of the force produced by muscle contraction. Compared to muscle, the tendon is stiffer, has higher tensile strength and can endure larger stresses. The tendon can support a large stress with only a small strain and thus makes muscle contraction more efficient as not much of the muscle action is wasted on movement of the tendon. This facilitates greater apposition of the bones. The properties of a tendon are dependent on the type and proportion of its fibres, as shown in Figure 5.10. The resultant strain of a tendon is also time dependent and the tissue exhibits a hysteresis loop, showing that deformation of the tendon will be permanent.

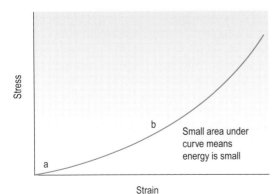

Figure 5.10   Stress/strain curve for a typical tendon. (a) Low strain (elastic fibres dominate and crimping straightens); (b) stiffer (viscoelastic matrix takes over).

This can be seen from Figure 5.11. Tendons have a low shear modulus so they can act as pulleys to redirect high forces.

Ligaments   Most ligaments contain a greater proportion of elastin than tendons and therefore have higher flexibility and lower strength and stiffness than tendons. Sometimes, however, ligaments have greater strength if resistance is applied quickly.

Muscle   Muscles vary in their reaction to stress, depending on which muscle is being studied and the age of that muscle (see Ch. 15). The structure of the muscle with its attendant tendon also has a role in the strain that occurs when stress is applied to the muscle–tendon–bone complex (Soderberg 1997).

Muscle, however, is an active tissue and the force produced within the muscle is due to its contraction. *Active tension* is developed in the muscle as a result of crossbridge formation and *passive tension* is developed as a result of the stress placed upon the connective tissue elements of the muscle when it is stretched past its resting length. Active tension is decreased, however, as the crossbridges are pulled apart. Therefore as muscle lengthens, passive tension increases.

Cartilage   Cartilage has a high fluid content so it has greater viscoelastic potential and becomes very variable in its properties.

Therapeutic stretching   Therapeutic stretching of soft tissue is a passive movement and is an important physiotherapeutic skill that can be carried out for a variety of reasons. The usual indications for performing stretching are to regain range of movement or to facilitate an increase in the available range of movement.

Changes in collagen that affect the stress/strain response

Immobilisation During immobilisation there will be a decrease in the collagen turnover rate with a consequent weak bonding between the new, non-stressed fibres. There will also be adhesion formation, with the consequent greater crosslinking between disorganised fibres, and ground substance will not retain its viscous properties.

Decrease in normal activity There will be a decrease in the size and amount of collagen fibres, leading to weakened tissues and possibly an increase in elastin with the consequent increase in compliance.

Effects of age One of the natural consequences of the ageing process is the decrease in tensile strength and elastic modulus of all soft tissues. This may lead to a decrease in the rate of adaption with the increased chance of overuse injury, fatigue and trauma (Cribb & Scott 1995).

Effects of drugs Corticosteroids cause a long-term decrease in tensile strength.

All the above effects must be taken into consideration when stretching is performed.

As has been described, stretching of collagen is due mainly to plastic deformation as the material is fairly inelastic. Connective tissue will reorganise itself in response to a sustained stretch provided the stress is not too great or applied for too long (Basmajian & Wolf 1990). Therefore, any stretch that does occur will be fairly permanent. It can be seen, then, that care must be taken not to reach the necking phase as this would compromise the integrity of the tissue being stretched and affect its function. This could lead to a decrease in stability and a greater risk of further injury to the joint.

To summarise, the effects of stretching are to:

* increase joint ROM
* increase soft tissue length
* relieve muscle spasm
* increase tissue compliance in preparation for an athletic event (Vujnovich & Dawson 1994).

Performing a stretch Passive stretching can, like passive movements, be performed as manual, auto- or mechanical stretching.

In manual (or auto) stretching, the therapist (or patient) produces the sustained stretch at the end of range with the patient relaxed. It is generally accepted that the stretch should be held for at least 15 seconds and repeated several times. When stretching a muscle tendon complex, it is important that the sarcomeres have an opportunity to 'give' before the tendon can be stretched. Sarcomere give occurs when the force applied to the muscle is sufficient to separate the actin and myosin filaments so that the non-elastic components of the complex can be stretched.

Mechanical stretching involves a low stress being applied by a machine over a prolonged period.

The above discussion refers to *static stretching*, which is defined as a slow sustained stretch at the end of range. This should be held, as stated, for up to 15 seconds but it is possible that a patient will be unable to tolerate a stretch held for this long and therefore the duration may have to be built up from a few seconds. This type of passive stretching is in contrast to *ballistic stretching*, which is defined as small end-of-range bounces. Despite having been used for many years, the ballistic method of stretching has been shown to increase the risk of injury and should not be performed (Vujnovich & Dawson 1994).

Accessory movements

As described earlier, Maitland (1986) defines accessory movements as those movements of the joints which a person cannot perform actively but that can be performed on that person by an external force. Although these movements form an integral part of the normal physiological movement, and occur throughout the ROM, they cannot be physically isolated by patients themselves. However, if the accessory movement was being performed by the physiotherapist, the patient would be able to stop the movement from taking place.

These movements take the form of glides (medially, laterally, longitudinally), compressions, distractions or rotations.

Anatomists group accessory movements into two categories: type one are those that cannot be performed unless resistance is provided to the active movement; and type two are movements that can be produced only when the subject's muscles are relaxed (Williams 1995). The latter are the type used for therapeutic purposes. Accessory movements are used to increase the range of movements at joints and also to decrease any pain that is present. These benefits are in addition to those of passive movements. The mechanism for decreasing pain depends, of course, on the cause of that pain. If the pain is caused by the decrease in ROM then the rationale of treatment will be the same as that for increasing the range. If not, then the usual effect of small-amplitude movements, applied rhythmically to the joints, is to inhibit the afferent impulse traffic from articular receptors, thus blocking the pain (Grieve 1988).

Twomey (1992) suggests that articular cartilage facilitates the ROM of joints. If there is joint immobility the articular cartilage will degenerate more quickly, as it requires movement and loading to ensure adequate nutrition. This nutrition is facilitated by the synovial fluid which is swept over the joint surface. As the stimulation of the synovial membrane declines, the amount of synovial fluid produced is decreased, becoming thicker with decreased osmolarity. Accessory movements assist in the maintenance of synovial production and, by the small oscillatory movements they make, produce the washing effect of the synovial fluid over the joint surfaces.

Twomey (1992) also suggests that movement is important for the nutrition of all collagenous tissue as well as the prevention of adaptive shortening. Small-amplitude movements at the end of range will elongate connective tissue, ligaments, joint capsule and other periarticular fascia via the processes described in the section dealing with stretching (p. 104). End-range movements will also break down any intra-articular adhesions that have been formed (Grieve 1988).

If joint stiffness is caused by fibrocartilaginous blocks and subsequent connective tissue short-ening, Threlkeld (1992) claims that the relative positions of the joint surfaces can be altered to regain normal accessory movement and restore displaced material.

Manipulation

Joint manipulations differ from all other types of therapeutic movement because the patient has no control over the procedure. These movements are potentially dangerous and should therefore only be performed by skilled professionals with much experience in the mobilisation of joints.

Manipulations are small-amplitude forceful movements that take the joint past the available physiological range. As Maitland (1986) states, manipulations are performed very quickly before the subject has time to prevent the movement from taking place. Lewit (1993) describes manipulation as a technique for treating end-range blocking of joints. Displaced intra-articular material may be one reason for the restriction of movement. Joint misalignment may be another. This blocking or restriction of movement, he claims, has two effects: one is the restriction of the subject's functional movement; the other is the effect on the accessory movement or joint play. Restrictions caused by meniscal or other material within the joint are termed 'loose bodies'.

Lack of movement of a joint may lead to adaptive shortening of the soft tissue structures sur-rounding it: capsule, ligaments, tendons or muscles, for example. This secondary consequence will in itself cause a restriction of movement and possibly pain when movement is attempted. Thus, a vicious circle is set up. The initial immobility may be a consequence of pain. If the pain is caused by trauma to the joint, then the problem may be compounded by the presence of adhesions within and around the joint that are the natural con-sequence of the inflammatory process.

Shortened soft tissue structures may also be manipulated to physically break the structures.

Effects   The primary effect of manipulating the joint is to restore its mobility. A secondary effect may be to decrease pain, if the pain was a direct result of abnormal tension on structures due to incorrect functioning of the joint.

These effects are brought about in a variety of ways. As the joint is manipulated, space is created between the surfaces. The movement of the surfaces, together with the greater space created, possibly causes any physical obstruction between the joint surfaces to be moved clear. Joint surfaces may then be realigned, causing the correct afferent information to be sent to the spinal cord. Fibrous adhesions, resulting from the inflammatory exudate, the organisation of the synovial fluid or the adaptive shortening of any soft tissue structure, will be physically torn. This takes the structure through the plastic phase and very rapidly past the breaking point. The intended consequence of this procedure is to free the joint to perform its full functional excursion.

Contraindications for the above technique are the same as those for relaxed passive movements.

Active movement

Active movement can be thought of as movements of the joint within the unrestricted range that are produced by the muscles that pass over that joint. The movements may be active assisted or free active. Therapeutically, these movements are performed as exercise.

Active assisted exercise is exercise carried out when the prime movers of a joint are not strong enough to perform the full ROM. The forces that need to be overcome are friction, gravity and the effects of the mechanical disadvantage of lever length. Assistance may be given by any external force but it is important that the external force provides assistance only so that the movement is simply augmented and does not become a passive movement. The external force has to be applied in the direction of the muscular action but not necessarily at the same point.

External assistance may be:

- manual assistance
- mechanical assistance
- auto-assistance.

Manual assisted exercise is where the subject's muscular effort is assisted by the therapist. The therapist changes the assistance as the muscles progress through their ROM, compensating for such factors as angle of pull and length–tension relationships. The amount of assistance may also be changed as the muscle strength increases.

Mechanical assistance may be provided by a variety of apparatus. Isokinetic equipment has the facility for active assisted movement provided the trigger forces are set low enough. The most useful

mechanical assistance is sling suspension, where the assistance is given in two ways. First, the resisting force of friction is reduced by physically lifting the segment clear of its resting surface, which also helps to counteract the force of gravity by supporting the segment. Second, depending on the point of fixation of the sling suspension, gravity may be used to assist the movement, provided the desired movement occurs on the downward arc of the curve produced by the segment within the sling suspension.

Auto-assisted exercise may be performed by the subject using the same principles as those of manual assistance. More common, however, is for the assistance to be a combined form of auto- and mechanical assistance. This is seen in the use of bicycle pedals for lower limb mobility or pulleys for upper limb mobility.

Free active exercise differs from assisted exercise in that the movement is carried out by the subject, with no assistance or resistance to the movement, except that of the force of gravity. There are many ways in which free active movements can be performed:

- *Rhythmical*: this uses momentum to help perform the movement taking place in one plane but in opposite directions.
- *Pendular*: these are movements performed in an arc and are useful for improving mobility as, on the downcurve of the arc, the movement is assisted by gravity.
- *Single or patterned*: depending on the aims of the intended movement, the choice of single or patterned movements is made. As a general rule, single movements are used to demonstrate or restore actions, whereas patterned movements are used for functional activities. The use of biceps brachii to flex the elbow as a pure movement is an example of a single movement. Reaching out to pick up an object (food) and taking it to the mouth also involves flexion of the elbow but this movement also uses other joint movements in a functional pattern (the feeding pattern).

These movements may also be classed by their effect.

- *Localised*: designed to produce a local or specific effect, such as mobilising a particular joint or strengthening a particular muscle.

- *General*: gives a widespread effect over many joints or muscles; running, for example (Gardiner 1981).

Exercise affects all the systems of the body and is covered elsewhere in this and many other textbooks. What must be remembered, however, is that the effects produced cannot be isolated to one particular system or even one effect within that system. Exercise, for example, will maintain muscle length and joint range but it may also alter the strength (aerobic and anaerobic capacity) of that muscle and have a more widespread effect on the cardiovascular system.

One of the major local effects of exercise is the increased rate of protein synthesis, thus producing more actin and myosin as a response and facilitating an increase in muscle length. Connective tissue also responds to increased exercise by becoming stronger in order to cope with the increase in function that is required of that muscle (Basmajian & Wolf 1990).

If active exercise is performed regularly and through the available physiological range, it has all the effects of passive exercise that were previously explained, including maintaining joint range, increasing joint nutrition and decreasing pain. Active movement has the advantage of strengthening muscles to some extent, thus providing stability for the joint with its increased

range. Another advantage of performing active movements is that, if they are performed in a rhythmical manner, they may promote relaxation of the muscles surrounding the joint. If this happens then the joint range may well be increased, especially if the restriction was due to muscle spasm.

CONCLUSION

Movement occurring at joints depends upon a variety of anatomical and biomechanical factors which can facilitate and/or limit the range of movement available. How movements are classified and described will depend on which discipline is being studied. For this text, movements are classified as either active or passive, with subdivisions of each. Restriction of movement, caused by pathological changes, can be successfully managed by the therapist using different forms of movement. This is achieved once the rationale of the chosen method is known and correctly applied to the fully assessed patient.

The preceding descriptions by no means represent an exhaustive survey of the therapeutic modalities available to improve joint range and muscle length. They are, however, representative of the basic principles of the techniques that are used based on normal joint movement.

REFERENCES

Basmajian J, Wolf S 1990 Therapeutic exercise, 5th edn. Williams and Wilkins, Baltimore

Basso D, Knapp L 1987 Comparison of two continuous passive motion protocols for patients with total knee implants. Physical Therapy 67: 360–363

Branch TP, Lawton RL, Iobst CA, Hutton WC 1995 The role of glenohumeral capsular ligaments in internal and external rotation of the humerus. American Journal of Sports Medicine 23(5): 632–637

Bromley I 1998 Tetraplegia and paraplegia: a guide for physiotherapists, 5th edn. Churchill Livingstone, Edinburgh

Cribb AM, Scott JE 1995 Tendon response to tensile stress: an ultrastructural investigation of collagen: proteoglycan interactions in stressed tendon. Journal of Anatomy 187 (part 2): 423–428

Cyr LM, Ross RG 1998 How controlled stress affects healing tissues. Journal of Hand Therapy 11(2): 125–130

Field LD, Bokor DJ, Savoie FH 1997 Humeral and glenoid detachment of the anterior inferior glenohumeral ligament: a cause of anterior shoulder instability. Journal of Shoulder and Elbow Surgery 6(1): 6–10

Gardiner MD 1981 The principles of exercise therapy, 4th edn. Bell and Hyman, London

Grieve G 1988 Contraindications to spinal manipulations and allied treatment. Physiotherapy 75(8): 445–453

Hall S 1995 Basic biomechanics, 2nd edn. Mosby, St Louis

Hardy M, Woodall W 1998 Therapeutic effects of heat, cold and stretch on connective tissue. Journal of Hand Therapy 11(2): 148–156

Hollis M 1989 Practical exercise therapy, 3rd edn. Blackwell Science, Oxford

Kisner C, Colby L 1990 Therapeutic exercise, foundations and techniques, 2nd edn. FA Davies, Philadelphia

Lewit K 1993 Manipulative therapy in rehabilitation of the locomotor system, 2nd edn. Butterworth-Heinemann, Oxford

Maitland G 1986 Vertebral manipulation, 5th edn. Butterworths, London

McCarthy M, Yates C, Anderson M, Yates-McCarthy J 1993 The effects of immediate continuous passive movement on pain during the inflammatory phase of soft tissue healing following anterior cruciate ligament reconstruction. Journal of Sport and Physical Therapy 17(2): 96–101

McMahon PJ, Tibone JE, Cawley PW et al 1998 The anterior band of the inferior glenohumeral ligament: biomechanical properties from tensile testing in the position of apprehension. Journal of Shoulder and Elbow Surgery 7(5): 467–471

Norkin C, Levangie P 1992 Joint structure and function: a comprehensive analysis, 2nd edn. FA Davies, Philadelphia

Norkin C, White J 1995 Measurement of joint motion: a guide to goniometry, 2nd edn. FA Davies, Philadelphia

O'Brien SJ, Schwarts RS, Warren RF, Torzilli PA 1995 Capsular restraints to anterior-posterior motion of the abducted shoulder: a biomechanical study. Journal of Shoulder and Elbow Surgery 4(4): 298–308

Palastanga N, Field D, Soames R 1998 Anatomy and human movement: structure and function, 3rd edn. Butterworth-Heinemann, Oxford

Soderberg GL 1997 Kinesiology – application to pathological motion, 2nd edn. Williams and Wilkins, Baltimore

Threlkeld J 1992 The effects of manual therapy on connective tissue. Physical Therapy 72(12): 61–70

Twomey L 1992 A rationale for the treatment of back pain and joint pain by manual therapy. Physical Therapy 72(12): 53–60

Vujnovich J, Dawson N 1994 The effect of therapeutic muscle stretch on neural processing. Journal of Sport and Physical Therapy 20(3): 145–153

Warner JJ, Deng XH, Warren RF, Torzilli PA 1999 Static capsuloligamentous restraints to superior-inferior translation of the glenohumeral joint. American Journal of Sports Medicine 20(6): 675–685

Williams P (ed) 1995 Gray's anatomy, 38th edn. Churchill Livingstone, Edinburgh

Wuelker N, Korell M, Thren K 1998 Dynamic glenohumeral joint stability. Journal of Shoulder and Elbow Surgery 7(1): 43–52

Chapter 6

Muscle work, strength, power and endurance

Tony Everett

LEARNING OUTCOMES

At the end of the chapter you should be able to:

1. Differentiate between muscle force and strength

2. Discuss muscle work

3. Differentiate between muscle strength and power

4. Discuss muscle endurance

5. Discuss the principles of measuring muscle strength and endurance

6. Describe the methods of increasing muscle strength and endurance.

INTRODUCTION

This chapter assumes knowledge of the human musculoskeletal system, particularly the myology. It is important that you can identify the position of the main muscle groups as well as being able to discuss the macroscopic and microscopic structure of muscles themselves. The physiology of the functioning musculoskeletal system is also important so you might find it beneficial to look up muscle contraction and the physiological processes associated with this. There are many standard texts in which you can find this information but it would also be useful to have read Chapters 2 and 3 of this book.

We know why muscles have to be developed in terms of strength and endurance when participating in sport at a high level. It is self-evident why a shot putter needs strong arms that can deliver a powerful thrust to propel an 8 kg shot 20 metres or a marathon runner needs muscle endurance to run over 26 miles. Although these athletes sometimes appear superhuman they actually function in the same way as you or I and the processes they need to build up their muscular systems are essentially the same as those for someone who has become weak and out of condition through trauma, disease or any other form of disuse.

Did you notice when undertaking Task 6.1 that movement was affected in many, if not all, of the diseases and traumas in your list? This decrease in movement occurs even when the disease or injury does not directly affect the muscles themselves. If a person does not move or moves incorrectly for any length of time, then the muscular and cardiovascular systems will deteriorate. This process is technically known as *deconditioning*. So just like the top-class athlete, deconditioned patients will need to improve their condition by increasing the strength, power and endurance of the muscles relevant to their functional needs.

In this chapter mechanisms by which muscle work produces increases in strength and endurance will be discussed. Basic definitions will be given as well as the physiological process and physical procedures required to produce these changes in condition.

THE DIFFERENCES BETWEEN MUSCLE FORCE AND MUSCLE STRENGTH

Muscle strength and muscle force are sometimes, erroneously, used as interchangeable terms. They are, however, two quite distinct concepts. As was demonstrated in Chapter 3, a force is an entity that is generated by an action, a push or a pull, for example, or imparted as a kick. The object to which the force is imparted may move or deform. Therefore a force can be defined as *an influence that changes the state of rest or motion of a body or object*. These forces are a product of the mass of the object producing them multiplied by its acceleration ($F = m \times a$). The unit of measurement is the newton (N).

Forces can be thought of as being either external or internal. External forces are those that happen outside the body, usually acting on the body, such as gravity, friction or other people. Internal forces are those mainly produced by the muscles. It is the *muscle's ability to produce force* that is a measure of the muscle strength. A fuller definition would be the *ability of a muscle or group of muscles to produce tension and a resulting force in one maximal effort, either dynamically or statically in relation to the demands placed upon it*. The production of the internal force was explained in Chapter 2. The sliding filament theory explains how the actin and myosin protein fibrils slide over one another and form a series of crossbridges that rotate and pull the sarcomeres closer together, thus shortening the muscle and producing the force (Hunter 2000).

MUSCLE WORK

A muscle has to contract to produce a force. The force it produces can either be very small, so that the resultant action is correspondingly fine (picking up a feather), or quite large, with a result of deforming, moving a large object or with a large movement (as in throwing a cricket ball across a field). As was discussed in Chapter 2, the shortening of the muscles (bringing the proximal and distal attachments closer together) produces the force. If this movement can be measured, i.e. the change in length of the muscle, then this can be multiplied by the force generated to give the work done by the muscle (work = force × distance). The unit of measurement of the work done is the joule (J).

From the definition, it can be seen that the muscle will only be doing work if there is a change in length. If the muscle is getting shorter as it is performing its task, it is said to be performing a *concentric contraction* and the work done is therefore *concentric work*. If, on the other hand, the muscle is getting longer as it is performing its task, it is said to be doing *eccentric work* as the contraction is eccentric. The former will be positive work and the latter negative. Paradoxically, if a muscle is producing an isometric contraction then mechanically no work is done as there is no movement. If you hold a weight in an outstretched upper limb you do feel as if you are doing some work! This is probably explained by the fact that there will be very small concentric and eccentric contractions of different groups of muscle fibres, giving an overall effect of no movement and thus technically no work being done.

The different amounts and types of muscle work which are due to the muscle's ability to alter the forces produced, and the direction of its action are important when we consider the activities which the human has to perform.

If you analyse the muscle activity in the first example in Task 6.2, it can be seen that biceps brachii appears to be doing most of the work throughout the movement. As you take the drink up to your mouth then the work being done by the muscle is concentric. As you lower the drink, the biceps again performs most of the work but this time the muscle work is eccentric. Energy is also used when the muscle has to contract isometrically to hold the drink to your mouth. As you drink more, the load which you have to move becomes less so although the type of work that the biceps produces does not change, the amount will decrease.

In the second example the muscles of the lower limb are working to produce walking. As you study gait in Chapter 10, you will see that there is a systematic and regular change between concentric and eccentric muscle work to produce the gait cycle. If you suddenly have to change the amount of muscle work in order to run for the bus then this is done by producing more force within the muscles.

These two examples show that there is a constant interplay between the type and quantity of muscle work that produces propulsion and control so that humans can perform the infinite variety of functional tasks that are needed throughout the day.

MUSCLE STRENGTH

The two activities in Task 6.2 show the amount of force that needs to be generated by a muscle or muscle group is used to carry out the functional activities of everyday life. The same muscles are used to walk and run and the biceps are capable of lifting a heavier weight than a pint. The shot putter, on the other hand, needs to use all the force that could be generated in his muscles to give impetus to the shot. Therefore it can be concluded that a muscle has the ability to change the force generation for different activities. In other words, each muscle has a range of strength available to it. How much strength has to be used to perform a task is dependent on many influences.

Recruitment

Past experience is a vital component. A full glass of fluid is often lifted so the brain has a good idea of how much strength is needed and therefore how much effort to use to lift the pint. On the other hand, if we lift a closed box expecting it to be heavy, the result may be that the box is thrown up in the air because it is, in fact, empty. The brain had been expecting a heavy load and the muscles had contracted accordingly.

The above scenarios are dependent on the number of motor units used during the muscle contraction. This process was explained in Chapter 2. The contraction of the motor unit is termed 'recruitment' and it is this recruitment which enables us to use our muscles to produce

---

Task 6.2

Think about these two activities:

1. Sitting in a bar lifting a full pint of fluid, taking a drink and lowering it back down to the table.
2. Whilst walking down the street, you see the bus standing at the bus stop so you have to run for the bus.

fine movements like writing, larger movements like picking up a glass or the whole of our strength in putting the shot. So the task itself or the load to be overcome is the main component in determining the strength exerted by the muscle.

However, as was seen in Chapter 2, the motor unit has an 'all-or-nothing' contraction. Therefore it is the number and size of the motor units which dictate the different strengths of contraction.

Length–tension relationship

As well as recruitment, other physical properties of the muscle are important in strength generation. Amongst these is the length–tension relationship of the contractile unit. It has been shown that the production of force in the muscle is proportional to the number of crossbridges that occur between the actin and myosin fibrils. If few myosin heads are in contact, as when the actin and myosin fibrils are stretched apart, for example, then force production will be decreased. If the fibrils are too contracted, the tapered ends of the myosin filaments push against the Z bands and again the force that can be generated is decreased. These length–tension characteristics are enhanced by the intracellular titin filaments which run through the length of the myosin protein filament, between the Z lines. These titin filaments have an intrinsic elastic property which can alter the propensity of the muscle to contract (Lakomy 1999).

Force–velocity relationship

Force–velocity relationship is another aspect that affects muscle strength. Different forces can be generated at different speeds. The force generated in a concentric contraction against a load is marginally greater when the contraction takes place at a fast speed as compared to slow speeds. Without a load, the strength generated by a fast contraction may be as much as three times greater than that generated at a slow speed. In eccentric contractions greater forces can be generated than in concentric contraction. This probably occurs because the muscle uses very little adenosine triphosphate (ATP) to break the bonds holding the crossbridges.

Angle of pull

Other anatomical and biomechanical aspects of muscle function will affect the strength generation. The angle of pull of a muscle at the time of its action will affect its strength. The angle of pull of a muscle is defined as *the angle between the segmental axis and the line of pull of the muscle*. An angle of pull that is nearer to 90° means that more of the resolved muscle force would rotate the segment (vertical component). If the angle of pull was greater or less than 90° then the distractive or compressive force (horizontal component) would increase. This is explained in Chapter 3. Luckily for us, the angle of pull never reaches 90°. If it did then all the muscle force would be used to move the segment and there would be no horizontal force to stabilise the joint. This would mean that the joint would actually be damaged along with other musculoskeletal structures!

Stability and sequencing

For the muscle to work efficiently, it should work from a stable base. The strength of the muscle will then be used for the intended task and not diverted to ensure a stable base is maintained. This is very important during early rehabilitation as the muscles are usually very weak. This is easily demonstrated if a weak person tries to throw a ball. The distance achieved would be greater if the starting position were sitting rather than standing. The base whilst sitting is larger (the chair and the feet) than it is during standing (just the feet). During many functional movements muscles are helped to achieve this stable base and work more efficiently by working in predefined sequences. These sequences are learned as movement is refined during the maturation process or we learn the pattern as a new skill. Chapter 7 explains these processes.

Anatomy

The gross structure of the muscle seems to be well adapted to provide the appropriate range, direction and force of contraction. The muscles that produce the precision movements appear to have fine fasciculi whereas the gluteus maximus, for example, has coarse fasciculi. How fasciculi are structured within the muscle is also important. They are usually parallel, oblique or spiral, relative to the direction of pull of the muscle. In parallel muscles the angle of pennation (the angle at which the fasciculi join the central spine of connective tissue) of the muscle itself will affect its ability to produce force. The greater the angle of pennation then the more sarcomeres there are in parallel. This will lead to an increase in strength but a decrease in shortening velocity (Hunter 2000).

The length–tension relationship, the angle of pull and the sequencing and patterning of muscle action are all most effective in producing greater strength when the muscle is in its middle range. Of course, these biomechanical factors only result in efficient strong muscle work if the neuromuscular and muscular systems are intact. The physiological systems, such as the circulatory system, must also be functioning optimally to initiate, maintain and terminate muscle action. If any of these systems malfunction, as in many pathologies, then muscle strength and subsequent efficient movement are decreased.

Age and gender

Age and gender also have an effect on absolute muscle strength. It will be seen from Chapter 15 that the changes due to ageing are complex and are a combination between the physiological process, disease and lifestyle. The general consequence, however, is that muscle strength decreases with age.

Psychological factors

It is also important to remember that as well as the physical and physiological aspects discussed above, there can also be a psychological element to muscle strength. The shot putter will only win the gold medal if all the psychological elements are right, if he has produced enough adrenaline and he believes that he is able to do it. Sometimes the apparent limit of physical ability to produce muscle strength is overcome by psychological influences. There is the tale of the mother who lifted a car under which her child was trapped. This was a feat which was obviously beyond her perceived physical ability.

MUSCLE POWER

In Chapter 3, power was defined as *the rate at which work is being done*. The unit of work is the watt (W). The rate at which a muscle works is termed muscle power and can be calculated by using the following formulae:

$$\text{Power} = \text{Force (of contraction)} \times \text{velocity (of contraction)}$$

where velocity = distance moved/unit time, i.e. distance of contraction, and:

$$\text{Power} = \text{net joint moment} \times \text{joint angular velocity.}$$

Positive power is generated in a concentric contraction and negative power is generated in an eccentric contraction.

In Chapter 2 it was explained that the velocity of muscle contraction is largely determined by the composition of that muscle, i.e. the fibre type(s) it contains. The type II (phasic fast twitch) fibres which generate large amounts of tension in a short time are geared towards anaerobic metabolic activity and tend to fatigue quickly. The power produced by these muscles will therefore be anaerobic and will produce high-intensity activity over short periods of time. Type I (tonic slow twitch) fibres generate a low level of muscle tension but can sustain contraction for a long time. These fibres are geared towards aerobic metabolism and are slow to fatigue. The power they produce is therefore aerobic power.

MUSCLE ENDURANCE

If activities that are carried out throughout the day are analysed there are very few occasions when

---

Task 6.3

For two examples of sporting extremes, for example a high jump and a marathon, and two examples of everyday activities, for example writing and opening a tight jam jar, analyse the differences between each upper and lower limb activity in terms of muscle strength, force, work and power.

maximum strength has to be used. Most activities that are performed will require the muscle action to be repetitive, as many activities will be carried out a number of times; just think of walking as an example. The muscle's ability to keep on working over long periods of time is a measure of its endurance and is defined as *the ability of a muscle to maintain isometric contraction or continue dynamic contractions.*

The muscular endurance can be thought of as the ability of a muscle not to tire; in other words, to resist fatigue.

In the preceding text strength was described in biomechanical and physical terms. Endurance, however, needs to be described with a more physiological perspective. As was described for aerobic power, endurance is dependent on the type of respiration performed by the working muscle, i.e. the aerobic energy systems. For the aerobic system to work there must be an adequate energy supply to the working muscle (Daniels 2001). This energy may be in the form of creatine phosphate and glycogen stored in the muscles themselves or the liver, which last for a short while (through anaerobic respiration). This is then replaced by energy that is brought to the area from the metabolism of foodstuffs derived from digestion (aerobic respiration). Since this foodstuff is being burned to produce energy aerobically, a key ingredient for the process is a constant supply of oxygen brought to the area. Thus oxygen transport from the lungs to the working muscle is a vital part of the muscle's respiratory function.

During continuous muscle respiration, waste products such as carbon dioxide, potassium, acetylcholine and lactic acid are being produced. It is just as important for the functioning of this system that this waste is removed from the area. If the waste is not removed then its build-up will cause the muscle to fatigue. The longer the muscle can resist fatigue then the greater is its aerobic capacity (Daniels 2001).

Fatigue

Everyone has felt tired at times where there seems to be a lack of energy at the end of a task or at the end of a long day at college. This must, however, be distinguished from true fatigue which means that there is an inability to carry on with the task. Fatigue can take two forms: *general body fatigue* or *local muscle fatigue.* The former involves the depletion of energy stores and/or the build-up of waste products in many regions and systems of the body. This is characterised by physical and mental exhaustion and is an extremely serious situation. Local muscle fatigue is caused by the depletion of energy and/or the build-up of waste products within the functioning muscle, a decrease in the availability of oxygen and any disturbances in the contractile mechanisms, such as inhibition by the central nervous system and a decrease in conduction at the neuromuscular junction. It is defined as a *diminished response to repeated stimuli characterised by a decrease in amplitude of the motor fibre units or the ability to sustain a force.* This is a much more common event than general fatigue and provides the biochemical and neurological stimuli necessary for the development of the aerobic capacity of the muscle. Local muscle fatigue is recognised by the inability to generate force and carry out the full range of movement of the task being undertaken, a decrease in the speed of contraction, shaking or fasciculation within the particular muscle, pain and a loss of coordination.

A full explanation of exercise physiology can be gained from many standard texts but from the brief description above and the preceding text, it can be seen that for the muscle to carry out its functions properly there have to be intact neuro-muscular, musculoskeletal and cardiorespiratory systems. Failure of any or all of these systems will lead to the muscle being unable to adequately perform its function (Wilmore & Costill 2004).

MEASURING STRENGTH AND ENDURANCE

To enable us to determine if a muscle is working to its maximum capacity for both strength and

---

Task 6.4

List the things that could affect the functioning of a muscle. For each of the items on your list, think of which component of muscle function could be impaired. Try also to analyse why this impairment is taking place.

endurance, it is important that both these components can be measured. For each of the problems you have listed from Task 6.4, you will need to measure the strength or endurance of the muscle or muscle groups used. This is important for several reasons: first, to determine if there is any deviation from the normal; second, to assess whether the condition is getting worse, better or remaining the same; third, to give a base measurement to the muscle condition; and lastly to assess whether any treatment you implement is having a positive or negative effect on the muscle.

Measuring strength

While studying the shot putter of the earlier example, it could be seen that the size of the muscle was important in producing strength. Those people with large muscles are usually stronger than those with smaller muscles. Thus it can be assumed that the larger the muscle, the greater the force that the muscle can generate. This would seem pretty obvious as the larger the muscle, the more actin and myosin would be present and thus the greater the propensity for the contractile unit to form crossbridges.

Physiological cross-sectional area

It has been described by many people (e.g. Jones & Round 1990) that the physiological cross-sectional area (PCSA) of the muscle is proportional to its strength. This, however, is not a convenient measure as only the anatomical cross-sectional area (ACSA) can be ascertained when measuring the girth of the limb using a tape measure. The true PCSA can only be found through dissection or modern scanning procedures. There is still a relationship, though, between size and strength. The results of measuring the girth of a limb to discover the ACSA must be read with caution as the whole of the limb may be asymmetrical when compared to the other side. This would mean that there is difficulty in distinguishing which component is responsible for the anomaly.

Atrophy and hypertrophy

When the muscle has decreased in size through injury, disease or disuse it will usually be weaker than normal. This decrease in size is termed 'atrophy'. When we build our muscles up in size we usually find that the muscle is stronger. This increase in size is termed 'hypertrophy' (Harris & Dudley 2000). Measurement of the PCSA is possible with the use of techniques such as MRI but these are not really practicable.

Indirect measures of strength, by measuring force, can be obtained using hand-held dynamometers but these are limited by the strength of the operator. Another valuable tool in measuring force production in the form of muscle torque (turning effect) is the isokinetic dynamometer, although this machine is often too expensive for general therapeutic departments. Chapter 8 gives a description of this and other devices used for measuring strength.

If the muscle is capable of performing its full range of movement, it is convenient to use the Medical Research Council Scale (the Oxford Grading Scale) to measure muscle strength. This is classified on a scale of 0–5 (Hollis & Fletcher-Cook 1999) where:

0 = no movement at all
1 = a flicker of movement
2 = full range of movement with the effect of gravity eliminated
3 = full range of movement against gravity
4 = full range of movement against gravity and resistance
5 = full range of movement with maximal resistance.

Although useful, the Oxford Grading Scale has many limitations and many variations of this scale have been developed (see Chapter 8). A more useful measure of strength in a wider context may be the 1 repetition maximum (1 RM), defined as *the maximum amount of weight a muscle can lift once only*. The 10 repetition maximum (10 RM) is a derivation of the 1 RM and is *the maximum weight a muscle can lift 10 times*. Both these quantities are found by trial and error. A more subjective measure that is frequently employed is isometric testing. This is carried out by manually resisting the muscle contraction in various positions within its range and not allowing any movement. The resistance that has to be used to prevent movement is compared to the unaffected side. This method is obviously only applicable if the problem is unilateral and the subject normally symmetrical.

Measuring endurance

As discussed earlier, there is a greater involvement of physiological processes in muscle endurance. Thus testing endurance is going to involve physiological testing. Measurements of expired air, heart rate, respiratory rate, blood gases and waste products after maximal and sub-maximal exercise on treadmills are the procedures usually used (McArdle et al 1996). These measurements would be fairly difficult in an ordinary department. Although it is difficult to measure muscle endurance directly, measuring the time to fatigue (or number of repetitions to fatigue) and the time to recovery will give an adequate estimate of the endurance of the muscle and how it is progressing and regressing. The isokinetic dynamometer described in Chapter 8 also has a facility to measure, indirectly, muscle endurance.

When things go wrong

There are times when muscle strength and endurance cannot be maintained. The most common causes of decrease in strength and endurance are injury, disease or disuse. Injury can be to the muscle itself, its nervous or vascular supply or the skeletal support. Direct trauma that disrupts the contractile unit, such as a muscle or ligament tear, will mechanically affect the ability of the muscle to either produce or transmit force. Disruption of nerve supply will mean that no recruitment is able to take place and hence no muscle contraction. Disruption of blood supply will mean that energy, in the form of foodstuff, and oxygen will not be delivered to the muscle and waste products will not be taken away. This will mean a decrease in the respiratory capacity of the muscle and hence a decrease in its endurance. There are many diseases that affect the muscle or its neurological supply. Muscular dystrophy is an example of a muscle wasting disease where the muscle protein is affected. A neuropathy would disrupt muscle stimulation, leading to a decreased contraction.

The examples above would lead to an inability of the muscle to function to its optimal capability. The muscle may also not be used if another body part, proximal or distal to the muscle, has to be kept immobile (as in a joint problem or bone fracture). Pain, muscle spasm, habit and certain psychological factors will lead to weakness caused by disuse. If the muscle is not used then the actin and myosin protein will be reabsorbed. This will diminish the ability to form crossbridges and hence the force production and strength will decrease. This decrease in strength is mirrored by a decrease in size, which is termed 'atrophy'. Therefore, the case above will be termed 'disuse atrophy'. Concurrent with the reabsorption of actin and myosin there will also be a collapse and eventual reabsorption of the small blood and lymph vessels. This, together with the decrease and inefficient use of energy stores, will cause a decrease in muscle endurance.

INCREASING STRENGTH AND ENDURANCE

For a muscle to perform any functional activity, it must be able to generate enough force to overcome the resistance of the task. This could be one maximal effort or a series of submaximal efforts over a time period. For the former, the muscle strength is paramount whilst the latter requires both strength and endurance.

Muscle strength

For a muscle to increase in strength, it has to work to fatigue with a load placed upon it which exceeds its usual metabolic work rate. This is known as the *overload principle*.

Physiological processes

If the muscle is stimulated to work hard then this information is relayed to the central nervous system, which in turn stimulates the ribosomes to replicate more actin and myosin protein. The myofibrils are therefore thickened and increased in length. There will be an increase in myocyte number and size and in the number of sarcomeres, which will increase the strength of the muscle. There will also be a change in the density of the mitochondria within the muscle tissue. More muscle glycogen, creatine phosphate and ATP substrate will be laid down. There will also be an increase in the concentration and activity of glycolytic enzymes, myokinase and creatine phosphate (the enzymes needed for growth) (Maughan & Gleeson 2004). This process usually takes about 4 weeks.

Increased vascularisation

If there is enough biochemical stimulation through activity then increased vascularisation of the area will also occur (up to 50%) and thus the supply and utilisation of oxygen and energy will also change so both strength and endurance will increase (Greenhaff & Hultman 1999).

Increase in size

As the muscle increases in strength it also increases in size, which is termed 'hypertrophy'. However, it must be noted that initially, increases in strength are not accompanied by a corresponding increase in size. It is thought that recruitment of motor units becomes more efficient and there is also an increase in the number of motor units that are recruited. There also appears to be an inhibition of the antagonist muscle groups together with a more efficient integration of synergists. The training effects described in Chapter 8 also play their part. Some authors believe that hyperplasia, or the splitting of developed fibres, takes place but there is debate concerning this (Conroy & Earle 2000).

Increasing strength

Muscle weakness is the inability to generate force. If a muscle is weak then the best method to increase strength is exercise in the form of training. Training can be defined as *the facilitation of biological adaptations that improve the performance of specific tasks*. There are three main categories of exercise that are used to increase muscle strength: *assisted exercise, free active exercise* and *resisted exercise*.

Assisted exercise could be manual or mechanical and is used when the muscle is so weak that the segment cannot be moved through a sufficient range against the force of gravity. Manual assistance may be given by the therapist (therapist assisted) or by the patient (auto-assisted). The assistance given may be just eliminating the effect of the force of gravity. The assisting force must be in the direction of the required movement and must only assist the movement. Care must be taken that the movement does not become passive. Mechanical assistance could be assisting the movement by eliminating or decreasing friction, by using a sliding board or sling suspension. Pulleys can also be used to facilitate the movement. Such assistance is useful for muscles that have been measured as grade 2 on the Oxford Grading Scale.

If the muscle has been measured at grade 3 or above then it can be strengthened by using free active exercise, defined as *exercise without the use of assistance or resistance except gravity* (some people make body weight the exception to this).

Fatigue, and therefore muscle strengthening, can be achieved with active exercise by changing the parameters of the exercise, such as repetition, speed, rhythm and leverage. The exercise can be progressed and regressed by altering the starting position.

Once a muscle is able to move a segment against gravity then the more usual form of exercise used to strengthen muscles is resisted exercise. To be most effective, the resistance must be directed against the movement of the muscle and if possible at 90° to the axis of the segment. The resistance may be given manually or mechanically. Manual resisted exercise can be defined as *active resistance exercise in which the resistance force is applied by the physiotherapist (therapist resisted) or the patient (auto-resisted) to either a dynamic or static muscular contraction.*

The position of resistance is an important consideration as the further away from the axis of rotation the resistance is given on the segment that

---

Task 6.5

Work in pairs. One of you sits over a plinth with your thigh supported, acting as the patient. The other one, acting as the therapist, gives resistance to the leg, beginning at the knee and moving down toward the ankle in increments. Think about the force required to resist maximal effort and the effect this has on the patient. What trick movements do you notice when the activity becomes more difficult? How could these be corrected?

is moving, the less effort has to be made by the therapist. This can be explained by considering leverage and the effect the length of the lever arm has on the effort required. As was seen in Chapter 3, the moment of force was defined as the force × the distance from the pivot. Therefore, if the distance from the pivot increased then to maintain the same moment, the force could decrease. The forward sliding force that causes the anterior glide at the knee joint is increased the further down the leg the resistance is given. This may have adverse consequences for the patient, so this has to be taken into consideration when performing the technique.

Mechanical resistance is any resistance against which the body can exercise. The main categories are weighted resistance, free weights (barbells, dumbbells, cuff weights, ankle weights, weighted boots or sandbags), multigyms, isokinetic dynamometer and springs, for example materials such as elastic latex. Exercise cycles, body weight or hydrotherapy may all be used as forms of mechanical resistance.

Strength training

When a muscle has to undergo exercise to improve strength it is usually because there has been a problem and it is very unusual for this problem to manifest itself as only a decrease in muscle strength. Many other systems may be involved so we need to approach rehabilitation holistically. Strength and endurance are closely linked and really should be treated together. Other factors such as muscle elasticity, joint range, coordination and balance and cardiovascular fitness must also be addressed. Although this text does not cover the skills involved in undertaking a training programme, it would be useful to cover the main principles even if there is an artificial separation between strength and endurance.

Assessment Muscle strength, joint range of movement and integrity, pain and functional ability all need to be assessed before any treatment is planned. This is a good time to work out the 1 RM and 10 RM of the muscle or the level of cardiovascular fitness or muscular endurance.

Overload As described earlier, the system must work at a level greater than normal function. For strength, this would mean moving a greater resistance and maintaining a contraction for a longer period.

Specificity It has been shown that training that mimics the activity for which the action is needed is more effective than if the conditions are different (Ackland & Bloomfield 1995). Conversely, training for one factor, for example strength, would not necessarily improve another factor, such as endurance. There is not necessarily an overlap. This is also true for different fibre types and possibly speed of activity.

Reversibility Strength gains will be lost or reversed more slowly than they were gained (Zatsiorsky 1995). Inevitably, though, if the demand is not placed on the muscle then the strength will only return to the level needed to carry out normal functional activities. It is interesting that the rate of decline is dependent on the type and length of exercise that was used to build up muscle strength. The longer the training period, the slower the decline. Concentric and eccentric work used to build strength will result in a longer deterioration period than concentric activity alone (Harris & Dudley 2000). It has also been suggested that fibre types decondition at differing rates.

Motivation and learning This is an important aspect of any exercise programme and is discussed in Chapter 8.

Progressive resistance exercise (PRE) These are specific exercise regimes that use weights in a strengthening programme. PRE is defined as *load or resistance to the muscle as applied by some mechanical means and quantitatively and progressively increased over time*. Below is a list of the variables that may be changed in addition to the load:

- Repetition: the number of a specific exercise, usually in sets
- Sets: a number of repetitions
- Frequency: the number of times the exercise session is performed
- Duration: the length of time of each session
- Speed: the speed at which the exercise is carried out

Table 6.1   The DeLorme and Watkins programme (DeLorme & Watkins 1948), the Oxford programme (Zinovieff 1951) and the MacQueen programme (MacQueen 1954, 1956)

Name	Regime	Effect	Conditions
DeLorme & Watkins	10 lifts at $\frac{1}{2}$ 10 RM 10 lifts at $\frac{3}{4}$ 10 RM 10 lifts at full 10 RM	Increases strength	× 3 each session, 4/5 per week, retest 10 RM weekly
Oxford	10 reps at 10 RM 10 reps at $\frac{3}{4}$ 10 RM 10 reps at $\frac{1}{2}$ 10 RM or 10 reps at 10 RM then reduced by 5 kg for 10 sets	Increases strength	× 5 sessions per week
MacQueen (1)	4 ×10 reps at 10 RM	Hypertrophy	
MacQueen (2)	10 reps at 10 RM 8 reps at 8 RM 6 reps at 6 RM	Power	

- Muscle action: concentric, eccentric or isometric
- Starting position: this is the position from which the exercise is performed.

Specific regimes   Many training regimes were developed during and just after the Second World War to treat the many injured soldiers. They were based on the fundamental principles given above and some are shown in Table 6.1.

Although these programmes are probably not used these days in their original form, derivations are used and the basic principles underlying them are certainly still valid.

Increasing endurance

Conditioning is the augmentation of the energy capacity of the muscle through an exercise programme. This is produced by exercise of sufficient *intensity, duration* and *frequency*. The methods used to increase endurance differ between the fit athlete and the patient who has become deconditioned, but the principles of treatment remain the same. The overriding consideration is the overload principle. As for strength training, the muscle must work above its usual metabolic function for adaptation to take place.

Intensity is the rate at which the exercise is carried out. Intensity is easier to quantify if we are trying to improve cardiovascular endurance. The maximum volume of oxygen uptake (VO_{2max}) is a function of the intensity and since heart rate and VO_{2max} are linearly related, heart rate can be considered as a function of intensity. So the intensity of the exercise could be described through the heart rate. Local muscle endurance is usually measured as the length of time the muscle can function or the number of repetitions of the activity before fatigue occurs. The muscle's ability to recover post exercise is also used as a measure of its endurance. General conditioning is said to take place when the heart rate is between 60% and 90% of maximum. For local muscle endurance to increase, the number of repetitions need to be high but against a low resistance.

The *duration* of an exercise is the length of time for which the exercise is carried out. The greater the intensity, the shorter will be the duration and vice versa.

Frequency is the number of times that the exercise programme is carried out per week. Although this will vary from patient to patient depending on the assessment, usually a minimum of three times per week is necessary to ensure that

---

Task 6.6

Choose a muscle or group of muscles, the shoulder abductors for example, and work out a strengthening regime as the muscle progresses from a grade 1 to a grade 5 on the Oxford Grading Scale. Set aims and objectives for each stage of the recovery and use assisted, free active and resisted exercise. Discuss how you would assess the condition and progress and regress the exercises as necessary.

Task 6.7

For the lower limb, devise a circuit that would improve local muscle endurance for the major groups of muscles.

---

the physiological adaptations take place (Watham & Roll 2000).

Endurance training

When training for endurance, the principles that were used for strengthening still apply. Exercise is still used but the repetitions have to be greater to ensure that the overload principle is met. Therefore it must be ensured that the aerobic system is utilised, so low or even no resistance is used. These exercises can be progressed or regressed with some degree of objectivity by either using numbers of repetitions, duration of exercise or a combination of both as markers. The rest or time interval between sets of exercise can also be used as a method of progression or regression. The rest interval can be shortened as the recovery from fatigue is speeded up.

For the earlier stages of rehabilitation, assisted and free active exercise can be used to increase endurance. As rehabilitation progresses, free active and resisted exercise are used.

Delivery of exercise The programme used to deliver the exercises for increasing strength or endurance could be either individual (patient and therapist) or in a group situation (therapist and class). Each has its advantages and disadvantages. In the one-to-one situation, the therapist could give individual encouragement and ensure that the exercise is being carried out properly. The exercise could be progressed and regressed as

soon as applicable as the therapist would be constantly assessing capability. In the group situation, however, the patient will be motivated by competition with others and the variety of exercise could be greater.

Circuit training as a group exercise is particularly effective when increasing cardiorespiratory endurance but is also very effective for increasing local muscle endurance as the delivery of oxygen and the ability of the muscle to use it are closely linked (Maughan & Gleeson 2004). The circuit is made up of a series of well-defined activities with a pre-described rest period between each. The circuit is usually repeated a set number of times with a rest period between each (usually enough time for recovery) (Astrand & Rohdal 1988).

CONCLUSION

Muscle strength, power and endurance, although described separately, can be seen to be closely integrated and should be thought of as equally important in affecting movement of the musculoskeletal system and ultimately locomotion of the human. We have seen through this chapter that the production of muscular force, movement initiation and control and continuation of useful integrated and functional movement require an intact neuromusculoskeletal system. These systems have to be studied through anatomical, physiological, biomechanical and psychological perspectives so that if any are disrupted through trauma or disease we can, after thorough assessment, return them to an optimal condition to perform functional human movement.

REFERENCES

Ackland TR, Bloomfield J 1995 Applied anatomy. In: Bloomfield J, Fricker PA, Fitch KD (eds) Science and medicine in sport. Blackwell Scientific Publications, Oxford

Astrand PE, Rohdal K 1988 Textbook of work physiology. Physiological basis of exercise. McGraw-Hill, Singapore

Conroy BP, Earl RW 2000 Bone, muscle and connective tissue adaptations to physical activity. In: Baechle TR, Earle RW (eds) Essentials of strength training and conditioning, 2nd edn. Human Kinetics, Champaign, Illinois

Daniels J 2001 Aerobic capacity for endurance. In: Foran B (ed) High performance sports conditioning. Human Kinetics, Champaign, Illinois

DeLorme TL, Watkins AL 1948 Techniques of progressive resistance exercises. Archives of Physical Medicine 29: 263–273

Greenhaff PL, Hultman E 1999 The biomechanical basis of exercise. In: Maughan RJ (ed) Basic and applied sciences for sports medicine. Butterworth Heinemann, Oxford

Harris RT, Dudley G 2000 Neuromuscular adaptations to conditioning. In: Baechle TR, Earle RW (eds) Essentials of strength training and conditioning. Human Kinetics, Champaign, Illinois

Hollis M, Fletcher-Cook P 1999 Practical exercise therapy, 4th edn. Blackwell Science, Oxford

Hunter GR 2000 Muscle physiology. In: Baechle TR, Earle RW (eds) Essentials of strength training and conditioning. Human Kinetics, Champaign, Illinois

Jones DA, Round JM 1990 Skeletal muscle in health and disease. Manchester University Press, Manchester

Lakomy HKA 1999 The biomechanics of human movement. In: Maughan RJ (ed) Basic and applied sciences for sports medicine. Butterworth Heinemann, Oxford

MacQueen IJ 1954 Recent advances in the techniques of progressive resistance exercise. British Medical Journal 2: 1193–1198

MacQueen IJ 1956 The application of progressive resistance exercise. Physiotherapy 40: 83–89

Maughan RJ, Gleeson M 2004 The biomechanical basis of sports performance. Oxford University Press, Oxford

McArdle WD, Katch FI, Katch VL 1996 Exercise physiology. Lea and Febiger, Philadelphia

Watham D, Roll F 2000 Training methods and modes. In: Baechle TR, Earle RW (eds) Essentials of strength training and conditioning. Human Kinetics, Champaign, Illinois

Wilmore JH, Costill DL 2004 Physiology of sport and exercise, 3rd edn. Human Kinetics, Champaign, Illinois

Zatsiorsky VM 1995 Science and promotion of strength training. Human Kinetics, Champaign, Illinois

Zinovieff AN 1951 Heavy resistance exercise. British Journal of Physical Medicine June: 129–133

Chapter 7

Motor learning

Nicola Phillips

CHAPTER CONTENTS

LEARNING OUTCOMES

At the end of this chapter you should be able to:

1. Define the term 'motor learning' and describe the limitations to motor control

2. Demonstrate an understanding of models of motor control

3. Define the term 'skill'

4. Discuss the main components involved in the skill acquisition process

5. Discuss how long- and short-term memory are involved in learning and performing a motor skill.

INTRODUCTION

Earlier chapters have explained some of the biomechanical principles of movement and the musculosketal and neurological bases of movement production and control. This chapter aims to explain how these human movements are learned and become the skilled coordinated patterns of activity necessary for function.

MOTOR LEARNING

Definition

Motor learning has been defined as a set process associated with practice or experience leading to relatively permanent changes in skilled behaviour (Schmidt 1988).

The set process mentioned in the above definition will be explained in this chapter. The other important term to note in the definition is 'relatively permanent changes'. A change in technique of carrying out a particular task is not considered learned if it just happens once or twice, possibly by chance. Vereijken et al (1992) described motor learning as the process of adjusting movement characteristics to a new task or challenge. This concept has a very similar meaning to Schmidt's definition but has an emphasis on observation of the movement characteristics as opposed to models of what might be happening in the brain. Again, this concept will also be explained later in the chapter.

Historical perspective

The field of movement control has historically been studied from two entirely different perspectives: those that provide models considering motor control as a 'top-down' process and those that describe it as a 'bottom-up' process. The psychology and neurophysiology researchers tend to describe a central nervous system (CNS) control of learning movement patterns. In contrast, the biomechanics researchers have adopted engineering principles to describe models of motor learning that are adapted to changes at the peripheries. It is very likely that motor learning is a combination of both schools of thought but unfortunately the language used by all these different groups can make comparison and integration of principles confusing.

Sherrington (1906) was an important early influence in neural control and his concept of reflex responses to stimuli causing movement of the extremities is still a foundation of many treatment approaches today. It was this formative work that highlighted some of the sensory receptors involved in proprioception and introduced the concept of reciprocal innervation of agonist and antagonist muscle. The term 'final common pathway' was also introduced at this time, indicating that the influences from reflexes, sensory sources and cognitive sources converge at spinal level.

Weiner first developed the information processing model in the 1940s and likened the brain to a computer in which information is received and processed, leading to an output to muscles, creating movement (Latash 1998). This approach was termed 'cybernetics'. Since then there has been a gradual progression in this line of thinking, towards a model of cognitive information processing (Schmidt 1975).

Bernstein (1967) was one of the formative authors on motor control and learning and was one of the first to attempt to integrate biomechanical, neural and psychological models of motor control. Much of his work has underpinned some of the current thinking of this subject.

Winstein (1991) stated that the acquisition of motor learning is fundamental to human life and consists of neural, physical and behavioural components. This statement conveniently encompasses many of the aspects which will be covered in this chapter and serves as a reminder of the different aspects that need to be considered in understanding the basic concepts of motor learning.

Types of movement

As described in Schmidt's (1988) definition, motor learning is a process which leads to changes in skilled behaviour. These motor skills are demonstrated by relatively predictable patterns of movement during performance of a particular task.

Before investigating motor learning any further, it is necessary to outline the categories of movement as it is the coordination of these movements which produces the learned motor skills described by Schmidt.

Movements can be broadly divided into two types:

1. *reflex*: these are usually inherited
2. *learned*: these do not appear to be inherited and therefore need practice.

Both these types of movement can be either simple or complex. For example, a simple reflex task would be blinking in response to an object near the eye. We might not be consciously aware that this has happened until after the response and quite possibly only then because the object, such as dust, might have caused some irritation. We certainly wouldn't remember ever having to learn how to blink at the right time.

Conversely, a simple learned task would be clapping your hands or reaching for a toy. Learning to clap requires conscious control and a number of attempts to bring the hands into contact at the right time to make a noise; the concentration on a young child's face is testament to this!

Similarly, breathing is a complex motor task subject to a great deal of variation but under reflex control. We are not consciously aware of the general rate or depth of our breathing unless it changes dramatically, such as after a fairly intense physical effort, but there is a high degree of coordination required to produce the optimum rate and depth of breathing for every circumstance. On the other hand, a gymnastic tumbling routine is a complex learned task which requires hours of practice and takes a great deal of conscious control throughout the learning process.

The learned movements described above are all tasks that have been refined through trial and error practice until they produce a successful outcome. This might be babies managing to clap their hands or grasp a toy after a few months of waving their arms around in a seemingly haphazard way. How these movements are learned is where the experts have differing views. Some believe that movements develop and become more refined as the central nervous system evolves and that more complex movements are not possible until the CNS has developed enough. On the other hand, the biomechanists believe that movement control arises as a response to the requirements made of the limbs, in which case the CNS develops as an adaptive mechanism and will therefore only adapt if those demands are made on the body.

Some of these models will be described later but in the meantime, the Schmidt (1988) model will be used to describe the main principles in this chapter as it is a relatively clear one to understand. This should then allow you to adapt this line of thinking to incorporate the other models.

MOTOR CONTROL

The schema theory

The coordination of movement, whether reflex or learned, can be termed 'motor control'. The dif-ferent areas of the CNS which deal with the reflex or learned responses have been highlighted previously and include spinal cord, brain stem, motor cortex and cerebellum. The study of this field covers how movements are selected in response to sensory information obtained from the environment and/or within the body, based on previous experience. The process, known as the *schema theory* (Schmidt 1975), is thought to be controlled by the long-term memory and then modified by other centres in the central nervous system. This process can be divided into three main parts for clearer explanation:

- *Stimulus identification*: input via interoceptors or exteroceptors is identified as stimuli at CNS level.
- *Response selection*: the appropriate movement pattern in response to the identified stimuli is chosen based on prior experience.
- *Response programming*: the motor experience is carried out with feedback to decide if it was the right choice.

Figure 7.1 is adapted from Schmidt's (1975) schema theory and shows how these stages are thought to work.

Let's take these processes step by step.

Stimulus identification

This stage can be subdivided into three separate steps.

Stimulus detection   First, it should be noted that there will be a tremendous amount of information being absorbed from various sources during any simple everyday activity. For example, when someone is walking downstairs the central nervous system is receiving information from the visual field, auditory input of the sound of each step, background noises and possibly continuing a conversation, as well as proprioceptive input from joint, muscles and tendons about the depth and width of the step. This amount of information would be far too much for anyone to cope with consciously so a *filtering process* takes place of what is important for that particular function and environment, based on prior experience. Any input considered irrelevant is discarded before continuing the process to conscious levels.

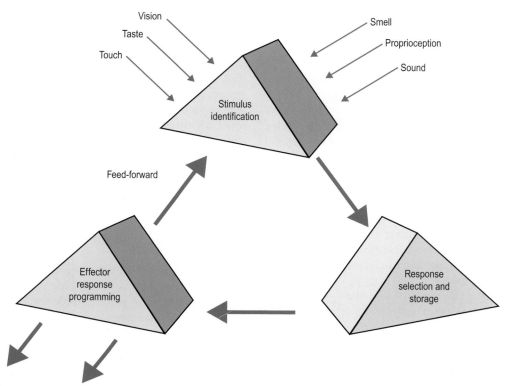

Figure 7.1   Information processing model (Schmidt & Lee 1999).

Consequently, there is not usually conscious awareness of this level of perception unless the brain receives input it does not recognise or is not expecting in comparison to previous similar functional tasks. For instance, during that normally familiar task of walking downstairs you don't notice the width and depth of each step, unless one step is suddenly different. You then become very aware of the steps beneath your feet. Your brain takes in the visual input and proprioceptive and tactile feedback but only alerts your conscious thought if there is a problem. How many times have you walked down a flight of steps and almost tripped because one step is slightly different from the others? You turn and look at the step and then, for a while, watch each step carefully to avoid stumbling again. Normally stimuli which have been received for a while are ignored whereas any new stimuli are passed on to the next stage of the process. This is a type of internal feedback and is termed 'knowledge of performance'.

Stimulus interpretation   How you interpret information will depend on what sort of stimulation is expected and any prior experience of similar situations. This is a form of pattern recognition which is stored in the long-term memory. The accuracy of this interpretation will depend on how efficiently the individual can retrieve previous experience from the long-term memory. For example, someone who has been on a rollercoaster many times will take in stimuli from the inner ear and the eyes but ignore input from the gut. Needless to say, the first-time rollercoaster rider is likely to feel quite sick if they pay more attention to the sensory information coming from their stomach.

A typical example in the sporting world would be two rugby union centres, one experienced player and one novice. The experienced player will recognise the body position and foot movements of an opponent who is about to make a dummy pass and react accordingly, successfully tackling the other player. The novice will probably

---

Task 7.1

If you can drive a car, think back to when you were learning.
How many different things did the instructor tell you to pay attention to at once?
How many different things did you have to do with your feet and your hands at the same time?
How many lessons did it take you to be able to cope with all those tasks at the same time?

---

miss the telltale visual signs allowing earlier re-action and feel very foolish lying on the floor, having missed the tackle as his opponent runs past him! In addition, the experienced player will be able to use a more parallel style of taking in external cues, which will be discussed later in the chapter. This means that instead of dealing with one stimulus at a time, which would result in quite a delay in some responses, the expert player could notice and react to a few things at once, allowing cues to be taken in at a glance. This would in turn allow concentration on other skills such as tactical decision making or ball retention skills.

The above is the difference between a learner having to deal with such challenges in a more *serial* manner whereas practice allows some challenges to be dealt with at the same time or in *parallel*.

Stimulus selection The type and amount of stimuli selected to be passed on to the next stage of the decision-making process will depend on how much attention is devoted to this particular function at the time. Selection of the most useful stimuli for that particular task requires the correct allocation of attention to ensure that the appropriate information is passed on. The breadth of attention needs to balance the focus of attention for the correct selection of movement. For example, consider attention to a beam of light – it can be a tightly focused spotlight or a diffused beam covering a large area. The focus needs to be tight enough to increase concentration but if it is concentrated too tightly it will create tunnel vision, therefore missing important cues around the periphery. People learning to ski have to concen-

trate on controlling the skis and are probably not able to take in the alpine scenery and stay on their feet at the same time. Therefore, they may not take in peripheral cues such as other skiers or trees in time to do anything about them!

Response selection

Once the afferent stimuli have been accepted and recognised, the brain must then decide what sort of response to make. A movement plan is assembled, based on identical or similar previous performances, which is tried out in the individual's head, usually at an unconscious level, to decide if the outcome of the movement is appropriate for the task. Any necessary modifications are then made before the movement plan is passed on to the effector stage.

Imagine you are about to assess a patient in an outpatient clinic, having been given a referral with a brief diagnosis of a condition you have not treated before. First, you look up the condition and different methods of treatment in a textbook (long-term memory). Then you make a rough plan of what you are going to do in the assessment (short-term memory). During your assessment, you modify what you do depending on what information you receive from your patient. Once you finish your assessment, you organise the subjective and objective information you have collected and formulate a treatment plan. This whole process is similar to the decision-making process involved with every motor task.

From this example you will see that if the emphasis is on a thoughtful or cognitive process as described in the schema theory, then there is likely to be a substantial delay which would be too slow for most functional tasks; even more so when considering complex skills. For instance, a tennis forehand takes around 200 ms to perform. Experienced tennis players do not need to consciously remember what sort of response a ball travelling towards their forehand requires but react to the ball immediately because the visual system is used to responding to this particular stimulus. This function is termed 'perception–action coupling' and allows for the faster reaction times needed in many activities. This is a type of triggered reaction and is thought to be the way in which practice can produce the speed of reaction needed in many activities where the stimulus is similar but not always identical.

Response programming

This is the stage in the process where the selected response is coordinated by recruiting the appropriate muscles with the right amount of effort, in the right direction at the right time. At first consideration, this would seem to be an insurmountable task to be performed within the time limits needed for almost all skilled movements. If every stage of all our movements had to be controlled by cognitive processes, how could we possibly think of other things or be able to speak or listen at the same time?

Central programming in the motor cortex allows unconscious performance of some skills once they have been learned, allowing an individual to divert cognitive processes to other areas which might be necessary at the time.

Constant monitoring of the movement through proprioceptive *feedback* allows knowledge of performance before knowledge of results. This means that we can be aware of how the movement is progressing by utilising sensory information from muscle spindles, and joint and tendon receptors without waiting for information from visual or auditory receptors on completion of the task. The frequency and timing of the feedback, as well as the nature, can have an influence on retention of a motor skill (Anderson et al 2001).

Continued monitoring each time a motor task is performed means that an expert in a particular skill will know if that movement was successful before viewing the outcome. For example, experienced weightlifters will know whether they have made a successful clean-and-jerk attempt before the referees pass or fail the lift. They can relate the current performance to previous attempts and compare the feel of that particular movement with previous successful and unsuccessful attempts as the movement is happening rather than waiting to view the outcome. Afferent information from joints and muscles is vital for the success of this function.

Engram

Coordination of a complex activation of different muscle groups for a specific task such as weight-lifting is known as a motor programme or *engram*. As mentioned earlier, for a coordinated movement to be accomplished there must be an optimal combination of agonists, antagonists, synergists and fixators at the right force, in the right direction and with the right timing. These patterns of movements are thought to be stored as action memory traces in the motor cortex once they have been refined through feedback mechanisms (Vansant 1995).

Feed–forward

However, some motor tasks are still too fast for this type of cognitive control, which has a refractory period of approximately 200 ms. A boxer's punch has a reaction time of 90 ms (Schmidt 1991). This is well below the reaction time necessary for a cognitive response. A *feed-forward* mechanism is thought to control this type of task which relies on more of a reflex reaction, as discussed earlier in the chapter. The memory trace in the motor cortex instigates preparatory muscle stimulation in order to respond at this speed. Although this mechanism allows a faster response, the boxer does not have time to think about altering the movement once the response has been initiated. This is why a boxer has to practise each different type of punch in his repertoire until the feed-forward mechanism is developed sufficiently for each response.

Realistically, the brain would never have the capacity to store individual movement programmes for each and every functional task. Schmidt (1975) described a schema theory that helps explain this phenomenon. He defined a motor scheme as a general motor programme that would be activated for all movements that are associated with a common task.

Limitations of motor control

Having discussed how this process of motor control works, we now need to look at the limitations within the whole mechanism:

- *Capacity*: how much information the system can process at any one time. Every individual has a

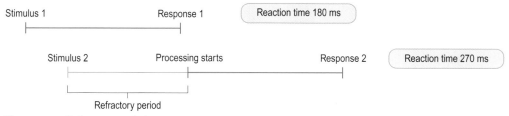

Figure 7.2   Refractory period.

limit to how much information can be coped with at once.

- *Speed*: how fast the system can process the information. This will depend on whether the individual has to deal with the information in series, i.e. one at a time if it is unfamiliar, or in parallel, i.e. at the same time if it is very familiar.
- *Distortion*: the extent to which information is lost or distorted during the process. This limitation will often depend on concentration or attention.

Refractory period

Schmidt's original information processing model assumed that all these processes happen in series, i.e. one after the other. In this form, the process would understandably involve a significant delay between stimulus and response, called the *refractory period* (Fig. 7.2). This delay would fit into the speed limitation of the control process described above.

In Figure 7.2 the top reaction shows the time taken for a response to a particular stimulus to be generated. If each stimulus were processed in series, processing of the second and subsequent stimuli would have to wait until the first response had been dealt with, hence increasing the reaction time necessary for the second and subsequent responses.

More recent thinking has led to the view that some of these processes can happen in parallel which would reduce the reaction time involved between impulse recognition and motor reaction, as in the earlier example of the rugby player. This would explain the ability of an expert to perform complicated decision-making processes, allowing motor skills to be performed more efficiently.

Dynamic systems theory

As suggested by its title, this approach attempts to explain motor control from a more mathematical point of view by observing and predicting patterns of multisegmental movement. The definition provided by Vereijken et al (1992) earlier in the chapter works on the principle of dynamic systems theory.

Some of the reasoning behind these theories is that individuals have been observed to perform specific tasks in similar ways, despite the opportunity to get to the endpoint by a variety of routes. This suggests that, for many tasks, there is likely to be an optimum way of moving that requires the least energy for that length and weight of limb as well as the sort of movement required.

A joint will have a certain number of degrees of freedom of movement. For example, a metacarpophalangeal joint will have one degree of freedom (flexion/extension), whilst the shoulder has three (flexion/extension, abduction/adduction and rotation). In addition to that, there are more muscles going over most joints than there are degrees of freedom, which gives us the choice of using different muscles to produce joint movement in a particular direction. Finally, each muscle has a number of different fibre types as well as different nerve endings that produce different qualities of muscle action and performance, such as power generators or stabilisers.

With all these parameters, we can perform a single movement in a host of different ways, yet we usually do familiar things in a similar way. For instance, a footballer will have a particular way of striking a ball that works best for him. That pattern still has to be flexible enough to accommodate slightly different circumstances but the pattern remains essentially similar for that skill. How much hip flexion compared to knee extension power is used to kick the ball will depend on the individual. Some players may include a different proportion of ankle movement or trunk rotation to put a spin on the ball or 'Bend it like Beckham'!

The more expert a person is at a skill, the more they are able, despite having well-practised movements, to utilise some of these degrees of freedom when needed so that movement can be subtly altered. This compares with the psychological models explained above, where experts can change their movements more easily in response to the environment, when the movement becomes more automatic.

Thelen (1998) described how babies learn to reach for objects depending on their initial, individual styles of early movement. The babies that tended to move quickly had to deal with trying to be more accurate to avoid missing the toy they were aiming at. On the other hand, the babies who moved more slowly were accurate but had to develop better anti-gravity control as their arms were held in the air for longer. They have to do all this with large heads, compared to the rest of the body, and narrow shoulders with weak muscles. Added to that, they have just spent 9 months floating around in an aquatic environment that didn't prepare them for dealing with the effects of gravity. The choice of which combinations of muscles and movement to use has to be made through trial and error. For instance, do they use the closest arm and abduct their shoulder or the other arm and adduct? Do they move the shoulder more and keep the elbow bent or vice versa? Do they need to have palm up or down? The list could go on forever and that is just reaching for a toy!

All the adaptations you would have tried in Task 7.2 would have required changing the degrees of freedom you used at different joints in the upper limb segments and probably in your trunk and lower limb as well. You increased the variety of movement at some joints whilst restricting the choice in others. This is called *recruitment* or suppression of biomechanical degrees of freedom (Kelso 1998).

SKILL

The term 'skill' has been mentioned frequently when discussing the process of motor learning. Before explaining how skills are learned and developed, it might help to define the word.

Skill is the accuracy, consistency and efficiency of movement deployment (Higgins 1991).

Accuracy, consistency, efficiency

In other words, the desired outcome of the motor task has to be achieved (accuracy) in a high proportion of the attempts (consistency or precision) and with the minimum amount of physical effort (efficiency). For example, beginners throwing a dart at a dart board might well hit the bull's-eye. Most people watching would put this success down to 'beginner's luck'. There would be a very slim chance of the lucky beginners reproducing their success consistently until they had learned which components of the combination of movements produced the first successful attempt.

Magill (2003) uses this sort of concept to explain the difference between accuracy and precision, using target shooters as an example. Figure 7.3

Task 7.2

Think of a task like reaching for a glass of water or throwing a ball.
How many different ways could you do this?
How would you do the same task if your shoulder movement was restricted?
How would you do the task if your elbow movement was restricted?
What alterations did the restricted movement attempts involve?

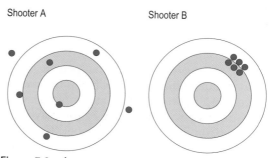

Figure 7.3   Accuracy versus precision.

illustrates the differences, where the target on the left (A) shows a widespread array of shots, some of which were over the centre, whereas the one on the right (B) shows a tight cluster but all of them a little way off the centre. Although both shooters might have achieved the same score in that particular attempt, which shooter do you think might be able to improve her scores more easily?

The answer is shooter B on the right. A simple adjustment of her sights would mean that the tight cluster she achieved could be moved over the centre of the target. This tight cluster reflects *precision*. Shooter A was equally as *accurate* as shooter B because she had the same score but not as *precise* because she could not reproduce the same performance consistently.

In addition to learning the optimal coordination of movements for a task, the beginner also has to learn the optimal amount of muscle work necessary. Usually people learning a new task will hold themselves very stiffly, only moving the limb sections absolutely necessary for the task in hand. Anyone who has ever tried out a new sport will remember the feeling of aching all over despite only needing to work certain areas for that activity. Students learning a new manual technique will have to consciously relax their shoulders as they gradually get closer to their ears and their arms begin to ache! This is known as freezing degrees of freedom (Vereijken et al 1992) and the principle was discussed earlier in the chapter. As the individual becomes more proficient, the limb and trunk segments are given a little more freedom of movement, making the functional task appear more fluid.

There are, once again, a variety of theories about how this learning process takes place. These fall into two main schools of thought; the maturation approach (Gessell et al 1974) and the perceptual cognitive approach (Bressan & Woollacott 1982).

Maturation approach

This approach describes alternating periods of stability and instability during maturation. The periods of instability are thought to be the times when new patterns of control are being learned and hence result in some instability or lack of control until the pattern becomes skilled. For example, toddlers learning to walk will make many attempts over a few months until they can control a walk without falling over. During this time the child's skill level in walking will be unpredictable, some days almost perfect and other days disastrous. Following this approach, each functional ability would develop in the same way throughout childhood, adolescence and adulthood.

Perceptual cognitive approach

The perceptual cognitive approach suggests that intellect may have a bearing on how well a motor skill is learned. Sensory input is regarded as having a significant impact on motor performance and feedback of the outcome of a particular movement. With this approach, trial and error plays an important part in the learning process. The learner consciously discards the motor patterns which produced an unsuccessful outcome and retains those that produced an outcome closer to the ideal.

Memory

Whichever approach is favoured, once a motor programme has been established, it then takes repeated practice to develop that pattern into a skilled movement. For any learning to occur, there must be a memory of that particular skill to allow repetition and refinement. This is thought to be controlled in the area of the cortex concerned with long-term memory.

Figure 7.4 illustrates a simplified version of how memory controls the learning process. First, sensory information is received via a variety of sources, as in the previous model of motor control. This might be a combination of sensory input such as kinaesthetic sensation, vision, sound, touch or pain. The relevant information is stored temporarily in the short-term memory. For something to be maintained in the short-term memory, it has to be constantly repeated, rather like remembering a telephone number from the directory when you haven't got a pen to hand. Once someone speaks to you the number is often forgotten. This is when information is lost by replacement with new sensory information which might be similar to or completely different from the previous information.

To be able to recall a telephone number, you would usually remember it in chunks of numbers

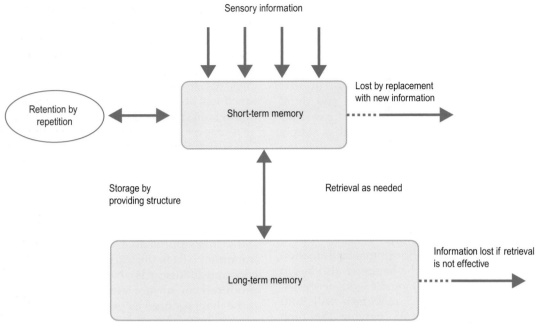

Figure 7.4 The memory process controlling learning of a new skill.

Task 7.3

Working in pairs, try two slightly different tasks.
1. The first person reads out any line from this book, letter by letter, backwards. To give the other person a chance, only use up to 20 letters.
   a. Ask them to repeat the sequence of letters (without writing them down!).
   b. Then get them to recite a nursery rhyme.
   c. Ask them to repeat the sequence of letters.
2. This time, read out the same letters forwards as complete words.
   a. Repeat the same process as above.
   b. Was the second attempt any different to the first?

---

and associate it with a particular name which allows it to be stored in the long-term memory. The first few times you need to use that number again, you still have to look it up. Eventually this number gets used frequently enough for you to remember it without looking it up. This is because you have practised retrieving the information from the long-term memory until this process becomes efficient by strengthening the memory trace of that particular skill.

Application in the rehabilitation setting

Transfer that model to a rehabilitation situation and it might explain why patients sometimes appear to retain improvement following treatment more than at other times. For example, imagine you have just spent some time trying to improve vastus medialis control in weight bearing during a gait rehabilitation session. Following repeated practice, the patient can eventually contract vastus medialis in a functional weight-bearing position. The patient is then sent home but on returning for the next treatment, appears to have forgotten everything that was taught in the previous session. This is possibly because the repetitions of the exercise were rehearsed to allow retention in the short-term memory but either not given enough structure to allow long-term memory storage or not given the practice of retrieval from long-term memory. The information then becomes lost or useless.

One way to improve this process would be to:

- explain why the exercise is being given to provide structure and assist with retention in long-term memory
- teach the particular motor skill required (vastus medialis control in standing)
- add in a new activity, possibly related to the first
- repeat the first skill/activity requiring recall of the taught skill.

Variable practice

Changing the activity will have the effect of distracting from information stored in short-term memory. This will encourage retrieval from long-term memory to facilitate retention of the new skill, which is control of knee extension in weight bearing. Repeated retention and retrieval will strengthen the memory trace. In addition to this, if the second activity performed is similar to the first, it is thought that some learning is transferred between skills, thus speeding up the learning process. This type of approach is called variable practice and there is some evidence demonstrating its efficacy (Eidson & Stadulis 1991, Lee et al 1985, Shea & Kohl 1990).

Closed and open skills

For the purposes of this chapter, skills are split into two broad categories:

- closed skills
- open skills.

Task 7.4

Think about how you would teach someone an exercise as part of a rehabilitation programme and how you could improve the skill acquisition process. Think of an example in each of the following cases:
- Improve understanding for more efficient storage in long-term memory.
- Provide better information on knowledge of performance.
- Progress to a more automatic movement.

A closed skill is movement that is repeated in the same way for each performance of the one task. Using the example of the weightlifter again, the technique for the clean and jerk will be identical for each attempt at the same weight. This skill requires a very high degree of spatial control with relatively little time limit, in comparison to something like catching a ball. To demonstrate what happens when a greater temporal (time) control is applied, imagine what happens in a competition when a lifter has to rush out to make his attempt because time is running out. It quite often fails because he has practised the movement skill many times but at the same speed. This type of skill is thus said to be performed in a *stable environment*. If any part of that environment is changed, the ability to perform that skill will be compromised. The fairly rigid sequencing that occurs in a movement such as this limits the performer to a relatively narrow choice of movements (degrees of freedom) compared to an open skill but allows very efficient performance (Browenstein 1997).

An open skill requires a combination of both spatial and temporal control. The movement has to be practised many times as in a closed skill but variation in speed and effort has to be applied to adapt to a changing environment. This time, refer back to the tackling rugby player as the example. Changes in the intended movement may have to take place depending on the actions of the opposing player and possibly the actions of players in the same team. This type of environment is said to be an *unstable environment*.

When re-educating a motor skill in a rehabilitation environment, both these principles need to be considered. To start progressing through a new skill, such as balancing on one leg following an ankle injury, a high degree of cognitive attention is required, using visual cues as well as input from mechanoreceptors in the limb. At this stage balancing can only be maintained as a closed skill and patients will usually attempt to freeze some degrees of freedom at selected joints in order to reduce the variable elements that have to be controlled for that activity. If any part of the environment changes, such as introducing an unstable base of support, balance reactions are challenged once more. Consequently patients will have to take a step onto their unaffected leg much earlier than an uninjured person, as they will have restricted themselves to a limited repertoire of balance reactions to be able to have better control. As balance improves, secondary activities are introduced. If balance has to be maintained whilst catching a ball or being pulled in one direction by elastic tubing, the balance strategies have to change with each different circumstance. Exercises such as this encourage skills learned as a conscious effort to become automatic and to adapt to a changing environment. They also encourage a gradual freeing up of the variation in degrees of freedom of movement. This same balance activity has now become an open skill in preparation for the functional mobility required of the ankle in everyday life.

Taylor et al (1998) highlight the effects of diverting attention on motor performance in their study investigating joint position error detection during concurrent cognitive distraction. Joint position sense was reduced in subjects who received an auditory distraction whilst performing the task. The authors point out that this can have a positive or negative effect depending on the timing of the distraction. For someone concentrating on mastering a very new task, distraction could reduce the safety of the activity. Conversely, appropriate distraction as a progression in later stages would supplement a rehabilitation programme.

Both types of skill need a significant amount of repetition to allow efficient retrieval from long-term memory and the development of a motor engram. For example:

- learning to walk (to age 6) – 3 million steps
- parade ground marching (end of army basic training) – 0.8 million steps
- hand knitting – 1.5 million stitches
- violin playing to a professional level – 2.5 million notes (4500 hours of practice)
- baseball throwing (pitcher) – 1.6 million throws
- basketball shot from any angle – 1 million throws (Kottke et al 1978).

Skill acquisition

Bressan and Woollacott (1982) describe a model of the stages of skill acquisition (Fig. 7.5).

Skill construction

The first stage involves organisation of the skill when an approximate estimation of the movement is constructed which will vary depending on prior experience of similar activity. Similar movement patterns used in other motor tasks can be transferred to the new skill and adapted as appropriate. For example, good basketball players could transfer their ball-handling skills to other sports, such as rugby. This would be called *positive transfer*. In this instance hand–eye coordination, wide visual field and manual dexterity skills would be similar enough in both to allow modification between the two activities.

However, a squash player would have problems on initially trying to play tennis as, despite the good hand–eye coordination, the racquet action required in squash has a detrimental effect on the technique used in tennis. This is called *negative transfer*.

The learner will need to devote a relatively high level of cognitive attention to the task to appreciate an overall picture of the required movement task. This would explain why a learner cannot always

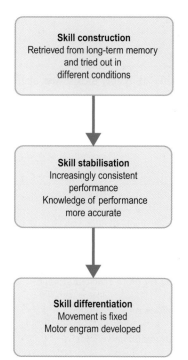

Figure 7.5 A model of the stages of skill acquisition (reprinted from Bressan & Woollacott 1982, p. 170, with permission from Elsevier).

Skill construction
Retrieved from long-term memory and tried out in different conditions

Skill stabilisation
Increasingly consistent performance
Knowledge of performance more accurate

Skill differentiation
Movement is fixed
Motor engram developed

listen to a teacher or coach at the same time as attempting to perform the new skill being taught. Watching a child learning to write illustrates this point quite well.

Skill stabilisation

As learning continues and the skill begins to stabilise, successful attempts will become more frequent and movement patterns will become more consistent. Feedback providing knowledge of results is important at this stage to correct minor faults as the motor engram is becoming established which will be difficult to change once the movement becomes automatic. In support of this, Prapavessis and McNair (1999) found that subjects who received verbal instruction and correction improved subsequent attempts at a jumping and landing task more quickly than those who used their own sensory feedback from each attempt. Hewett et al (1996) had similar findings where subjects taken through a programme designed to improve neuromuscular control in addition to strength in the lower limb were able to reduce landing forces on the knee more efficiently than those who progressed through a strengthening programme alone.

A typical example of this would be someone progressing through a gait re-education rehabilitation following a lower limb fracture being encouraged to continue using a stick or crutches after the fracture has healed enough to bear weight. This is not just a safety aspect but it prevents an abnormal gait pattern becoming automatic, making progression to a more normal gait easier once the appropriate joint range and muscle strength have been achieved. Feedback on correct gait patterns can then be reinforced before full weight bearing is encouraged.

Skill differentiation

By the final stage the movement pattern has been established. Knowledge of performance is now being monitored and the proprioceptive feedback is routinely being filtered out from conscious awareness unless there is any significant change. This change in allocation of attention means that more can be devoted to higher processes, within the individual's capacity, during the task. Think

back to the earlier example of the experienced rugby player who is able to time the tackle more appropriately and also be more aware of tactical considerations. This ability has become possible because the actual movement skill has become automatic, freeing up more attention for anticipation or communication with team mates.

Think back to Task 7.1 about driving a car. Once you have learned to drive, you can probably listen to music, talk to a passenger, read road signs and be aware of other traffic and pedestrians whilst performing the task of driving automatically. What happens if you suddenly have to drive in another country on the other side of the road? What sort of things do you do to be able to perform the task? Suddenly the task changes and cannot be dealt with automatically. The sorts of things you might do would be to turn the music off, stop talking and ask people to look for road signs and landmarks. You have thus reduced some of the sensory input and additional cognitive tasks being performed at the same time in order to make more capacity for a motor task that now requires cognitive attention rather than being automatic.

Any change in sensory input involved with a learned stabilised skill will have a similar effect. Injury is no exception to this. For instance, if a joint has less range of movement after an injury, the kinaesthetic input from joint and muscle proprioceptors will be different. The cognitive process of relearning a motor skill, whether it be walking, running or climbing stairs, will need to be repeated, albeit with some prior experience for comparison, until the task becomes automatic again.

CONCLUSION

Motor learning requires a combination of factors to be successful. This chapter has outlined many of the principles involved but the reader is

Task 7.5
Think of ways in which the experience of some pain or discomfort following injury would affect the control process in a functional movement that had been automatic prior to injury.

directed to some of the texts solely devoted to this subject, listed in the reference section, for more in-depth information. The main factors to consider in the field of motor learning are short- and long-term memory, transfer of skills, modifying degrees of freedom of a movement, knowledge of both performance and results and, finally, practice. How we use these principles in the clinical setting will have a significant impact on the success of a rehabilitation programme, whether the ultimate goal is to walk unaided, transfer from bed to chair or return to a highly skilled activity.

You should now have an understanding about how an individual controls movement for both simpler repetitive movements and more complex skilled tasks. You should understand how these skills are learned and how the learning environment can be manipulated to facilitate this process.

REFERENCES

Anderson DI, Magill RA, Sekiya H 2001 Motor learning as a function of KR schedule and characteristics of task-intrinsic feedback. Journal of Motor Behaviour 33(1): 59–66

Bernstein NA 1967 The coordination and regulation of movements. Pergamon Press, New York

Bressan ES, Woollacott MH 1982 A prescriptive paradigm for sequencing instruction in physical education. Human Movement Science 1: 155–175

Browenstein B 1997 In: Browenstein B, Shaw B (eds) Functional movement in orthopaedic and sports physical therapy: evaluation, treatment and outcomes. Churchill Livingstone, Edinburgh

Eidson TA, Stadulis RE 1991 Effects of variability of practice on the transfer and performance of open and closed motor skills. Adapted Physical Activity Quarterly 8(4): 342–356

Gessell A, Ilg FL, Ames LB 1974 Infant and child in the culture of today. Harper and Row, New York

Hewett TE, Stroupe AL, Nance TA, Noyes FR 1996 Plyometric training in female athletes. Decreased impact forces and increased hamstring torques. American Journal of Sports Medicine 24(6): 765–773

Higgins S 1991 Motor control acquisition. Physical Therapy 71(2): 123–129

Kelso JAS 1998 Coordination dynamics. In: Latash ML (ed) Progress in motor control, vol 1. Human Kinetics, Leeds

Kottke FJ, Halpern D, Easton JKM, Ozel AT, Burrill CA 1978 The training of coordination. Archives of Physical Medicine and Rehabilitation 59: 567–572

Latash ML 1998 Progress in motor control, vol. 1. Human Kinetics, Leeds

Lee TD, Magill RA, Weeks DJ 1985 Influence of practice schedule on testing schema theory predictions in adults. Journal of Motor Behaviour 17(3): 283–299

Magill RA 2003 Motor learning: concepts and applications. McGraw-Hill, Columbus, Ohio

Prapavessis H, McNair PJ 1999 Effects of instruction in jumping technique and experience jumping on ground reaction forces. Journal of Orthopaedic and Sports Physical Therapy 29: 352–356

Schmidt RA 1975 A schema theory of discrete motor skill learning. Psychological Review 82: 225–260

Schmidt RA 1988 Motor control and learning. A behavioural emphasis, 2nd edn. Human Kinetics, Champaign, Illinois

Schmidt RA 1991 Motor learning and performance. Human Kinetics, Champaign, Illinois

Schmidt RA, Lee TL 1999 Motor control and learning, 3rd edn. Human Kinetics, Champaign, Illinois

Shea CH, Kohl RM 1990 Specificity and variability of practice. Research Quarterly for Exercise and Sport 61(12): 169–177

Sherrington CS 1906 On the proprioceptive system, particularly in its reflect aspects. Brain 29: 467–482

Taylor RA, Marshall PH, Dunlap RD, Gable CD, Sizer PS 1998 Knee position error detection in closed and open kinetic chain tasks during concurrent cognitive distraction. Journal of Orthopaedic and Sports Physical Therapy 28(2): 81–87

Thelen E 1998 How infants learn to reach. In: Latash ML (ed) Progress in motor control, vol 1. Human Kinetics, Leeds

Vansant A 1995 Motor control and motor learning. In: Cech D, Martin S (eds) Functional movement development across the lifespan. WB Saunders, Philadelphia

Vereijken B, van Emmerik RE, Whiting HTA, Newell KM 1992 Free(z)ing degrees of freedom in skill acquisition. Journal of Motor Behaviour 24(1): 133–142

Winstein CJ 1991 Knowledge of results in motor learning: implications for physiotherapy. Physical Therapy 71(2): 140–149

Chapter **8**

Measuring and analysing human movement

Tony Everett

LEARNING OUTCOMES

When you have completed this chapter you should
be able to:

1. Understand why the measurement of human
   movement is difficult

2. Discuss the range of measurement techniques
   available

3. Choose the appropriate tool for analysing and
   measuring movement

4. Evaluate the different measurement techniques.

INTRODUCTION

When considering human movement, it is
immediately evident that each movement performed is complex. This complexity involves not
just the degree and sequence of joint motion or the
amount and type of muscle work but a host of
other parameters as well. Some of these include
initiation, control and stopping; voluntary or
involuntary components; intentional or non-
intentional movement; speed; direction; balance
and equilibrium; patterned or isolated. There are
also other dimensions to movement such as the
social context, the environment and the health
status of the mover. Some of these are considered
within this book and some are not.

It is relatively straightforward to measure some of the physical aspects of movement such as joint range or muscle strength in a non-functional context but difficulty arises when quality of movement must also be considered. Some aspects of quality and health status are considered in the next chapter but on the whole there is no consensus as to what constitutes quality of movement. The task of measuring and analysing movement therefore seems very daunting. Until there is consensus on what constitutes movement and what its components are, absolute measurement and analysis will be difficult.

Throughout this book there have been attempts to define aspects and components of human movement and the increasing sophistication of technology means that progress in analysis is being made. This chapter will explore methods of measuring some of the components of movement and suggest ways in which movement can be analysed.

Task 8.1

Working in small groups, share your ideas of what you think movement is. What are the areas of life in which movement is involved?

Working in your small groups, choose an activity, walking or throwing a ball for example, and discuss the parameters you would have to consider to enable you to describe this activity.

ANALYSIS OF MOVEMENT

The method of analysing movement will depend on the purpose for which the analysis is taking place. A judgement will have to be made as to the required accuracy, validity and reliability of the result obtained. Will the results be used to determine what normal movement is, to establish deviations due to pathologies, to measure the outcome of interventions, as a research tool or to inform the patient? Each of these will require subtly different uses of the results as well as possibly different methods to obtain the outcomes.

In your discussion in Task 8.1 of what we mean by movement, you may have included topics like mobility, function, occupation, communication and leisure. I am sure that you have come up with a lot more. This shows the complexity of human movement and you can begin to appreciate the difficulty in analysing it. In the second question you might have come up with a list which probably included muscle activity, strength and endurance, joint range, balance and posture, coordination and a goal. How you discussed the quality of movement would be interesting!

Despite all the difficulties, we still need to try to analyse movement with the most accurate results. Movement analysis may be defined as the subjective and objective measurement of:

- the activity
- its components
- goals obtained.

METHODS OF ANALYSIS

There are a variety of methods that can be used to analyse movement or to measure the components of the movement. Measuring these components will be considered later in this chapter, although it is difficult to separate the analysis of movement from the measurement of its components.

The methods of analysis can be split into two broad categories:

- observational
- mechanical/instrumental.

Observational analysis

Observational analysis is what most therapists, ergonomists or coaches have at their disposal.

As you will see from Task 8.2, describing an observed movement is very difficult. After the movement has been performed several times then you can begin to see trends occurring. The problem is that the more the subject repeats the

---

Task 8.2

Using the parameters that you have listed from Task 8.1 and those suggested in the text, try and describe the activity being performed by one of the group.

---

movement, the more tired they will become so the initial movement may change. This will make analysis very difficult. A method of limiting this problem could be the use of video recording. Video recording reproduces the movement but it becomes two-dimensional and this in itself will cause difficulties. Video recording will be discussed later.

To enable us to optimise the use of visual analysis it is important to develop a framework on which to build the analysis. A suggested framework could be:

- the starting position
- the movement
- the finishing position.

The starting position

The starting position can be defined as a position of readiness from which the movement can take place. It can be used as:

- a foundation for the activity
- a point of fixation for one part of the body
- a training for posture and balance.

There are four functional *fundamental starting positions*. These are:

- lying
- kneeling
- sitting
- standing.

All other starting positions are termed *derived starting positions*. Analysis of the starting position can take place by considering the following criteria:

- Joint position – position in degrees (visual estimation)
- Muscle work – name the muscle, type of work (static usually) and range (inner, outer or middle).

The movement

This is analysed sequentially in time and order:

1. Segment movement
   a. type of movement
   b. plane in which the movement takes place
   c. axis around which the movement takes place

2. Joint action
   a. type (flexion, extension, etc.)
   b. approximate range (in degrees)
   c. sequence
3. Muscle work
   a. function
   b. range (inner, middle or outer)
   c. type (concentric, eccentric or static)
   d. sequence.

The finishing position

- Return to the original position
- Beginning of a new phase
- Starting position for a new movement
- A position of rest.

Using something like the above list allows us to get some order into our movement analysis and we can optimise our success by repetition, breaking down the components and being systematic.

Mechanical analysis

Use of film for analysis of movement

Whilst experienced observers can obtain a substantial amount of subjective information about human movement, they do not have the ability to observe and remember all the complex, multijoint movement patterns that occur in even the simplest functional activities. The unassisted eye functions at the equivalent of 1/30th of a second exposure time and can only see details of slow motion; the brain, too, despite its amazing ability, has a limit on the amount of information it can absorb and remember. As a consequence, when observing complex movement only a limited amount of the detail is actually seen (Terauds 1984). The other major drawback to unaided visual observation is that only subjective information can be obtained and without baseline data, reliable measurement of change is impossible.

Task 8.3

Working in your small groups and using the same activity that you have previously discussed, use the suggested list to describe the activity.

Film has been used to enhance understanding of human movement for more than a hundred years. Cine, video and still photography are all valuable as they all enable movement to be observed in much more detail than is possible on unaided visual analysis; they also permit measurement and provide a permanent record. Whilst cine is the most accurate of these methods, it is expensive and difficult to use and the process of developing films is time-consuming. Still photography is limited by the fact that it only captures one instant in time and the totality of movement cannot be seen. Video is cheap, easy to use and very portable and the results are immediately available. These advantages outweigh the limitations of only being able to sample data 50 or 60 times a second and it is now used in preference to all other methods.

Cine film and video tape can be stored over many years and replayed repeatedly. This is particularly valuable as it allows the analysis of movement after the patient or subject has left, when there is time for uninterrupted observation and analysis. Visual analysis of film is enhanced by the use of freeze-frame, slow motion facilities and computer-aided analysis software. Video and cine film of human movement enhance the acquisition of qualitative information and quantitative data and can also be used as feedback to the patient or athlete.

The qualitative and quantitative use of film   A vast amount of qualitative information can be obtained from film. Human movement as a total pattern can be observed and reobserved. The relationship of all body parts to each other can be seen, as can the quality of the movement – whether it is fast or slow, uncoordinated or smooth. The patient can be shown the film as part of the rehabilitation process and this greatly facilitates understanding of movement difficulties. Patients who have seen their own films are frequently able to formulate their own recovery objectives and monitor their own progress. Though there is no research in this area, it is likely that this greatly improves compliance and as such is a tool that ought to be used frequently. Finally, the film can be kept and used for subjective comparison with films taken at a later date, enabling judgements to be made about progression or deterioration.

Quantitative data can be obtained by digitising the video image and subjecting the data to computer processing and analysis. Digitisation is the process whereby the image or parts of the image are converted to digital form so that the data can be manipulated by a computer. In order to be able to digitise film, skin markers must be placed over major landmarks prior to filming. The film is then either manually or automatically digitised. This process involves viewing each frame (or field) of the video tape and identifying and storing the coordinates for each of the skin markers, in each of the frames of the film. The data thus obtained can be called upon when calculations are required. The process of digitising can be undertaken either manually or by use of a computer program. Direct measurements of an image taken from the video screen are subject to considerable error and should not be used as a method of quantifying human movement.

Computer-aided analysis of video tape can give a wide range of information and most systems now allow the analysis of movement in more than one plane. The computer analysis software makes it possible to plot body coordinates (centre of gravity, etc.). Knowledge of the position of the centre of gravity is important when considering the efficiency of movement. For example, smooth displacements of the centre of gravity tend to indicate a more efficient movement than those where the centre of gravity is subjected to extensive vertical displacement. Figure 10.4 in Chapter 10 illustrates the displacement of the centre of gravity and the original information that enabled this figure to be drawn was taken from computer analysis of video tape. The computer can also generate stick diagrams and these are valuable as an initial qualitative analysis of the sequence of movement. A stick diagram of a jump is shown in Figure 8.1.

Data on joint angles in one or more planes of movement can be collected and the pattern of movement at a joint can be graphically represented and related to other joints or the whole body. Joint angle data are available for any instance in the movement sequence.

The velocity and acceleration of limb segments can be measured and the data give useful information about patterns of movement, for example when comparing the acceleration of the tibia in the

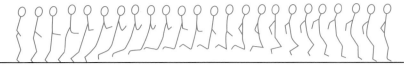

Figure 8.1   A stick diagram of a jump. This was generated from data obtained by digitising a video film and gives an overall, subjective impression of the movement.

swing phase of normal gait with the acceleration of the shank of an artificial limb in amputee gait.

Using video tape, it is also possible to calculate cadence, stride length and velocity in gait but to do this it is necessary to provide some form of scaling in the filming area (Whittle 1991). Filming with video is a relatively simple and cheap technique that can be undertaken almost anywhere and, because it does not require measuring equipment to be attached to the subject, it does not disrupt the movement being analysed. (Whether there is a psychological effect on movement patterns brought about by the self-consciousness of being filmed is not known but this should not be discounted.)

The value of film as a movement analysis tool has long been recognised by sport scientists but the health-care professions appear to have been less enthusiastic about its use. Film has been used to analyse human movement in a limited range of activities, for example the ability of paraplegic subjects to reach from their wheelchairs (Curtis et al 1995); the measurement of angular velocity of the leg in a patient with cerebral palsy (Winter 1982); the biomechanical analysis of swing-through gait (Noreau et al 1995); and the energy transfers of children walking with crutches (McGill & Dainty 1984).

For meaningful data collection, great care must be taken in setting up the filming site and arranging the camera. For accurate spatial and temporal measurements, the camera must be positioned carefully in relation to the subject and timing and scale devices must be included in the field of view.

Computerised kinetic analysis system   Systems are now being developed that enable valid and reliable data from movement analysis to be collected and analysed. These systems can collect three-dimensional movement data from many

Case Study 8.1

Mrs Wilson, 59, had had rheumatoid arthritis for approximately 20 years when she suddenly noticed an increased clumsiness when undertaking functional activities using her hands. She had learned to cope with limited movement and pain at both shoulder and elbow joints and severe ulnar deviation of her metacarpophalangeal joints. For many years she had managed most activities of daily living despite her substantial problems but now she found she was knocking over items as she went to pick them up and her accuracy at putting down objects like cups or a vase of flowers was seriously compromised. She reported that she had noted no change or deterioration in her physical condition so it was decided to evaluate the total upper limb joint movement patterns by use of video. When viewed in slow motion the tape revealed an inability to fully extend the joints of her index finger beyond the resting position. As she performed grip activities, the index finger became caught on the object she wished to pick up and, because of the lack of extension, she was unable to let go of objects at the end of a task. A physical examination subsequently showed total rupture of the extensor indices tendon.

joints and body segments simultaneously. The systems use high-resolution cameras which capture infrared light reflected from markers placed at predefined points on the subject. Strobe lights are situated around the cameras and as the subject moves, the reflected light is captured by the cameras. The data are then digitised and processed through specifically designed software and displayed as movement diagrams and as calibrated data. Such systems are very sophisticated but therefore expensive and usually only available in specialised centres.

The difficulties in obtaining quantitative data when analysing movement have been discussed.

Collecting data on the individual parameters is easier and thus more technically advanced. It must be remembered, however, that many of these measurements are taken when the parameter is isolated and not within the functional activity.

Measuring joint range

Hand–held goniometers

Traditionally, joint motion has been investigated by measuring the maximum range of movement available at individual joints. This is a static measurement of the end-of-range position and a hand-held goniometer is used for the purpose. These simple goniometers have to be aligned over the joint axis and this introduces a potential source of error if the instantaneous centre of rotation changes throughout the movement or if the goniometer becomes misaligned. Nevertheless, the reliability and validity of hand-held goniometers have been shown to be fairly good (Gajdosik & Bohannon 1987) although their usefulness is limited by the fact that they can only record static position and therefore have little value in the description of continuous or functional movement. Despite being used as objective measures for testing the efficacy of therapeutic intervention, they give no indication of the functional range of joint movement.

Normally, static goniometric measurements are taken with the joint in a non-weight bearing position that allows full range of active or passive movement to be measured. However, very few functional activities of the lower limb are performed in a non-weight bearing position and few upper limb functions are performed without the limb holding a weight, so the results obtained are not an accurate reflection of the subject's capabilities in a functional activity.

Electrogoniometers

Electrogoniometers have opened up the possibility of measuring joint movement during a functional activity. The electrogoniometer, which was introduced by Karpovitch in the 1950s, can take a number of forms (Rothstein 1985). At its most simple, it can consist of two endblocks joined by an electronic potentiometer which is encased within a protective spring. More sophisticated devices may use up to three potentiometers for each joint, thus allowing simultaneous measurement of movement in three planes.

Two different types of goniometer are shown in Figure 8.2. In both cases the way in which they are designed allows measurement to take place regardless of whether the centre of rotation of the goniometer coincides with the centre of rotation of the joint. Figure 8.3 illustrates how this is possible. With these types of electrogoniometers, movement of a joint will result in movement of the potentiometer and the resultant strain on the potentiometer generates electrical signals, i.e. the resistance in the potentiometer is changed. These signals, in the form of voltage and, less commonly, current, are plotted and, after calibration, represent the angular displacement of the joint. Only angular displacements are measured. Linear movements that result in telescoping of the potentiometer do not produce strain and consequently no voltage is recorded. The joint displacement curves for the hip, knee and ankle joint which are shown in Chapter 10 were taken from data obtained from an electrogoniometer (see Fig. 10.6).

Electrogoniometers are lightweight and do not interfere to any great extent with the activity being tested. Only a small force is needed to distort the potentiometer, making the instrument very sensitive. Error associated with the use of electrogoniometers comes mainly from the means by which they are fixed to the subject and the method by which data are relayed to the computer for analysis. Fixation has proved to be a problem over many years as human limbs are normally conical in shape and, unless the goniometer is stuck directly to the skin, it is in danger of sliding down or round the limb during movement. When straps or bands are used to hold the goniometer onto the limb, they normally need to be so tightly fastened that they are uncomfortable and restrict movement. Using adhesive tape to affix the electrogoniometer directly to the skin is a more satisfactory means, although skin movement over the joint may present a problem. Reliability of results using this method of fixation is reasonably good (Troke et al 1998).

Some electrogoniometers relay the joint positional data to the computer via leads and subjects can find this both offputting and restrictive, especially

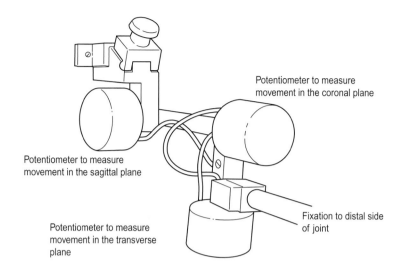

Figure 8.2   Two different types of electrogoniometers.

Potentiometer to measure
movement in the coronal plane

Potentiometer to measure
movement in the sagittal plane

Potentiometer to measure
movement in the transverse
plane

Fixation to distal side
of joint

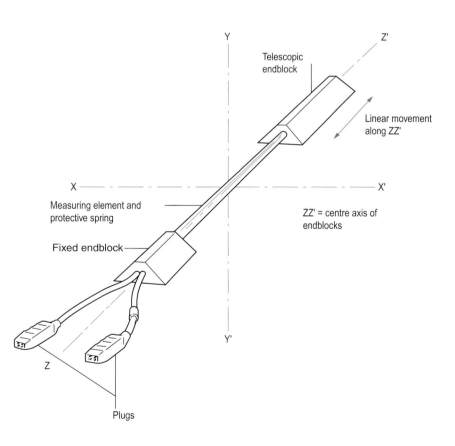

Y

Z'

Telescopic
endblock

Linear movement
along ZZ'

X

X'

Measuring element and
protective spring

ZZ' = centre axis of
endblocks

Fixed endblock

Y'

Z

Plugs

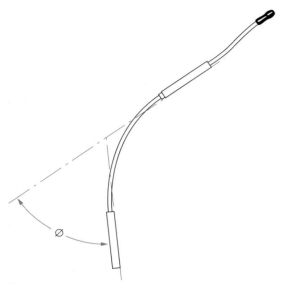

Figure 8.3 This electrogoniometer does not need to be aligned over the axis of the joint. Movement of one endblock in relation to the other enables calculation of the position of the joint.

on fast movements or when they are covering a substantial distance. The swinging of the leads may also introduce movement artefacts, resulting in the normal data becoming distorted by false signals caused by the movement. Telemetry is one solution to the problem of movement artefact; in this case the electrical signal caused by the joint movement is relayed to a storage device some distance from the subject (Whittle 1991). Alternatively, some electrogoniometers have a small data logger which can be placed somewhere convenient, like the subject's waistband. The data logger records data during the activity and this information can later be downloaded onto a computer and the results analysed at the researcher's convenience.

Many researchers have demonstrated the reliability of electrogoniometers (Rowe et al 1989, Troke et al 1998). Rome and Cowieson (1996) investigated the reliability of electrogoniometers when measuring the full range of movement at the ankle joint and found that there was no significant difference in the results obtained on separate days, thus suggesting that the goniometer was highly reliable. Myles et al (1995) found the

hysteresis effect to be 3.6° with a residual error of 2.9° for repeated measurements of large ranges. Smaller joint ranges, however, showed discrepancy only in the order of 1° for hip and knee flexion during walking. Hazelwood et al (1995) tested the construct validity of the electrogoniometer and found the measures to be highly repeatable with little variation. All these errors can be kept to a minimum if the operational definition is implemented with care. Whilst the intra- and inter-tester reliability are reasonably good, the accuracy of measurement of electrogoniometers is still questionable, with different systems giving significantly different results when measuring the same subject.

Electrogoniometers have been found to be valid, reliable and easy to use. They help to measure joint ranges during activity and, therefore, represent a good picture of the functional capabilities of that joint. Although electrogoniometers are mostly used within the field of research, it is hoped that the costs will decrease, bringing them within the price range of clinical therapists and sport scientists.

Optoelectronic devices and polarised light goniometers

These devices use the radiation of light in the measurement of movement. Light is either reflected from or transmitted from markers placed on the subject's skin. These devices come in several forms and tend to be costly but can produce detailed and highly accurate information relating to the movement of segments of the human body. Opto-electronic devices are based on the same principle as cine and video in that they require markers to be placed on the body; the coordinates of the markers are tracked throughout the movement and calculations can then be made. Unlike cine and video, the systems do not give a visual image of the subject but simply a frame-by-frame representation of the position and change in position of each marker. From this it is normally possible to produce computer-generated stick figures or graphs of the position of a joint showing range plotted against time. This gives good quantitative information but does not address the issue of quality of movement as there is no visual representation of the actual subject. The markers can either be active or passive.

Systems using passive markers rely on reflective markers placed on the subject's skin. Some form of light, often infrared, is transmitted towards the subject and the rays are reflected back off the markers to a series of 'cameras' that record the marker position. Sufficient 'cameras' need to be placed around the subject so that each marker is visible to a minimum of two 'cameras'. Sampling frequency is normally 50 Hz which enables the system to track the change in position of the markers and produce a reasonable record of the gross pattern of movement. The markers have no identity, leaving the system vulnerable if crossover of markers occurs. This is commonly seen when, for example, the marker on the wrist crosses the marker on the greater trochanter during the stance phase of gait. The accuracy of the system relies on human input to ensure that the computer accurately identifies which is the wrist marker and which is the marker on the greater trochanter or it is dependent on a good-quality computer program that is able to correctly process the incoming data.

The more expensive systems use active skin markers each of which has its own small power pack that enables it to actively transmit infrared rays to a receiving system of several 'cameras'. Because each marker has its own transmitting signal, the receiver not only picks up the position and displacement of the marker but can identify which marker it has picked up. This gives the advantage of differentiating between markers and removes the potential source of error that can occur when two markers cross over each other.

For both the active and passive systems, it is necessary to identify a ground reference point before measurement takes place. This enables the computer to calculate the absolute and relative positions of the markers in three dimensions.

If only one marker is placed on a segment of the body, the system can measure and record displacement of that segment in three dimensions, giving the segment's absolute and relative position. The application of two markers enables the system to calculate the distance between them relative to time and this enables calculations of velocity and acceleration. If the two markers are placed to represent the two ends of a long bone then the computer can calculate the displacement of that bone relative to the floor or another reference point. With three or more markers, the angles at joints can be measured as well as the accelerations and velocities of limb segments.

Measuring the force generated by muscles

At this point it would be worth referring back to Chapter 6 and reading the discussion on muscle strength, force and torque.

Manual testing

Many therapists and coaches test muscle strength manually. This will give a crude and subjective description of the force that can be generated by the muscle. Manual muscle testing can be carried out on an individual muscle or a group of muscles. The therapist or coach has to resist the action of the muscle being tested throughout its range (isotonic or concentric strength) or in a fixed position (isometric strength). The result obtained is purely subjective on behalf of the tester and this places obvious limitations on the usefulness of this measure. If the muscle or muscle group is bilateral then the tester can test it against the other side. This is more useful as there is a baseline to test against although the result is still fairly subjective and not so useful if there is a bilateral problem!

Mechanical testing

Use of free weights　As was discussed in Chapter 6, finding the 1 repetition maximum (1 RM) by calculating the maximum weight that can be lifted for one repetition only is a useful quantitative measure. It gives an objective measurement and involves the use of equipment that is readily available within most departments or sporting areas. The drawback is that it takes a long time to elicit the measurement as it has to be done by trial and error. This has implications for inducing fatigue in the patient, safety issues and time constraints. Once obtained, it gives an objective baseline of muscle strength that can be used in rehabilitation or in a sporting context.

Isokinetic dynamometry　There are no direct methods of measuring the work undertaken or force generated by individual muscles during functional movements, though there are mathematical

Case Study 8.2

Mr G, a keen motorcyclist, was struck from the side by a car which joined a main road without stopping. Apart from the injuries received as a consequence of the impact, Mr G was then run over by an oncoming bus. He suffered multiple fractures and avulsion of soft tissue but despite his injuries made a remarkable recovery.

During his rehabilitation, force traces taken from a Kistler force plate showed considerable variation from the ground reaction forces that would normally be expected in walking (a normal trace taken from a force plate is shown later in the chapter, see Fig. 8.5). His trace indicated a marked reduction in initial foot-to-floor contact force and also in the force that should have been generated on push-off. Mr G was reluctant to approach heel strike at normal velocity because the forces generated caused him considerable pain at the tibial fracture sites. He also experienced difficulty in generating force at push-off because of tissue damage to the plantarflexor muscles.

approaches which can be employed to provide data on the net muscle moment at a joint (Winter 1990). Isokinetic dynamometers can record the variation in muscle torque throughout a range of joint movement and this is a major advance on manual assessment of force or hand-held dynamometry.

Unfortunately, isokinetic dynamometers are large machines and in order for measurements to take place, the subject has to be attached to the machine; clearly this is not going to permit the measurement of muscle torque in functional activity. The isokinetic dynamometer requires the subject to be seated, with the axis of the joint to be tested aligned with the axis of the machine. The limb must be strapped tightly to the dynamometer chair to ensure that misalignment of these two axes does not occur and movement can only occur through the range permitted by the fixation.

Modern isokinetic dynamometers are able to measure muscular torque, work, power, the rate of torque production (explosiveness) and endurance in movements that involve the muscle concentrically and eccentrically. The force generated in isometric muscle activity can also be measured.

Information gained from the static testing position is then used to extrapolate to the moving human being.

Peak torque   This is measured in newton.metres (N.m) and represents the highest torque output achieved by a muscle as it moves its joint through range of motion. It would appear to be an accurate and reproducible measure and the most commonly collected data using the isokinetic dynamometer (Kannus 1994).

The peak torque generated by a muscle varies according to the velocity of the movement and this is known as the torque–velocity relationship. It is greatest at the lower velocities and declines as the velocity increases.

Angle to peak torque   Kannus (1994) suggests that with increasing angular velocity, the point at which peak torque is achieved occurs later in the range. In normal muscle there is an optimum part of the range when muscles are able to generate maximum force (mid-range). It is speculated that on the faster angular velocities, the muscle may not have recruited all possible fibres by mid-range and the angle to peak torque may be changed. If peak torque is to be considered at different velocities then angle to peak torque should also be taken into consideration.

Angle-specific torque   Torque can be measured anywhere within the range of movement and this is called angle-specific torque. When angle-specific torque is measured in inner or outer range, the accuracy of the measurement decreases and may fall below an acceptable level, making results inconsistent (Kannus 1994).

Figure 8.4 shows the traces taken from a normal subject who was measured during concentric contractions of the shoulder joint abductors and adductors. The traces clearly indicate that peak torque for both abduction and adduction was achieved towards the early part of the measured range. As the torque recordings do not start until the preset velocity has been achieved, the actual joint and muscle range is greater than that shown on the traces.

Work and power measurements   These can be obtained from the isokinetic dynamometer. In isokinetics, work is defined as the area under the

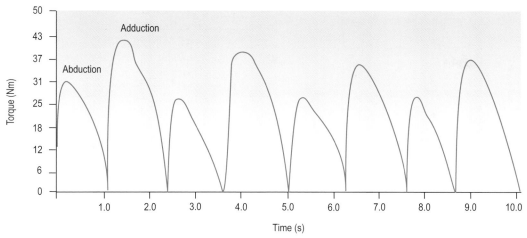

Figure 8.4 Torque curves of repeated concentric activity of the shoulder abductor and adductor muscles. Data were obtained using an isokinetic dynamometer.

torque curve where the torque curve is torque against angular displacement (work is torque ∞ angular displacement). Work is measured in joules. Power is the rate of muscular work and increases with angular velocity. Average power is total work for a given contraction divided by the time taken and is measured in joules per second or watts.

It is also possible to measure peak torque acceleration energy, which is the greatest amount of work performed in the first 125 ms of a contraction. It is measured in joules and it is suggested that this measurement is indicative of explosive ability as it gives the rate of torque production. There is some doubt about the reliability of these data and their repeatability, especially at low speeds (Kannus 1994).

Endurance indices can be defined as the ability of muscle to perform repeated contractions against a load. An endurance index is supposed to indicate the rate of fatigue. There appears to be no agreement as to the best way to test for endurance, though most tests work on a reduction from peak torque over a specified period of time. Isokinetic dynamometers can provide this information.

The isokinetic dynamometer as a measure of human function   The isokinetic dynamometer is a popular tool because it provides information about muscle groups which may be functioning isometrically,

isotonically and isokinetically. It is the only device that makes concentric and eccentric measurements possible. Unfortunately, the data obtained do not relate to human function because they have been collected from a single joint/single muscle group activity. Extrapolating from isokinetic dynamometry data to function must therefore be viewed with caution.

FORCE AND PRESSURE MEASUREMENTS

Ground reaction forces

It is possible to measure reaction forces between the human being and the supporting surface in a number of functional activities. Chapter 3 introduced the mechanics that underpin this method of measurement. This technique is most commonly seen in the evaluation of activities such as locomotion, getting out of a chair and postural sway in standing.

There are a number of different ways in which ground reaction forces can be measured; the most complex methods measure vertical forces and shear forces in the horizontal plane. In the horizontal plane they measure forces both in an anterior/posterior direction and also in a medial/lateral direction. From these three forces it is possible to calculate a single point about which

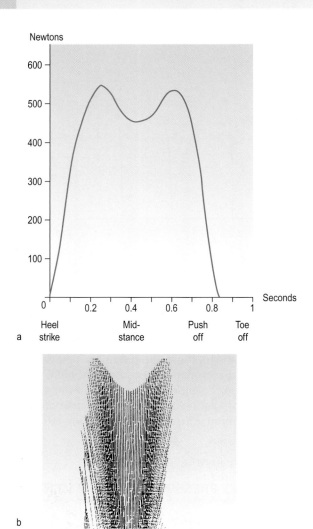

Figure 8.5   Normal force traces taken from the stance phase of walking: (a) a force curve; (b) a vector diagram.

Task 8.4

In Figure 8.6, the effects of abnormal gait are illustrated. Work out how the normal gait pattern has been changed in order to produce the two force traces. What might be the possible causes of these two changes in gait pattern?

detailed examination of a force trace (Fig. 8.6). The advantage of using a force plate is that the data obtained enable quantification of change over time. Force plates are, however, very expensive and their use as a clinical tool is likely to remain limited.

Pure pressure measurements

These can be made via pressure plates or in-shoe devices. In both cases pressure sensors are distributed across the whole load-bearing surface of the measuring device. This enables measurements of pressure to be made over the whole of the area that is in contact with the device. Figure 8.7 shows a printout from a Musgrave footprint pressure plate. The printout is colour coded to indicate different levels of pressure and the load during any part of the stance phase can be obtained.

Pressure plates take a variety of forms and different models are available to measure foot pressures and the pressures in sitting and lying. Floor-mounted pressure plates provide information about standing and the different forms of locomotion but they are restrictive in that they may have to be set into the floor or into a walkway and are normally directly linked to a computer. Pressure distribution in sitting and lying has proved useful in the design and evaluation of beds and chairs and has also provided an insight into how pathologies can alter the distribution of pressure.

If a device is placed inside a shoe, the foot–shoe interface pressures can be measured and these provide information on pressure distribution across the foot in all functional situations (see Fig. 8.8). These in-shoe devices enable data to be collected both on pressure distribution across the whole of the plantar surface of the foot and also across time. Most of these devices are connected by a short lead to a data logger that is normally worn on the

these forces are said to act and also to represent these forces by a single ground reaction vector of given magnitude and angle.

Typically, force plate data are plotted against time, showing the patterns of change of force during the period of time that the foot is in contact with the supporting surface. Figure 8.5 shows the normal vertical reaction forces seen in walking plotted in two different ways.

The clinical value of force plate data is debatable. Major movement abnormalities are apparent both on visual observation and on

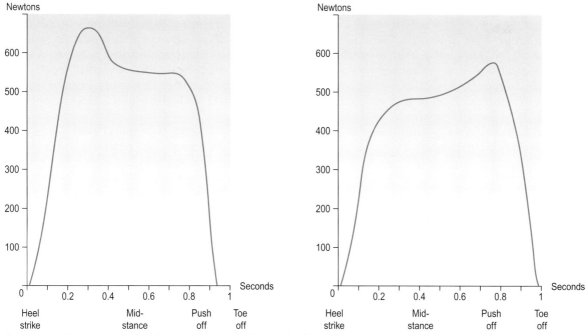

Figure 8.6   Force traces taken from patients with abnormal gait patterns.

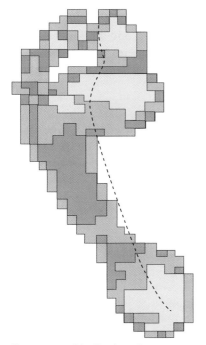

Figure 8.7   Distribution of pressure across the sole of the foot during walking. The light areas represent the greatest pressure.

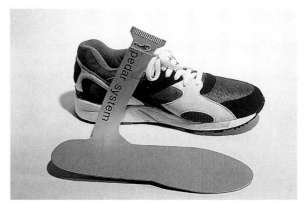

Figure 8.8   An in-shoe pressure device.

waist belt and the data can be downloaded onto a computer for analysis at a later date.

ELECTROMYOGRAPHY (EMG)

EMG is the term used to describe not only the electrical signals produced as a result of the contraction of a muscle but also the method of collecting these signals and the data that are produced.

When a muscle is quiescent there is little electrical activity. However, during muscular activity, electrical signals are produced and can be recorded. Electromyography will show if a muscle is active or not, the duration of that activity and, as the EMG increases in magnitude with tension, the signals will also give an indication of how much torque is being generated.

The basis of EMG

At a cellular level, the muscle fibre or cell is the unit of contraction. During muscle activity there is an electrical potential change and depolarisation and repolarisation of the surface membrane of the cell. There is transmission of impulse across the sarcolemma to the interior of the muscle cell via a complex system of tubules.

When a neural impulse reaches the motor end-plate, a wave of depolarisation spreads across the cell, resulting in a twitch followed by relaxation. This twitch can last from a few milliseconds to 0.25 s. The depolarisation is followed by a wave of repolarisation.

The muscle electrical potentials, called muscle action potentials (MAPs), will result in a small amount of the electrical current spreading away from the muscle in the direction of the skin, where electrodes can be used to record the electrical activity. The nearer the electrode is to the muscle, the larger the recorded signal. If muscle fibres some distance from the electrodes are conducting electrical current, the MAPs recorded will be smaller than they would be for similar sized motor units closer to the electrodes.

Values actually obtained from muscle vary between 100 µV (microvolts) to 5 mV (millivolts). The signal can be very small and a problem may exist because electrical activity from sources other than the muscle can overwhelm the desired signal. This unwanted electrical activity is called 'noise' and a number of strategies have to be adopted to eliminate unwanted noise.

Types of electrodes

Either surface or indwelling needle electrodes can be used, though surface electrode EMG is most common in the analysis of human movement. Both types of electrodes not only pick up electrical activity which passes over their conducting surface but can also register electrical currents nearby. Surface electrodes are normally small metal discs of about 1 cm diameter, though they can be smaller if tiny muscles are being tested. The electrodes are usually made of silver/silver chloride and are sensitive to electrical signals from superficial muscles. They give a reading corresponding to the average electrical activity.

Needle electrodes are normally fine hypodermic needles containing a conductor which is insulated except for its protruding end. As two electrodes are needed, the outer part of the hypodermic forms one and the conductor inside the hypodermic forms the other. Otherwise fine wires can be used and these are less intrusive.

There is some evidence that the surface electrodes are more likely to give reliable data and, as a non-invasive technique, they are preferable (Arokoski et al 1999, Winter 1990). Subjective reports indicate that, despite the use of local anaesthetics, there is a degree of discomfort from needle electrodes and the movement of the contracting muscle in relation to the overlying skin, when pierced by the electrode, produces some inhibition to normal movement.

Recording the EMG

In order to be able to use the data collected from muscle, the signal must be 'clean', i.e. free from noise, artefacts and distortion (Winter 1990).

Noise may come from a variety of sources. These include:

- other muscles, especially the heart
- nearby electrical machinery, including the EMG recording equipment
- radio waves, e.g. ambulance/police/CB radios
- power lines, domestic electrical supply
- fluorescent lights.

Artefacts are 'false signals' which are generated or caused by the EMG machine or its cabling. Some are difficult to distinguish from the true signal coming from the muscle but others can easily be identified. Into this latter category come movement artefacts that occur when the cables or the electrodes are moved and touched. The movement artefacts are usually at the upper and lower ends of the frequency range and can therefore be filtered out.

Distortion of EMG signals usually results as a consequence of the signals needing to be amplified before they can be of use. Distortion may occur if the signal is amplified in a way that is not linear over the whole range of the system. It is important that the larger signals are amplified to the same degree as the smaller signals.

EMG processing

After the EMG signal has been amplified, it can be viewed as a raw signal or processed to enable it to be compared or correlated with other physiological and biomechanical signals (Winter 1990). Computers are used for this purpose and it is important to be aware that the original signals will have been subjected to a number of manipulations before the final data are produced. This should not normally be a problem but where the output is not what was expected then the signal processing should be checked.

Raw EMG

This is illustrated in Figure 8.9 and EMG in this form enables judgements about the onset and cessation of muscle contraction. This can provide information about the sequence of muscle activation and current thought suggests that there may be a 'normal' pattern of muscle activation which, if altered, can lead to movement problems and pain. The traces in Figure 8.9 were taken from a normal shoulder during the movement of flexion and extension and were part of a study to identify the sequence of activation of the various shoulder muscles. The trace illustrates the difficulty often experienced when trying to identify the instant of muscle activation.

Processed EMG

The first stage of processing the EMG signal involves rectification. Normally raw EMG has both negative and positive polarity which means that the mean of the spikes above and below the zero line will be zero. Clearly this is of little value. Rectification converts the signal to a positive polarity so that the mean amplitude of the spikes

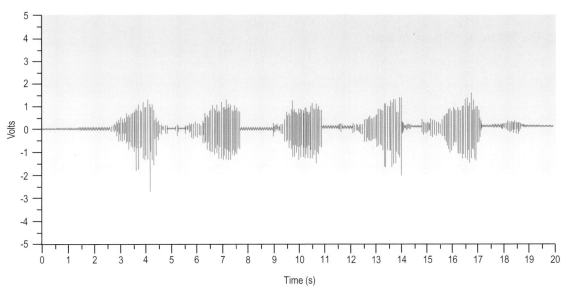

Figure 8.9 A raw EMG trace taken from supraspinatus during repeated repetitions of shoulder joint flexion at 608/s.

becomes meaningful. As the mean amplitude varies with the strength of the muscle contraction, it enables judgements about whether there is more or less muscle activity in a given situation. In addition to rectification, the signal can also be subjected to a low-pass filter, called a linear envelope, which cuts out high-frequency signals. It can also be integrated and this can take several forms. For more details a specialist EMG textbook should be consulted.

Clinical significance of EMG for measuring human movement

A question that has been puzzling researchers for at least 25 years is 'how valuable is EMG in reflecting and predicting muscle function and can findings be extrapolated to total body function?'. EMG surface electrodes are non-invasive and the method is cheap and simple to apply. Various authors have suggested that EMG will provide information on muscle power, muscle sequencing, fatigue, composition of fibre type and metabolism. The simplicity and inexpensive nature of EMG ought to make it an important method of evaluating function but the fact that the value of EMG is still being questioned after so long indicates its limitations. There are still sufficient doubts about what EMG can reliably do to suggest that it must be used with caution.

EMG and the phasic activity of muscles

EMG can provide information on whether or not a muscle is active and for how long the period of activity or inactivity continues. There is always a small lag between the onset of electrical activity in a muscle and perceived movement of the limb; this is in the region of 30 ms and is probably not significant in terms of analysis of the phasic activity of muscles. The lag is due partially to the chemical changes which must take place before the muscle can contract and partially to the need for the muscle to 'take up slack' before joint movement can occur.

A similar lag occurs at the end of muscle activity. With the cessation of electrical activity, the muscle continues to contract for a short period whilst the chemical changes stabilise and the muscle is able to relax. It is likely that the period between the end of electrical activity and the cessation of contraction will vary between muscle groups and will also be dependent on the type of muscle contraction. In the normal human being, the quadriceps has been studied most often and it shows a lag period of between 250 ms and 300 ms (Inman et al 1981).

It is valuable to know the duration of involvement of various muscle groups during movement but there can be practical problems. It is not always clear from the EMG traces when a muscle starts to contract and when contraction ends. Figure 8.9 illustrates this well. All current information on the phasing or sequencing of muscles in functional activity is taken from EMG studies. These studies show when the muscles are activated and when they cease activity but EMG is not able to provide information on whether the activity is isometric, concentric or eccentric. EMG studies of muscles involved in normal walking have shown that the input of individual muscles may only last for a very short time, often in the region of 0.2 s. As this would not give the muscle sufficient time to produce a movement at a joint, it leads to speculation that these muscles are doing no more than producing an isometric action (Inman et al 1981). With such minor involvement of muscles in normal gait, it is no wonder that people are able to walk for many hours before experiencing fatigue.

EMG and force production

There is considerable controversy about whether EMG can give reliable, quantifiable information on the magnitude of muscle activity, the recruitment of contractile elements and muscle metabolism and fatigue. Whilst it is commonly agreed that EMG can distinguish between a working muscle and a quiescent muscle, there is disagreement about whether the relationship between EMG activity and torque is consistent and linear. If the relationship is linear, EMG can be used to calculate the forces generated by muscles during functional activities. If, however, the EMG signal has an inconsistent, non-linear relationship with muscle torque, then it has little value as a measurement tool.

EMG and isometric tension

Early experiments by Lippold (1952) found that for the gastrocnemius muscle, a linear relationship could be shown between the average amplitude of EMG and the tension developed in muscle. This appeared to indicate that EMG could be used to measure the force generated but unfortunately, in subsequent decades other workers found different results. Although the EMG increased, it did not do so in direct relationship to the actual amount of force generated by the muscle (Lawrence & De Luca 1983, Rau & Vredenbregt 1973, Zuniga & Simons 1969). Winter (1990) suggests that there is no more than a 'reasonable relationship' between isometric force generation and EMG activity. If this is true, the results from EMG can only be used to give a general prediction of muscle tension.

EMG and isotonic tension

Much less experimental activity has been undertaken in the field of EMG–isotonic force relationships than that of EMG–isometric relationships. On low-velocity contractions there is an identifiable but inconsistent relationship between EMG and muscle torque and the faster the contraction, the more difficult it becomes to see any relationship (Komi 1973).

Mathematical calculations of muscle moment, based on force plate and joint angle data, can be made. Information gained from these calculations and from simultaneous EMG correlates very closely, suggesting that EMG is an accurate method of collecting information about whether a muscle is contracting or not during a functional activity (Olney & Winter 1985). EMG will also give some indication of the magnitude of the force being generated by that muscle, though no detail.

ENERGY EXPENDITURE ANALYSIS

There are a number of approaches which can be used to calculate energy expenditure during movement; the details are beyond the scope of this book but can be found in any advanced physiology text. Direct calorimetry produces highly accurate and repeatable results but is largely impractical as it requires the use of an airtight insulated chamber in which the activity is performed. Indirect calorimetry most commonly relies on the analysis of the oxygen and carbon dioxide content of expired air and is valuable and reasonably practical but still requires the subject to be attached to some form of device in which expired air can be collected. The need to wear a noseclip and to breathe through a fairly large mouthpiece can be rather daunting and needs quite lengthy acclimatisation. In addition, upper limb activities may be restricted by the tube leaving the mouthpiece (McArdle et al 1997, Whittle 1991).

Consideration of energy expenditure is important in patients who are frail or disabled. When individuals are already functioning at the limit of their ability, it is essential that they are encouraged to undertake activities in the most energy-efficient way possible. Analysis of human movement in terms of energy expenditure provides essential information that will then inform treatment approaches.

CONCLUSION

This chapter has shown that technological advances have made it possible to get good objective data for many of the individual parameters involved in human movement. These data have a variety of uses in many aspects of movement analysis. The fact that many of these take place in isolation from the functional activity is a drawback and caution must be used when the results are extrapolated to the movement itself. The increasing use of video and computerised kinematic systems is making an impact on the understanding of human movement and leading to some exciting areas of research into human movement.

REFERENCES

Arokoski JPA, Kankaanpaa M, Valta T et al 1999 Back and hip extensor muscle function during therapeutic exercise. Archives of Physical Medicine and Rehabilitation 80(7): 842–850

Curtis KA, Kindlin CM, Reich KM, White DE 1995 Functional reach in wheelchair users: the effects of trunk and lower extremity stabilisation. Archives of Physical Medicine and Rehabilitation 76: 360–367

Gajdosik RL, Bohannon RW 1987 Clinical measurement of range of motion: review of goniometry emphasising reliability and validity. Physical Therapy 67: 1867–1872

Hazelwood ME, Rowe PJ, Salter PM 1995 The use of electrogoniometers as a measurement tool for passive movement and gait analysis. Physiotherapy 81(10): 639

Inman VT, Ralston HJ, Todd F 1981 Human walking. Williams and Wilkins, Baltimore, Maryland

Kannus P 1994 Isokinetic evaluation of muscular performance: implications for muscle testing and rehabilitation. International Journal of Sports Medicine 15: S11–S18

Komi PV 1973 Relationship between muscle tension, EMG and velocity of contraction under concentric and eccentric work. In: Desmedt JE (ed) New developments in electromyography and clinical neurophysiology, vol. 1. Karger, Basel

Lawrence JH, De Luca CJ 1983 Myoelectric signal versus force relationship in different human muscles. Journal of Applied Physiology 54(6): 1653–1659

Lippold OCJ 1952 The relationship between integrated action potentials in a human muscle and its isometric tension. Journal of Physiology 117: 492–499

McArdle WD, Katch FI, Katch VL 1997 Exercise physiology, energy, nutrition and human performance, 4th edn. Lea and Febiger, Philadelphia

McGill SM, Dainty DA 1984 Computer analysis of energy transfers in children walking with crutches. Archives of Physical Medicine and Rehabilitation 65: 115–120

Myles C, Rowe PJ, Salter P, Nicol A 1995 An electrogoniometry system used to investigate the ability of the elderly to ascend and descend stairs. Physiotherapy 81(10): 640

Noreau L, Richards CL, Comeau F, Tardif D 1995 Biomechanical analysis of swing-through gait in paraplegic and non-disabled individuals. Journal of Biomechanics 28: 689–700

Rau G, Vredenbregt J 1973 EMG force relationship during voluntary static contractions (M. biceps). Medicine and Sport Biomechanics III(8): 270–274

Rome K, Cowieson F 1996 A reliability study of the universal goniometer, fluid goniometer and electrogoniometer for the measurement of ankle dorsiflexion. Foot and Ankle 17: 28–32

Rothstein JM (ed) 1985 Measurement in physical therapy. Churchill Livingstone, Edinburgh

Rowe PJ, Nicol AC, Kelly IG 1989 Flexible goniometer computer system for the assessment of hip function. Clinical Biomechanics 4: 68–72

Terauds J 1984 Sports biomechanics. Proceedings of the International Symposium of Biomechanics in Sport. Academic Publishers, Del Mar, California

Troke M, Moore AP, Cheek E 1998 Reliability of the OSI CA 6000 spine motion analyzer with a new skin fixation system when used on the thoracic spine. Manual Therapy 3(1): 27–33

Whittle M 1991 Gait analysis, an introduction. Butterworth-Heinemann, Oxford

Winter DA 1982 Camera speeds for normal and pathological gait analyses. Medical and Biological Engineering and Computing 20: 408–412

Winter DA 1990 Biomechanics and motor control of human movement, 2nd edn. Wiley Inter-science, New York

Zuniga EN, Simons DG 1969 Non-linear relationship between averaged electromyogram potential and muscle tension in normal subjects. Archives of Physical Medicine and Rehabilitation 50: 613–620

Chapter 9

Scales of measurement

Susan Corr

LEARNING OUTCOMES

When you have completed this chapter you should be able to:

1. Understand that loss of movement has an impact on an individual's ability to carry out everyday activities

2. Recognise that loss of movement can affect functional status and quality of life

3. Understand that measuring the effect movement loss has on mobility, function and quality of life is difficult

4. Identify appropriate measurement scales needed to measure the impact of movement loss.

INTRODUCTION

Previous chapters have outlined common methods of measuring human movement. When considering human movement, it is important to be aware that a loss of movement, minimal or severe, potentially has an impact on the wider aspects of an individual's life. This chapter will outline two areas that could be affected when looking at movement in a more global context. As a consequence, it is necessary to consider movement as a multifactorial, multidimensional complex concept. It is important to know how the loss of movement affects an individual's ability to carry out everyday activities and the effect loss of movement has on how individuals perceive their quality of life. In essence, this type of measurement is moving away from measuring impairment to measuring disability or handicap. Identifying symptoms is not enough to establish how an illness, disorder or injury actually affects a person's life (Üstün et al 2003). The World Health Organisation's *International Classification of Functioning, Disability and Health* (ICF) reflects a change towards considering functioning and disability (WHO 2001).

There are many measurement scales to choose from and it is important to consider these when deciding how to measure the impact of loss of movement. It is critical that therapists choose one designed for the purpose for which it is required (Fisher 1992). A lot of measurement scales can also be used to assess the outcome of treatment and therefore are suitable to measure the impact of loss on more than one occasion. Gompertz et al (1993) suggest that in stroke rehabilitation, for example, broader issues such as mood and perceived health should be measured and not just movement loss or functional status.

GENERAL PRINCIPLES OF MEASUREMENT SCALES

Validity and reliability

Whichever measurement scale is selected, it is essential to consider its reliability and validity. Validity relates to whether a measurement scale measures what it is intended to measure (Bowling & Normand 1998). A scale needs to appear relevant and clear (face validity) and to examine comprehensively the concept that it intends to measure (content validity) (Bowling 2002). Scales also need to be reliable, i.e. consistent at producing the same results whether at repeated intervals (test-retest), by the same rater at different times (intrarater) or by different raters (interrater) (Gompertz et al 1993). If a measurement scale has high interrater reliability, different raters when measuring the same individual will produce the same results (Burton 1989).

It is also important to question the sensitivity of the measurement scale. This addresses whether the measure is able to identify changes that may

occur over time (Bowling & Normand 1998). A further issue to consider is whether the scale is relevant to every person being measured (McDowell & Newell 1996). Measurement scales that have been developed for specific client groups include the Glasgow Assessment Schedule for Head Injuries (Livingstone & Livingstone 1985), Parkinson's Disease Disability Index (McDowell et al 1970) and Robinson-Bashall Functional Assessment for Arthritis Patients (McCloy & Jongbloed 1987).

If a measurement scale is shown to be reliable and valid, then it is considered to be standardised. This standardisation process allows scales to be used to compare individuals (McDowell & Newell 1996). Once a measurement scale is standardised, the process of conducting it will be formalised, meaning that there will be procedural instructions outlining in what environment the scale should be conducted, what materials are required and the sequencing of the scale. These procedural arrangements should be clear and concise and, if followed strictly, ensure that the scale remains reliable and valid (Burton 1989, Law & Letts 1989).

The King's Fund (1988) recommends that measurement, using standard scales, should be undertaken on all patients. Although this is desirable, it is important to consider Barer's (1989) suggestion that formal measurement scales used by a therapist may show what patients can do under test conditions but informal measurements made by carers are more likely to indicate what patients do in real life. Barer goes on to suggest that postal surveys or interviews of patients at home may reveal what they think they can do.

Methods of scoring

There are several different ways in which a measurement scale may be scored. The types of scales being described in this chapter are not interval or ratio measurements where the distance between two numbers on the scale is of a known size, like exact degrees of movement or length in centimetres (Bowling & Normand 1998). On the whole, a verbal description will be used to identify how able an individual is to carry out an activity or to provide a continuum of agreement based on verbal expressions such as 'disagree, unsure,

Task 9.1

Try to identify some examples of each of the three different types of scales. You may find some examples in everyday situations such as in supermarkets or questionnaires in magazines. For interval scales there needs to be an equal gap between two scores; for nominal scales numbers are used to label the items in the scales but there is no relationship between the numbers; and for ordinal scales there is a grading system although the intervals are not equal.

agree'. Scales using verbal definitions like this are ordinal scales, i.e. the options for responses are in some kind of order and have a relationship to each other (Bowling & Normand 1998). A third type of scale is the nominal scale where numbers are used just for labels, such as male or female, and have no value in relation to each other. However, nominal scales are not commonly used in the type of measures being discussed in this chapter.

It is necessary to be able to identify how a scale is measured in order to understand the appropriateness of the measurement to the question being asked. Regardless of which scoring system is used, it should be straightforward and quick. Also it needs to be easy to interpret so that the results can be used for treatment planning or measuring the outcome of treatment (Law & Letts 1989).

Data collection methods

Further consideration needs to be given to how information is gathered when using measurement scales. There are several options including observation, interview or self-rating. Each method has strengths and limitations.

Observation

When observing, it is possible to see exactly how able an individual is to carry out an activity. However, a limitation may be that 'being watched' affects individuals as they demonstrate their ability to perform a task. This may be positive or negative: they may make greater efforts or alternatively they may feel more anxious and lack confidence if being observed. A key to using observation as an assessment method is being clear about what is to be observed and how to match what is seen with possible scores. For example, it is important to know exactly what needs to be observed in order to rate an individual as 'able to manage most of the task'.

Interview

Interviews are another mechanism for gathering information. Often the interview is structured, which means there are particular questions to ask and possibly even suggestions as to how they should be phrased. One limitation of interviews is the reliance placed on the individual's perception of their ability, rather than actually observing their ability. Alternatively, if it is very difficult for an individual to carry out an activity, it may be easier for them to inform you of this rather than struggle to demonstrate their difficulties.

Self-rating

Similarly self-rating methods of gathering information are usually very structured. The measurement scale is most likely to be in questionnaire format. It may be valid and reliable for use by post, which makes it a useful tool for research as a well as clinical practice. To be used in this way it will need to be easy to complete, have clear instructions and should not take long to fill in.

Some measurement scales are reliable for use by observation, interview or self-rating. The Barthel Activities of Daily Living Index, which is an example of this, is outlined in the next section.

Task 9.2

Draw the following table on a sheet of paper and use it to consider the strengths and limitations of using interviews, observation and self-rating scales to measure an individual's ability to ride a bicycle.

Method	Strengths	Limitations
Interviews		
Observation		
Self-rating		

MEASUREMENT SCALES FOR MOBILITY

Defining mobility

The ability to move around with ease, i.e. to mobilise, enables individuals to carry out everyday activities. However, this requires the consideration of a range of concepts including lying to sitting, sitting to standing, turning, stopping, gait, walking speed, balance and functional reach (Smith 1994, Wall 2000). Independent mobility incorporates all of these critical tasks.

Mobility scales

A wide range of mobility scales are available for use in clinical settings. Some have been developed to measure a particular aspect of mobility, such as balance; the Berg Balance Scale (BBS) (Berg et al 1992) is an example of this. Others measure the impact of diseases such as cardiovascular disease and lung disease on the exercise capacity of older people. An example of this is the 6-minute walk test (Enright el al 2003).

More commonly, mobility scales have been developed to measure mobility as a global concept. Two such scales that will be outlined further in this section are the Get Up and Go Test (GUGT) (Mathias et al 1986) and the Elderly Mobility Scale (EMS) (Smith 1994).

Get Up and Go Test (GUGT)

The GUGT was developed in the UK by Mathias et al (1986). It was designed to challenge an elderly person's sense of balance and it requires the individual to stand up from a chair, walk a short distance, turn around, return and sit down again. It is considered a simple test to administer and uses a five-point ordinal scale where 1 equals normal (patient is not at risk of falling), 2 equals very slightly abnormal, 3 equals mildly abnormal, 4 equals moderately abnormal and 5 equals severely abnormal. Face, content and concurrent validity have been established for this measure as have interrater and test-retest reliability (Nakamura et al 1998). It is considered as a good tool for use with the elderly (Nakamura et al 1998). More recently, Wall (2000) has revised this measure and developed the Expanded Timed Get

Up and Go (ETGUG). The ETGUG uses a multi-memory stopwatch and an extended walkway, resulting in a more sensitive and clinically useful measure of mobility. It requires minimal equipment, professional expertise and training to administer.

Elderly Mobility Scale (EMS)

The EMS was developed by Smith (1994) to assess mobility in elderly patients. It tests lying to sitting, sitting to lying, sitting to standing, standing, gait, walking speed and functional reach (see Table 9.1). Therefore it covers locomotion, balance and key position changes which are components of more complex activities of daily living (ADL). The maximum score possible, which represents independent mobility, is 20 and the minimum score is 0.

The concurrent validity and interrater reliability of the scale have been established and it is easy to use in practice (Prosser & Canby 1997, Smith 1994). Smith (1994) suggests that individuals scoring under 10 on the EMS are likely to need help with mobility and ADL, while those scoring 14 or more are likely to be independent in mobility.

It provides an effective and ready objective measure of the change in the individual's mobility (Prosser & Canby 1997, Spilg et al 2001). It can be useful in determining the effectiveness of differing approaches to rehabilitation although it must always be remembered that for those requiring rehabilitation, mobility is not the only factor determining need and outcome. The EMS can also predict the probability of a patient having two or more falls (Spilg et al 2003).

MEASUREMENT SCALES FOR FUNCTIONAL STATUS

Defining function

There are several different interpretations of functional status. According to the Collins Dictionary (Harper Collins 1987), function means a natural action. This can be interpreted in humans to be the natural everyday actions carried out by individuals such as walking, toileting and eating. The perspective taken on function can also be influenced by the different philosophies of the professions within multidisciplinary teams. Fisher

Table 9.1   Elderly Mobility Scale showing the interpretation of the scores (after Smith 1994, with permission)

Concept	0	1	2	3	4
Lying to sitting	Needs help of 2+ people	Needs help of 1 person	Independent	N/A	N/A
Sit to stand	Needs help of 2+ people	Needs help of 1 person (verbal or physical)	Independent in over 3 seconds	Independent in under 3 seconds	N/A
Stand	Stands only with physical support* (i.e. help of another person)	Stands but needs support*	Stands without support* but needs support to reach	Stands without support* and able to reach	N/A
Gait	Needs physical help to walk or constant supervision	Mobile with walking aid but erratic/unsafe turning	Independent with frame	Independent (including use of sticks)	N/A
Timed walk	Unable to cover 6 metres	Over 30 seconds to cover 6 m	16–30 seconds to cover 6 m	Under 15 seconds to cover 6 m	N/A
Functional reach	Under 8 cm or unable	N/A	8–16 cm	N/A	Over 16 cm

*Support means needs to use upper limbs to steady self

Task 9.3

Using your local workplace or academic library, conduct a search for mobility scales that may be of use to you. Before you start, establish what criteria you are looking for in the scale, for example suitable for use with a particular population, standardised, developed in the last 5 years. Use these criteria to help you draw up relevant keywords for your search.

(1994) outlines them in relation to the goal of intervention (see Table 9.2). There are, of course, many overlaps between the professions but Table 9.2 highlights the unique aspects of each profession.

All the disciplines share concerns related to function and functional independence; they differ on how they frame the patient's problems and the goal of treatment. These differences may have an influence when choosing a measurement scale. Also, it is important to be aware of the interpretation of function that may have been adopted

by those who have developed scales for measuring function. By developing scales to measure an individual's functional status, the expectation is that it will be possible to get a current picture of the individual's abilities to carry out the actions that are natural to all. According to McDowell & Newell (1996), an individual is healthy if he or she is physically and mentally able to do the things he or she wishes and needs to do.

Activities of daily living (ADL) scales

Many scales have been developed over the last few decades, mainly in rehabilitation medicine. This section describes two in detail: the Barthel ADL Index, which measures ADL, and the Nottingham Extended ADL Scale, which measures extended activities, i.e. more community-based activities which also require movement in order for them to be carried out. These scales have been selected to illustrate the types available and are by no means the only ones that should be considered when identifying a measurement scale to assess function. Health-care professionals need to carefully consider

Table 9.2 Unique perspectives of medicine, nursing, occupational therapy, physiotherapy and social work (after Fisher 1994, with permission)

Profession	Frame	Methods	Goal
Medicine	Illness	Pharmacology Surgery	Symptom elimination
Nursing	Health	Helping/Caring Interprofessional interactions	Healthy function Wellness
Occupational therapy	Occupation	Therapeutic activity Adaptation	Occupational function
Physiotherapy	Physical capacity	Therapeutic exercise and agents	Physical function Mobility
Social work	Systems	System change Helping process	Social function

Table 9.3 Barthel ADL Index showing the interpretation of the scores (after Wade 1992, with permission)

Concept	0	1	2	3
Bowels	Incontinent	Occasional accident	Continent	–
Bladder	Incontinent	Occasional accident	Continent	–
Grooming	Dependent	Independent	–	–
Toilet use	Dependent	Needs some help	Independent	–
Feeding	Unable	Needs help	Independent	–
Transfer	Unable	Major help	Minor help	Independent
Mobility	Dependent	Wheelchair independent	Walks with one person	Independent
Dressing	Dependent	Needs help but can do half	Independent	–
Stairs	Unable	Needs help	Independent	–
Bathing	Dependent	Independent	–	–

the options available when they are selecting a measurement scale. The choice will depend on why it is being used. It may be needed to measure ability, to evaluate the amount of help patients may need on discharge, to identify treatment goals or as an outcome measure.

Barthel Activity of Daily Living Index (BI)

One of the most widely known and used measures of ADL is the BI. It was developed in 1965 by Mahoney and Barthel as a simple index of independence to score the ability of patients to care for themselves and, by repeating the test, to assess their improvement (Mahoney & Barthel 1965). It contains 10 items and has both a self-care and a mobility component. This scale does not measure movement in isolation but the output of movement; that is, the ability to carry out activities. The mobility component contains items related to transfers and ambulation. The original scoring system was from 0 to 100 but this has been modified so that scores range from 0 to 20 with higher scores signifying better functioning (Bacher et al 1990, Collin et al 1988). This modified version is most commonly used in practice. Table 9.3 shows the 10 items in the scales and the scoring system used. Two items, transfer and mobility, can be scored 0, 1, 2 or 3 while the remainder just 0, 1 and 2. The table indicates the interpretation of each score for all the items. A total score is then calculated.

The BI is not hierarchical, meaning that it does not result in a total score that gives a clear indication of the level of disability (Gibbon 1991). This means that two people may score the same, for example 10, but it would not be possible to assume that both are independent in the same activities. The items are not in an order that reflects the complexity and difficulty of carrying out particular activities. As can be seen from Table 9.3, the BI also has different interpretations for the score values. For example, for bathing, being independent scores only 1 where being independent in transfers scores 3. This does not necessarily reflect the complex movements and skills required to carry out each of these activities. Wade (1992) provides working definitions for the scores so that therapists are clear about what the individual needs to be able to do in order to be scored as independent. These will ensure a standardised use and understanding of the scale.

There is no single way of interpreting the total score. Granger & Hamilton (1990) found that no specific total score could be regarded as adequately specific or sensitive to be used as the criterion for admission to rehabilitation services or as an indication of readiness for discharge. Rodgers et al (1993) suggest that the BI is most useful in assessing patients who are moderately or severely disabled. There is a ceiling and flooring effect, meaning that those scoring the maximum (20) may still be significantly handicapped but with the potential of improvement beyond the limits of the scale. As a result the BI lacks sensitivity to change in its upper range (Rodgers et al 1993). The same occurs at the lower end. To overcome this, patients with high BI scores should subsequently be assessed with an ADL scale, i.e. a scale that assesses a broader range of activities.

The BI is most frequently used in clinical practice by therapists and other members of the multidisciplinary team. It has been shown to be reliable for use in this format and also for use in formal research, by post and over the telephone (Wade 1992). Law and Letts (1989) indicated that, more specifically, it has been shown to have adequate observer and test-retest reliability. It is a valid measurement scale for function in ADL and is sensitive to measure changes in ADL after treatment in controlled research settings.

Eakin (1993) suggests that the appeal of the BI lies in the fact that it is simple and quick to use; its results can be easily understood and communicated between different professions; and its content is perceived as relevant to both clinicians and patients. However, it has also been thought not to have enough items to account for the impact of rehabilitation and that the grading system is not sufficiently sensitive to reflect change, particularly in the short term.

Task 9.4

Read the two case studies below. Using the information given, calculate the subjects' scores using the Barthel ADL Index. Once you have completed this, consider the usefulness of the index in establishing levels of function.

Mrs Smith is a 45-year-old teacher who recently had a right cerebrovascular accident (stroke). She has been discharged back to her two-storey house and is beginning to settle into some routine at home. She manages to wash and dress independently. With the aids provided by the social services occupational therapists, she is independent going up and down stairs and getting in and out of the bath. Although she can manage to make a hot drink, she is unable to cook a meal or cut up her food. At the moment her husband does the cooking and shopping. Mrs Smith manages to walk around the house but is unable to walk on uneven ground. She has not been outside and does not feel confident to go to the shops. She is glad that they have a downstairs toilet, which she can manage to get to and use independently.

Mr Jones is a 55-year-old car mechanic who runs his own small business. He has rheumatoid arthritis. He is currently unable to work or tend his garden due to pain and stiffness mainly in his hands. He walks to his local shop daily to get the paper. He has always been a casual dresser (T-shirts and deck shoes rather than shirt and tie or suits) and can get dressed if wearing his normal clothes. His is unable to drive at the moment but uses public transport. He has difficulty turning on the taps but can make a cup of tea if the kettle is filled for him. He can also shower independently as he has a walk-in shower rather than a bath. He is independent going up and down the stairs. Mr Jones recently bought an electric shaver and manages to shave independently with this.

Table 9.4   Extended Activities of Daily Living Scale (Adapted from Nouri & Lincoln 1987, with permission Lippincott, Williams & Wilkins)

Concept	No (0)	With help (0)	On my own with difficulty (1)	On my own (1)
Mobility Do you: Walk around outside? Climb stairs? Get in and out of the car? Walk over uneven ground? Cross roads? Travel on public transport?				
In the kitchen Do you: Manage to feed yourself? Manage to make yourself a hot drink? Take hot drinks from one room to another? Do the washing up? Make yourself a hot snack?				
Domestic tasks Do you: Manage your own money when you are out? Wash small items of clothing? Do your own housework? Do your own shopping? Do a full clothes wash?				
Leisure activities Do you: Read newspapers or books? Use the telephone? Write letters? Go out socially? Manage your own garden? Drive a car?				

Extended activities of daily living (EADL) scale

The EADL scale was developed in Nottingham by Nouri and Lincoln (1987) to assess the activities which may be important to stroke patients living in the community. It includes activities that relate to carrying out domestic tasks and other activities that take place outside the home environment. It has been validated for administration by interview and post (Lincoln & Gladman 1992, Nouri & Lincoln 1987, Wade 1992). It consists of a questionnaire of 22 activities divided into four groups: mobility, kitchen, domestic and leisure.

The EADL scale is a ranked scale, meaning that all patients with the same scores are independent in the same items. Lincoln and Gladman (1992) found that an overall total score could provide an indication of overall independence in the activities if comparing groups of people. They recommend that with individual patients, section scores, for example mobility or leisure scores, rather than overall totals should be used when identifying a patient's progress or change over time. They recommend this as they found discrepancies when using the total score. The scale is appropriate to use in research into the evaluation of rehabilitation.

Table 9.4 outlines the items in each of the four sections of the scale. The response options are the

---

Task 9.5

Here is some additional information about Mrs Smith and Mr Jones. Use this information along with what you already know about them to calculate their scores using the Nottingham Extended ADL scale.

Mrs Smith loves reading but finds she takes a long time to read the newspaper. She feels her concentration is too poor to read books. She has yet to go out anywhere mainly because she is unsteady walking and lacks confidence. She is anxious about whether she may ever return to work. She has been overwhelmed with the good wishes from her pupils and colleagues and has written several thank you notes.

Mr Jones is anxious about his business, which his son is currently running. He has been struggling of late to hold a pen to write and has done most of his communication over the telephone. His wife has traditionally done all the household tasks with the garden being his domain. He has needed help with the garden lately. At the moment his wife drives when they go out shopping or visiting friends.

Task 9.6

Ask a number of friends and family of different ages to sum up what issues contribute to their definition of quality of life. If they include health as one issue, ask them to clarify what they mean by this. Also find out what level of 'ill health' they need to experience in order for their quality of life to be affected. Are there differences in views between people of different age groups?

---

same for each item. The score 1 is given if activities are performed by patients on their own or on their own with difficulty. For activities which patients are unable to perform or for which they require help, the score is 0.

MEASUREMENT SCALES FOR QUALITY OF LIFE

Defining quality of life

Like functional status, quality of life is not easy to define. There are a number of different views on the scope of what should be included in the broad consideration of quality of life. Fallowfield (1990) and De Haan et al (1993) suggest that four domains make up quality of life: physical, functional, psychological and social health. The physical health dimension refers to disease-related and treatment-related symptoms as well as pain and sleep. The functional dimension comprises self-care, mobility and physical activity level, as well as the capacity to carry out various roles in relation to family and work. The psychological dimension includes issues such as depression, anxiety and adjustment to illness, cognitive functioning, well-

being, life satisfaction and happiness. Finally, the social health dimension includes qualitative and quantitative aspects of social contacts and interactions such as relationships and participation in leisure and social activities. The inclusion of these dimensions reflects the need to ensure that when thinking of quality of life as a concept, it is seen as a broad spectrum of consequences of disease, including elements of impairment, disabilities and handicaps, as well as the patient's perceived health status and well-being. Quality of life relating to health is distinct from quality of life as a whole, which would also include adequacy of housing and income and perceptions of the local environment (Bowling & Normand 1998).

What is not clear is the balance of the four dimensions required in order to ensure quality of life. Diener (1984) suggests that the influence of health on quality of life is not simply the direct effect on how people feel physically but also on what their health allows them to do. For example, in two separate studies of stroke patients, Niemei et al (1988) and Wyller et al (1997) found that even when patients had a good recovery in terms of physical movement, they reported a poor quality of life. This shows that the impact of a disease on health-related quality of life is important but can be difficult to understand and to measure.

Quality of life measures

Quality of life measures range from broad general health profiles (generic) to disease-specific scales. The broad health profiles are those which have not been developed for specific target populations or patient groups. A strength of these is that quality of life results can be compared across patient populations. A limitation is that they do not always focus on the specific problems of a given patient group. Two examples of these are the SF-36 and the Nottingham Health Profile (NHP). Both of these will be discussed later in this section. Disease-specific quality of life scales exist for a range of specific patient groups, including those who have had strokes (Holbrook & Skilbeck 1983), who have rheumatic disorders (Liang et al 1990), cardiovascular diseases (Wenger & Furberg 1990) and cancer (Van Knippenberg & de Haes 1985). Disease-specific scales do not allow cross-disease comparisons but are often more sensitive to the quality of life issues particularly relevant to specific populations of patients.

Most of the available quality of life scales depend on patients to rate themselves. Quality of life is a very personal issue and therefore getting individuals to rate themselves is the preferred method of administration. It is also possible to use structured interviews or written questionnaires. It can be difficult for patients with serious cognitive, speech and language disorders to complete these (De Haan et al 1993).

Quality of life measures can be used for a number of reasons. They may be useful for patients with chronic conditions where recovery is not expected and where success of treatments may best be measured in terms of maintaining an acceptable quality of life for the patient as the disease progresses (Talamo et al 1997). They can also be used to facilitate the process of identifying which patients will likely benefit from which type of rehabilitative procedure (Mathias et al 1997). Treatment from a multidisciplinary team may include a range of interventions which individually are difficult to measure directly or for which there is no sensitive measure. In these situations a quality of life measure may be the most appropriate option to demonstrate outcome from the treatment. Quality of life measures can also be used to evaluate treatment programmes. Baker & Intagliata (1982) suggest that if a patient's life situation is not improved in some way and they are not happier or more satisfied after participating in treatment then it is difficult to ultimately justify the treatment.

The Short Form 36 (SF-36)

The SF-36 health survey is an example of a measurement scale for quality of life that includes physical functioning as a component of the measurement. It has been developed from a longer medical outcomes study questionnaire, which has had the number of items reduced to 36, hence the title Short Form 36 (SF-36). The aim of reducing the items was to develop a scale that could be conducted in a short period of time and therefore be used in a broad range of settings (Ware & Sherbourne 1992).

The SF-36 is an indicator of quality of life for population studies as well as an outcome measure in clinical practice and research (McDowell & Newell 1996). It is suitable for use with all patients as the measure addresses aspects of health that are important to all patients, rather than just those with a particular condition. It is a questionnaire that can be completed by anyone over 14 years of age in a clinical setting or at home. It can also be administered in an interview. It is easy to use and takes between 5 and 10 minutes to complete, which has made it popular (Larson 1997).

The SF-36 categorises the 36 items into eight areas relating to health concepts. These are physical functioning (10 items), role limitations due to physical problems (four items), social functioning (two items), bodily pain (two items), general mental health (five items), role limitation due to emotional problems (three items), vitality (four items) and general health (five items) perceptions (Larson 1997) and health change over the past year. The inclusion of bodily pain and vitality as concepts of health is unique to the SF-36 scale (Ware & Sherbourne 1992). The items relating to movement (see Tables 9.5, 9.6 and 9.7) ask about levels and types of limitations when lifting and carrying groceries, climbing stairs, bending, kneeling and walking moderate distances.

Each of the eight different sections produces an individual section score ranging from 0 to 54. For each item, there is a choice of responses on a Likert scale, ranging from 'limited a lot' to 'not limited at all' or 'all of the time' to 'none of the time' (Brazier 1995). These are not combined to form an overall score and therefore it is hard to make comparisons (Bowling & Normand 1998). It is possible to identify the scores relating to movement separately from those indicating other concepts relating to health. Like all scales that contain sections, it is important to carry out the

Table 9.5   The 10 items of the SF-36 that relate to physical functioning (Adapted from Ware 2000 with permission from Lippincott, Williams & Wilkins). The following questions are about activities you might do during a typical day. Does your health now limit you in these activities? If so, how much?

Activities	Yes, limited a lot	Yes, limited a little	No, not limited at all
Vigorous activities such as running, lifting heavy objects, participating in sport	1	2	3
Moderate activities such as moving a table, pushing a vacuum cleaner	1	2	3
Lifting or carrying groceries	1	2	3
Climbing several flights of stairs	1	2	3
Climbing one flight of stairs	1	2	3
Bending, kneeling or stooping	1	2	3
Walking more than a mile	1	2	3
Walking half a mile	1	2	3
Walking 100 yards	1	2	3
Bathing and dressing yourself	1	2	3

Table 9.6   The four items of the SF-36 that relate to role limitations due to physical problems and pain (Adapted from Ware 2000, www.qmetric.com with permission from Lippincott, Williams & Wilkins). During the past four weeks have you had any of the following problems with your work or regular daily activities as a result of your physical health?

	Yes	No
Cut down on the amount of time you spent on work or other activities	1	2
Accomplished less than you would like	1	2
Were limited in the kind of work or other activities	1	2
Had difficulty performing the work or other activities (for example, it took extra effort)	1	2

whole scale and not just select the aspects relating to movement. These sections are not validated to be used in isolation. Higher scores indicate a perception of good quality of life (Talamo et al 1997).

There is considerable evidence for the validity and reliability of the SF-36 and its ability to measure changes in health status over time (Brazier et al 1992, Garratt et al 1994, Jenkinson et al 1994, Ware & Sherbourne 1992). This supports its use as a routine scale for monitoring and assessing quality of life in both clinical practice and research. Anderson et al (1996) found it to be valid for use in stroke rehabilitation and Talamo et al (1997) with patients with rheumatoid arthritis. However,

as with other measurement scales, ceiling and flooring effects can occur.

Nottingham Health Profile (NHP)

Hunt, McEwen and McKenna developed the NHP in 1980 as a scale to measure health status (Hunt et al 1985). To develop it, 768 patients with a variety of health problems generated over 2000 statements. These statements were then reduced to 38. The profile has two parts, the first consisting of 38 statements addressing the following areas: energy, pain, emotional reactions, sleep, social isolation and physical mobility. The second part has seven

Table 9.7   The two items of the SF-36 that relate to pain (Adapted from Ware 2000, www.qmetric.com with permission from Lippincott, Williams & Wilkins)

How much bodily pain during the past four weeks?	
None	1
Very mild	2
Mild	3
Moderate	4
Severe	5
Very severe	6
During the past four weeks, how much did pain interfere with your normal work (including work both outside the home and housework)?	
Not at all	1
A little bit	2
Moderately	3
Quite a bit	4
Extremely	5

Table 9.8   Examples of statements (reproduced with permission from McKenna 2000, spm@galen.eng.net)

I can only walk about indoors
I find it hard to bend
I'm unable to walk at all
I have trouble getting up and down stairs or steps
I find it hard to reach for things
I find it hard to dress myself
I find it hard to stand for long (e.g. at the kitchen sink, waiting for a bus)
I need help to walk about outside (e.g. a walking aid or someone to support me)

statements concerning paid employment, jobs around the house, social life, personal relationships, sex life, hobbies and interests and holidays. Table 9.8 includes examples of statements that address issues relating to movement used in the profile and again, like the SF-36, these examples should not be used out of the context of the whole measure.

The NHP is short, simple and can be self-administered or carried out by interview. It takes about 5 minutes to complete. It is sensitive to change and has been tested extensively for reliability and validity (Bowling 1991). Scores range from 0, indicating no problem, to 100, where problems in all areas have been identified. As a result, a higher score reflects severe problems.

There are different views on whether the NHP is actually measuring quality of life. Wade (1992) suggests that it may be recording mood rather than global quality of life. Ebrahim et al (1986) suggest it is an indicator of depressed mood while Bowling (1991) suggests that it is identifying how people feel when they are experiencing various states of ill health.

CONCLUSION

Movement cannot be considered as an isolated component of life. If there is a loss of movement for any reason, this will affect how everyday activities are carried out and how quality of life is perceived. The difficulty is in quantifying or measuring these implications. Scales have been developed to try and measure these issues. When selecting a measurement scale, careful consideration is required to ensure it fulfils the purpose for which it is needed.

REFERENCES

Anderson C, Laubscher S, Burns R 1996 Validation of the Short Form 36 (SF36) Health Survey Questionnaire among stroke patients. Stroke 27:1812–1816

Bacher Y, Korner-Bitensky N, Mayo N et al 1990 A longitudinal study of depression among stroke patients participating in a rehabilitation program. Canadian Journal of Rehabilitation 4:27–37

Baker F, Intagliata J 1982 Quality of life in the evaluation of community support systems. Evaluation and Program Planning 5:69–79

Barer DH 1989 Use of the Nottingham ADL scale in stroke: relationships between functional recovery and length of stay in hospital. Journal of Royal College of Physicians of London 23(4):242–247

Berg KO, Maki BE, Williams JI et al 1992 Clinical and laboratory measures of postural balance in an elderly population. Archives of Physical Medicine and Rehabilitation 73:1073–1080

Bowling A 1991 Measuring health. A review of quality of life measurement scales. Open University Press, Milton Keynes

Bowling A 2002 Research methods in health. Investigating health and health services. Open University Press, Buckingham

Bowling A, Normand C 1998 Definition and measurement of outcome. In: Swash M (ed) Outcome in neurological and neurosurgical disorders. Cambridge University Press, Cambridge

Brazier J 1995 The Short-Form 36 (SF-36) Health Survey and its use in pharmacoeconomic evaluation. PharmacoEconomics 7:403–415

Brazier J, Harper R, Jones N et al 1992 Validating the SF-36 health survey questionnaire: new outcome measure for primary care. British Medical Journal 305:160–164

Burton J 1989 The model of human occupation and occupational therapy practice with elderly patients. Part 2 application. British Journal of Occupational Therapy 52:219–221

Collin C, Wade DT, Davies S et al 1988 The Barthel ADL Index: a reliability study. International Disability Studies 10:61–63

De Haan R, Aaronson N, Limburg M et al 1993 Measuring quality of life in stroke. Stroke 24:320–327

Diener E 1984 Subjective well-being. Psychological Bulletin 95:542–575

Eakin P 1993 The Barthel Index: confidence limits. British Journal of Occupational Therapy 56(5):184–185

Ebrahim S, Barer D, Nouri F 1986 Use of the Nottingham Health Profile with patients after a stroke. Journal of Epidemiological Community Health 40:166–169

Enright P, McBurnie M, Bittner V et al 2003 The 6-min walk test, a quick measure of functional status in elderly adults. Chest 123:387–398

Fallowfield L 1990 The quality of life. The missing measurement of health care. Souvenir Press, London

Fisher AG 1992 Functional measures, part 2: selecting the right test, minimising the limitations. American Journal of Occupational Therapy 46(3):278–281

Fisher AG 1994 Functional assessment and occupation: critical issues for occupational therapy. Key note address at Annual Conference of New Zealand Association of Occupational Therapists

Garratt A, Ruta D, Abdalla M et al 1994 SF-36 Health Survey Questionnaire: II. responsiveness to changes in health status in four common clinical conditions. Quality in Health Care 3:186–192

Gibbon B 1991 Measuring stroke recovery. Nursing Times 87(44):32–34

Gompertz P, Pound P, Ebrahim S 1993 The reliability of stroke outcome measures. Clinical Rehabilitation 7:290–296

Granger CV, Hamilton BB 1990 Measurement of stroke rehabilitation outcome in 1980's. Stroke 21(suppl):II-46–47

Harper Collins 1987 The new Collins dictionary and thesaurus in one volume. Harper Collins Publishers, Glasgow

Holbrook M, Skilbeck CE 1993 An activities index for use with stroke patients. Age and Ageing 12:166–170

Hunt SM, McEwen J, McKenna SP 1985 Measuring health status: a new tool for clinicians and epidemiologists. Journal of the Royal College of General Practitioners 35:185–188

Jenkinson C, Wright L, Coulter A 1994 Criterion validity and reliability of the SF-36 in a population sample. Quality of Life Research 3:7–12

King's Fund 1988 Treatment of stroke. British Medical Journal 297:126–128

Larson J 1997 The MOS 36-Item Short Form Health Survey. A conceptual analysis. Evaluation and the Health Professions 20:14–27

Law M, Letts L 1989 A critical review of scales of activities of daily living. American Journal of Occupational Therapy 43(8):522–528

Liang MH, Katz JN, Ginsburg KS 1990 Chronic rheumatic disease. In: Spiller B (ed) Quality of life assessments in clinical trials. Raven Press, New York

Lincoln N, Gladman J 1992 The Extended Activities of Daily Living Scale: a further validation. Disability and Rehabilitation 14:41–43

Livingstone MG, Livingstone HM 1985 The Glasgow Assessment Schedule: clinical and research assessment of head injury outcome. International Rehabilitation Medicine 7:146–149

Mahoney FI, Barthel DW 1965 Functional evaluation: the Barthel Index. Maryland State Medical Journal 14:61–65

Mathias S, Nayak USL, Isaacs B 1986 Balance in elderly patients: The "Get-up and Go" test. Archives of Physical Medicine and Rehabilitation 67:383–389

Mathias S, Bates M, Pasta D et al 1997 Use of Health Utilities Index with stroke patients and their caregivers. Stroke 28:1888–1894

McCloy L, Jongbloed L 1987 Robinson-Bashall Functional Assessment for arthritis patients: reliability and validity. Archives of Physical Medicine and Rehabilitation 68:486–489

McDowell F, Lee JE, Swift T 1970 Treatment of Parkinson's syndrome with L dihydroxyphenylalanine (levodopa). Annals of Internal Medicine 72:29–35

McDowell I, Newell C 1996 Measuring health. A guide to rating scales and questionnaires, 2nd edn. Oxford University Press, Oxford

Nakamura D, Holm M, Wilson A 1998 Measures of balance and fear of falling in the elderly: a review. Physical and Occupational Therapy in Geriatrics 15:17–32

Niemi M, Laaksonen R, Kotila M et al 1988 Quality of life four years after stroke. Stroke 19(9):1101–1106

Nouri F, Lincoln N 1987 An extended activities of daily living scale for stroke patients. Clinical Rehabilitation 1:301–305

Prosser L, Canby A 1997 Further validation of the Elderly Mobility Scale for measurement of mobility of hospitalised elderly people. Clinical Rehabilitation 11:338–343

Rodgers H, Curless R, James OFW 1993 Standardised functional assessment scales for elderly patients. Age and Ageing 22:161–163

Smith R 1994 Validation and reliability of the Elderly Mobility Scale. Physiotherapy 80:744–747

Spilg E, Martin B, Mitchell S et al 2001 A comparison of mobility assessments in a geriatric day hospital. Clinical Rehabilitation 15:296–300

Spilg E, Martin B, Mitchell S et al 2003 Falls risk following discharge from a geriatric day hospital. Clinical Rehabilitation 17:334–340

Talamo J, Frater A, Gallivan S et al 1997 Use of the Short Form 36 (SF36) for health status measurement in rheumatoid arthritis. British Journal of Rheumatology 36:463–469

Üstün T, Chatterji S, Bickenbach J et al 2003 The international classification of functioning, disability and health: a new tool for understanding disability and health. Disability and Rehabilitation 25:565–571

Van Knippenberg FCE, de Haes JCJM 1985 The quality of life of cancer patients: a review of the literature. Social Science and Medicine 20:809–817

Wade DT 1992 Measurement in neurological rehabilitation. Oxford University Press, Oxford

Wall J 2000 The timed get up and go test revisited: measurement of the component tasks. Journal of Rehabilitation Research and Development 37(1):109–114

Ware J, Sherbourne C 1992 The MOS 36-Item Short Form Health Survey (SF36). 1. Conceptual framework and item selection. Medical Care 30:473–481

Wenger NK, Furberg CD 1990 Cardiovascular disorders. In: Spiller B (ed) Quality of life assessments in clinical trials. Raven Press, New York

World Health Organisation 2001 International classification of functioning, disability and health. World Health Organisation, Geneva

Wyller T, Sveen U, Sodring K et al 1997 Subjective well-being one year after stroke. Clinical Rehabilitation 11:139–145

Chapter 10

Function of the lower limb

Marion Trew

LEARNING OUTCOMES

When you have completed this chapter you should be able to:

1. Recognise the normal patterns of movement for rising from a chair

2. Discuss the importance of walking

3. Identify the characteristics of normal gait

4. Describe the gait cycle

5. Recognise the joint movements and muscle activity that occur in normal gait

6. Recognise the normal patterns of movement for ascending and descending stairs.

INTRODUCTION

The main functions of the lower limbs are to support the body when standing and to enable locomotion. To be able to stand and move is a key part of normal, active life and it is important to have a detailed understanding of the normal function of the lower limbs in order to plan purposeful activity or rehabilitation programmes. In this chapter getting out of a chair, walking and stair climbing are considered in some detail as they represent major functions of the lower limb. There are interesting similarities in the patterns of movement between these apparently different activities and these patterns are repeated in other activities not covered by this book. Although this chapter is primarily concerned with lower limb function, it is impossible to ignore the movement patterns that occur in the rest of the body during sitting, standing and stair climbing. Some consideration will be given to patterns of movement in the upper limbs and spine, though not in as much detail as the lower limbs. This is partially because it is beyond the scope of this chapter but also because it is an aspect of human movement that has not attracted the attention of the research scientists and as a consequence our knowledge is somewhat limited.

MOVING FROM SITTING TO STANDING

The ability to rise from sitting to standing is essential for the achievement of many everyday activities. It is the key that opens the door to movement and without this ability, standing and locomotor activities are virtually unattainable. Given its importance, it is surprising that the movement has not been studied in greater depth. It is also noticeable that in some therapy departments considerable emphasis is placed on re-educating walking and little time is expended on guiding the patients towards independence in standing up. The importance of being able to stand up from the seated position cannot be denied and the maintenance of this ability or its re-education must be a primary rehabilitation goal.

There are patterns of joint movement and muscle activity during rising from a chair that are

---

Task 10.1

It is important to be aware of the different ways in which people get out of chairs. Watch people, particularly in relaxed situations, and note the different ways in which they rise from a chair. Work out what abilities they need (joint range, muscle function, balance) in order to stand up in both a 'conventional' and a 'non-conventional' manner.

Are you able to notice any differences in the way older and younger people rise from chairs?

---

normally stored as motor programmes in the motor cortex of the brain. Consequently, for the majority of the population, getting out of a chair is an automatic activity requiring no thought. It is only when the chair is particularly low or deep or the individual is feeling tired or weak that the activity requires conscious thought in order to complete. Varying the seat height or depth will change the range of lower limb joint movement and the amount of energy but the pattern of movement remains essentially the same (Janssen et al 2002). For older people a seat height of no less than 120% of leg length is recommended, though it should not be forgotten that some fit older people can rise from the squatting position.

Whether the upper limbs are involved in the process of getting out of a chair depends on the strength of the individual, the height of the chair and the presence of armrests. Under normal circumstances the upper limbs are not essential to the activity and can be used for carrying or manipulating objects during the activity of standing up or sitting down. However, if weakness, balance problems or pain are factors then the upper limbs will be used to assist. It is estimated that the force production by the hip and knee extensor muscles can be reduced by about 50% if armrests are used (Janssen et al 2002).

The movement of sitting to standing can be divided into two phases – a seated phase and a stance phase – both of which occur whether or not armrests are used (Fig. 10.1). In the seated phase, the subject prepares for standing by adjusting the position of the limbs and trunk to cause the centre of gravity to move forward until it is almost over the feet. In the stance phase, weight is taken through the lower limbs as the centre of gravity is transferred forwards and upwards. There are two main subdivisions to the stance phase: first, the transfer component as the centre of gravity is transferred forwards until it is slightly in front of the ankle joint and then the extension component when the lower limbs extend until the erect posture is achieved.

The period of time needed to complete the seated and stance phases is very variable but takes on average 1–3 seconds (Baer & Ashburn 1995, Kerr et al 1991). The seated phase consists of about 30% of the total movement time and in the stance

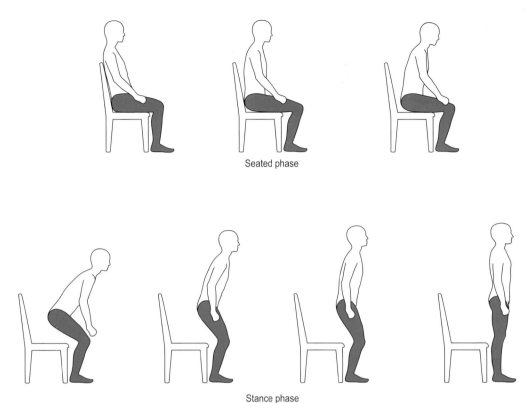

Seated phase

Stance phase

Figure 10.1   The pattern of movement when rising from a chair.

phase the transfer and extension components take 20% and 50% respectively.

Seated phase

Usually people sitting in a relaxed manner lean against the back of the chair with their centre of gravity well behind their feet. This is a very stable position as the whole chair forms the base of support. As the person stands, the feet become the base of support and for balance to be achieved, the centre of gravity must be moved horizontally until it is directly above them. The seated phase has two important components: first, that of positioning the body correctly in anticipation of weight transfer from the seat to the feet and second, the development of momentum to assist the muscles in achieving the upright position.

The ideal preparatory position for standing up is with the knees flexed between 90° and 115° so that the feet are placed under, or slightly behind, the knee joints. By having the feet well back, energy is conserved because the horizontal distance that the centre of gravity has to travel is minimised. Conversely if the feet are placed too far back the knee extensors will be in a lengthened position and may not be at their optimum length to generate force. It is suggested that the feet should not be placed more than 10 cm behind an imaginary perpendicular line dropped from the knee (Ikeda et al 1991, Shepherd & Koh 1996). If the person has been sitting in a chair with the knees relatively extended, then a substantial amount of knee flexion has to occur before a successful attempt at standing up can begin. This usually occurs simultaneously with the initiation of forward movement of the trunk; as the feet move backwards, the head moves forwards.

By the start of the stance phase the centre of gravity needs to be about 2 cm anterior to the ankle joints. To achieve this position the hips have to be flexed to about 120° and as the hips flex the head and trunk move anteriorly (Mak et al 2003, Shepherd & Koh 1996). In normal subjects there is an initial contraction of the hip flexors in order to initiate the movement and the anterior abdominal muscles contract isometrically to ensure that the trunk follows the hip movement. Once the hip joints have passed 90°, the flexors relax and momentum and the force of gravity cause the movement to continue. Towards the end of the hip flexion phase there may be slight eccentric activity of the hip extensors to control the forward movement (Ikeda et al 1991, Kelly et al 1976). In obese people where the flesh of the abdomen comes into contact with the thighs, or in people who have 'stiffness' of the hip joint, the activity of the hip flexors will need to continue throughout the movement. In these cases, considerable effort may be needed to achieve the required amount of hip flexion. Some further knee flexion may occur at the end of this phase and this will in turn cause slight passive dorsiflexion.

Task 10.2

Here are three small tasks that will enable you to test the importance of transferring the centre of gravity over the feet before standing up:

1. Sit comfortably in an easy chair. Move your bottom slightly towards the front of the chair, lean back and relax. Now try and stand up without leaning forward; you may use your arms if you wish.
2. To make it easier, now sit upright towards the front of the chair; don't lean back against the chair. Your hips should be at a right angle. Concentrate hard on your hip angle and see if you can stand up without allowing that angle to decrease (without leaning forwards).
3. Finally sit well back on the chair. In this position, look carefully at how much flexion you have at your hip joints. If you lean forward your centre of gravity will translate anteriorly, so you can use changes in hip angle to judge if you are leaning forward. So, stand up naturally and note, or get a friend to note, what happens to your hip angle in a normal movement.

Very little motion is seen in the joints of the vertebral column. Schenkman (1990) reported between 0° and 16° of trunk flexion in this phase and Baer and Ashburn (1995) found negligible trunk lateral flexion and rotation. The greatest ranges of movement occur in the cervical spine, which appears to have two functions. Initially in the seated phase it flexes, carrying the head forwards as part of the process of developing the momentum that will translate the centre of gravity over the feet. Then as the seated phase comes to an end and the stance phase commences, the function of the cervical spine appears to be to keep the vertex of the skull uppermost and the eyes horizontal. A pattern of movement at the cervical spine is identifiable and the overall range of movement is, on average, about 30° (Fig. 10.2).

If the upper limbs are not being used to push up from the chair arms, they usually flex between 11° and 53° at the shoulder joint. This combination of trunk and shoulder movement serves to move the centre of gravity forwards and also provides horizontal momentum which will contribute to the transfer of body weight onto the feet and be translated into a vertical movement as the lower limbs extend (Riley et al 1991).

The seated phase ends with the lift-off from the chair. There is considerable variation in the degree of flexion at the hip and shoulder joints during this phase and also in the exact position of the head. The velocity of the movement also varies between individuals and under different circumstances. The height of the chair relative to the subject's leg length, the age of the subject and the

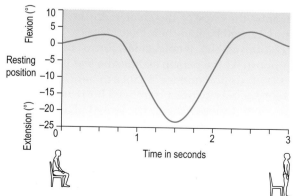

Figure 10.2 The pattern of cervical flexion and extension when rising from a chair.

degree of joint mobility and muscle strength all have effects on the velocity of movement (Kerr et al 1991). Despite this variability, there is an optimum speed for rising from a chair. Too fast is likely to induce loss of balance and require excessive muscle force to prevent an unwanted step or fall. If the speed is too slow the momentum needed to assist the transfer of weight from the seat to the lower limbs will not be achieved and either the activity will fail or excessive amounts of energy will be required for successful completion. In older people the ability to develop momentum is often lost and when this is combined with age-related joint stiffness and muscle weakness, it is quite obvious why they find rising from a chair very difficult.

Stance phase

The stance phase can be subdivided into transfer and extension components.

Transfer

This begins on lift-off from the seat and continues until the centre of gravity is about 7 cm anterior to the ankle joints, where it will remain until the erect posture is achieved (Ikeda et al 1991, Kelly et al 1976). The transfer component takes about 20% of the total time needed to rise from a chair and is completed in advance of hip and knee joint extension. There is peak quadriceps and hip extensor activity at the instant of lift-off when the knees and hips extend to raise the body off the seat. Dorsiflexion of the ankle joints reaches its maximum during this phase.

The trunk and upper limbs continue the horizontal movement begun in the seated phase and the momentum developed in the seated phase carries the centre of gravity forwards until it is substantially in front of the ankle joints. As the trunk moves forwards, the cervical spine extends through a range of about 25° in order that the head can be positioned appropriately and the eyes can look straight ahead (see Fig. 10.2).

The forward transfer of weight is completed relatively quickly but it is vital to the whole process as standing is not possible until the centre of gravity is positioned over the feet. It is a time of peak muscle activity in the knee and hip extensors and also a time of instability because the body is no longer supported by the seat and the centre of gravity is moving forwards. Failure to complete the transfer phase is one of the main reasons why people are unable to stand up from a chair.

Extension

Once the centre of gravity is positioned over the feet, vertical movement replaces horizontal. Extension of the hips and knees begins in earnest and there is also slight plantarflexion of the ankle joints. As the joints become progressively extended, the trunk also starts to extend and the cervical spine flexes to keep the vertex of the skull uppermost. The upper limbs relax and return to their normal resting position. The very last part of this activity again involves the cervical spine. Once the lower limbs and the trunk are vertical there is a small phase of flexion and extension in the cervical spine as final head position is adjusted.

Rising from a chair is an important functional activity that requires greater joint range and muscle torque than walking and most stair climbing (Kelly et al 1976). To be successful, it is necessary to have more than 100° of flexion at the hip and knee joints and virtually full-range dorsiflexion. It is also necessary to have good balance because the centre of gravity is moving in relation to the base of support. If the relationship of the centre of gravity to the feet is not correct, the individual is likely to lose balance and fall. Flexibility of the cervical spine is particularly important because balance requires correct head positioning and, if the vertebral column is stiff, then the appropriate positions may not be achieved.

The individual must also have the strength and the balance ability to complete the transfer phase, which is arguably the most crucial part of the whole process.

Forces required to rise from a chair

The energy requirements for rising from a chair are higher than for walking because the muscles have to raise most of the body weight vertically through a distance of about a metre. The greatest force production is found immediately upon lift-

10.1 Clinical considerations

Failure of one or more muscle groups to work can result in quite dramatic gait abnormalities. Weakness of the hip abductor muscles is quite common and will make it difficult for patients to keep their pelvis level during the stance phase. Under these circumstances the pelvis may drop to the unsupported side producing a 'Trendelenburg gait'. Such a gait is often quite uncomfortable for patients; to avoid discomfort, they may laterally flex their trunk towards the stance side. This shifts their centre of gravity over the stance limb and the pelvis no longer drops painfully to the unsupported side. A very obvious lateral movement of the upper trunk is apparent when observing this sort of gait.

Paralysis of the dorsiflexors will lead to a high stepping gait. Dorsiflexion is normally needed to ensure that the toes will clear the floor in the swing phase and dorsiflexion is also needed to facilitate heel strike. When patients cannot dorsiflex, they have to increase the range of hip and knee flexion in the swing phase in order to avoid dragging their toes on the ground. Under these circumstances, heel strike is not possible and the patient's toes hit the ground first with the heel slapping down immediately afterwards. If you look at the shoes of a patient who has paralysis of the dorsiflexors, you will find that the toe area on the affected side is excessively scuffed and worn.

Task 10.3

It is important to develop good observational abilities. Most people are better at observing human movement than they realise. Interestingly, the general population can recognise someone they know well even when that person is too far away to make out facial details. It is likely that at a subconscious level we are aware of the small differences in the ways that people move. In the case of walking we probably store information about the transverse and coronal plane movements and use this to distinguish between different individuals when we are too far away from them to see their faces. Next time you are in a suitable place, watch the way in which people walk and see if you can work out how the gait of one individual differs from another. In particular, you should observe the degree of knee flexion and extension in the stance phase and the rotation and lateral flexion of the trunk. Are the differences in gait between individuals simply a consequence of different walking velocities?

off from the seat with quadriceps torque being around 1.1 Nm/kg/m and hip extensor torque of approximately 0.9 Nm/kg/m (Mak et al 2003). Differences have been found between the forces generated by the hip flexors and the ankle dorsiflexors in younger and older adults. It appears that younger adults produce substantially more hip flexor torque in the seated phase than do elderly subjects. This may be explained by the fact that younger adults have good balance and are comfortable with generating substantial momentum when rising from a chair as they are not in danger of falling. Older people not only have poorer balance but also have a fear of falling and may tend to avoid rapid movements when they are changing position (Mak et al 2003, Pai & Rogers 1991).

WALKING

Human beings can perform many types of locomotion including walking, running and, less commonly, crawling, hopping, jumping and even rolling. The diversity of locomotion is even greater when you consider that each of these movements can be performed in a variety of ways and directions. Despite this variety, all these methods of locomotion have common patterns of movement and by studying normal walking in detail, it becomes easier to understand the rest.

Walking is a highly energy-efficient method of progression involving rhythmical, reciprocal movements of the lower limbs where one foot is always in contact with the floor. People normally walk for a purpose, perhaps because they want to reach a certain place at a certain time but they may also walk for pleasure and for health. Increasingly, walking is being advocated as a safe and effective way of maintaining fitness, particularly in the later years of life (Arakawa 1993, Hardman & Hudson 1994, Pereira et al 1998) and in many countries walking for pleasure and health is a popular pastime. Providing walking speeds of more than 6 km/h are achieved and hills are incorporated into the route, walking maintains reasonable ranges of lower limb joint motion and a functional level of cardiorespiratory fitness.

Although to most people walking is fully automatic and requires no thought, it actually comprises complex patterns of movement involving all lower limb joints. In addition, there is movement of the joints of the vertebral column, from lumbar to cervical spine and, when unrestricted, the upper limbs swing in a reciprocal pattern. This involvement of all the body segments requires considerable neural control and this explains why, at birth when the nervous system is not fully developed, walking is impossible. It is not until the infant has gained control over all body parts and is able to balance that the first uncertain steps can be taken. Even then, the child is unable to walk while carrying objects and may be 7 or 8 years old before the activity becomes mature and fully automatic.

In the health-care professions it is quite common for the term 'gait' to be used in preference to walking. 'Gait' means the manner or way in which walking takes place and implies a detailed consideration of the kinetics and kinematics of the activity.

Basically, all people walk in the same way, with the lower limbs moving reciprocally to provide alternate support and propulsion, and if the upper limbs are unencumbered, they demonstrate a stereotyped pattern of reciprocal movement in phase with the lower limbs. The joint movements that occur in the sagittal plane (flexion and extension) are very similar in both range and direction of movement between individuals (Murray et al 1964). The differences that set one person's gait apart from another's occur mainly in movements in the coronal and transverse planes. For example, the amount of hip rotation and therefore foot angle can vary dramatically between individuals and noticeable variation also occurs in trunk lateral flexion. The range of trunk rotation in the transverse plane is variable, with some people having almost imperceptible rotation and others rotating through such a wide range that they appear to be swaggering (Murray et al 1964, Smidt 1990).

Walking is a smooth, highly coordinated, rhythmical movement by which the body moves step by step in the required direction. The forces that cause this movement are a combination of muscle activity to accelerate or decelerate the body segments and the effects of gravity and momentum.

Walking has often been described as a fall followed by a reflex recovery of balance and, to a certain extent, this is true. To initiate the first step the anterior muscles at the ankle contract to move the centre of gravity forwards in relation to the feet and this causes a loss of balance anteriorly. Once the centre of gravity has been displaced, gravity and momentum continue the movement initiated by the muscles. In order to avoid a fall, there is a reflex stepping reaction which causes one of the lower limbs to be moved forwards so that one foot can be placed in front of the other. This alters the base so that the centre of gravity is once again above the feet. If walking is to continue, the centre of gravity must again be displaced anteriorly. However, once inertia has been overcome by muscle action on the first step, all subsequent steps benefit from the momentum accrued and only a minor amount of propulsion comes from the calf muscles. For each step, balance is disturbed so that a subsequent, reflex step will occur. This continues until the purpose of walking has been achieved and, because the momentum involved in walking removes the need for much muscle activity, the whole process is remarkably energy efficient.

Once a steady walking velocity has been reached, the actual process of walking requires low energy expenditure and it is possible to walk for long periods of time with surprisingly little fatigue (McArdle et al 2001, Smidt 1990). As would be expected, the least energy is expended when walking at a moderate speed on level ground but an increase in velocity or a change from a firm surface to a surface such as soft sand would immediately increase energy expenditure. There are two other instances in walking on level ground when energy expenditure is relatively high. Energy expenditure is higher on the initiation of movement, when inertia has to be overcome so that the body weight can be displaced forwards, than it is during a continuous sequence of steps. Conversely, at the end of walking an increase in energy expen-

Task 10.4

Analyse the effects of using a walking frame. Consider the gait of a patient using a quadruped walking frame. Is the smooth, rhythmical, reciprocal movement of normal gait preserved? Will using a walking frame conserve or increase energy expenditure? How do you think the energy expenditure needed for walking with a frame would compare with the energy needed for walking, fully weight bearing, with crutches?

diture is required to stop forward movement of the limbs and trunk. The faster an individual walks, the more difficult it is to stop suddenly and this causes a greater expenditure of energy.

Understanding the role of inertia and momentum in walking is important as the energy-efficient nature of the activity is lost if momentum is restricted and the walker is constantly having to overcome inertia either to initiate or stop the movement. You are probably already aware of this as you must have noticed that you feel disproportionately tired after a day wandering around the shops. When people go shopping, particularly when they are not strongly focused on what they need to buy, they constantly stop to look at goods and then move on. The repeated stopping and starting involved in shopping can be surprisingly

tiring. Re-education programmes for weak people should aim to develop the rhythm of gait and the smooth swinging motion of the upper and lower limbs so that they can benefit fully from an energy-efficient gait. As they develop strength then walking can be made more difficult by introducing stairs and slopes and by disrupting the normal rhythmical patterns.

Terminology of gait

Walking is a complex activity and if it is to be fully understood, it needs to be broken down into phases. There are a number of ways in which gait can be described and the most commonly used international terminology is given here. It is useful to consider gait in terms of both the temporal and spatial components. The temporal components are those periods of time during which events take place and are often measured in seconds. For example, the stance phase of walking is a temporal component and relates to the period of time that the foot is in contact with the floor. The spatial components refer to the position or distances covered by the limbs and an example of this would be step length. When analysing gait it is essential to consider both the temporal and spatial components because disease or trauma can affect either. The temporal components are illustrated in Figure 10.3.

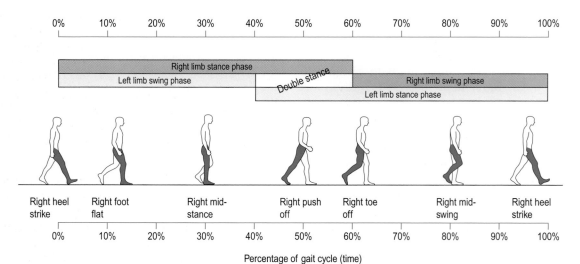

Figure 10.3 Terminology and timing of the gait cycle.

Table 10.1   Alternative terminologies used to describe gait

Terminology suitable for describing the temporal components of normal gait	Terminology suitable for describing the temporal components of pathological gait
Stance phase	Stance phase
Heel strike	Initial foot–floor contact
Foot flat	Loading phase
Mid stance	Mid stance
Heel-off	Propulsive phase
Push-off	Propulsive phase
Toe-off	Pre-swing
Swing phase	Swing phase
Acceleration	Acceleration
Mid swing	Mid swing
Deceleration	Deceleration

Table 10.1 illustrates two common approaches to the terminology of gait. Most of the descriptors for normal gait refer to events in the gait cycle which may be absent in pathological gait and so alternative terminology is needed. For example, a person with a painful, sprained ankle is unlikely to demonstrate heel strike but to make initial foot–floor contact with the whole foot. A person with increased tone in the lower limbs may be unable to move out of plantarflexion and so never achieves foot flat. For these reasons some authorities like to use gait terminology which is equally applicable for normal or pathological gaits.

Gait cycle

This is the period of time during which a complete sequence of events takes place. Whilst it is usual to consider the gait cycle as beginning when the heel of one foot strikes the floor and continuing until the same heel strikes the floor again, it may be measured from any moment in the gait cycle. The gait cycle is subdivided into a stance phase and a swing phase and these terms describe the periods of time when the foot is either in contact with the floor or swinging forward in preparation for the next step. The swing phase is the period of time when the limb under consideration is not in contact with the floor. The stance phase is the period of time when the limb under consideration is in contact with the floor. In walking there is always a period of time when both feet are in contact with the floor simultaneously and this is called 'double stance' (see Fig. 10.3).

Stance phase

The stance phase is the most complex and arguably the most important phase of gait. During the stance phase the lower limb has to provide a semi-rigid support for the body weight, facilitate balance and allow forward propulsion. The stance limb also has a role in compensating for uneven ground and when positioned correctly, it enables an accurate swing phase on the contralateral limb to take place. The stance phase can be subdivided into the following stages.

Heel strike or initial foot–floor contact   In normal walking the leading limb initially contacts the floor by heel strike. At the moment of heel strike the following limb is also in contact with the floor, giving a position of double stance. This is the moment when the whole-body centre of gravity is at its lowest and the walker is most stable (Fig. 10.4).

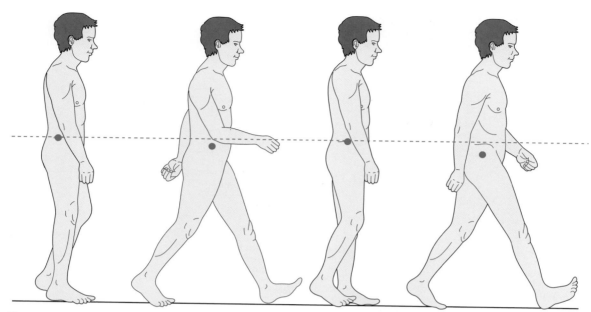

Figure 10.4 Vertical displacement of the centre of gravity when walking with an extended stride.

Foot flat or loading phase Immediately on coming into contact with the floor, the stance limb takes the body weight. To be effective in supporting the body weight, the foot has to move rapidly to plantigrade from the position of dorsiflexion at heel strike. At foot flat the whole foot comes into contact with the floor, allowing it to accept the weight of the body as the mid-stance phase takes place. During heel strike and foot flat there is rapid loading of the limb and it is important that during this phase strategies exist to absorb the sudden imposition of ground reaction forces.

Mid stance In mid stance the body is carried forward over the stance limb and the opposite limb is in the swing phase. The whole-body centre of gravity passes from behind to in front of the stance foot and it is in mid stance that the centre of gravity rises to its highest position in relation to the supporting surface. This is the position when the walker is least stable due to the small base of support and the relatively high centre of gravity.

Heel–off, push–off and toe–off or the propulsive phase There are now several events that happen in quick succession, all of which are designed to propel the body forwards and terminate the stance phase. Initially, the heel lifts off the ground, an event which is passive in slow gait but may require a small degree of muscle activity from the plantarflexor muscles at faster velocities. This is usually followed by a propulsive stage when the same muscles contract to plantarflex the forefoot against the floor and this is called 'push-off'. Finally there is the moment of 'toe-off' when propulsion ends, the contact between the toes and the floor is lost and the swing phase for that limb starts.

At an average speed, the stance phase takes about 60% of the gait cycle and the swing phase about 40% (Murray 1967) but the relative percentages vary as the speed of walking increases or decreases. In slow walking the stance phase can constitute more than 70% of the gait cycle with the swing phase being less than 30%. As the velocity of walking increases, the length of time in the stance phase decreases until on very fast walking, the stance phase may be reduced below 57% of the cycle (Smidt 1990). The period of double stance also decreases with increasing velocity. When walking very slowly, the double stance may last as long as 46% of the total gait cycle; on very fast walking the double-stance period may be reduced to 14%, and when walking develops into a run, there is no double-stance period.

Swing phase

During the swing phase, the swinging limb moves in front of the stance limb so that forward progression may take place. In order to swing successfully, the limb must be shortened sufficiently to enable the foot to clear the ground and this is normally achieved by flexion of the hip and knee joints and dorsiflexion of the ankle. Clearing the ground is key to a successful swing phase, but to conserve energy it is important that the limb is not lifted further than is necessary. In normal adult gait the average clearance of the foot from the ground in mid-swing phase is around 2 cm and with so little leeway for error, it is quite remarkable that people do not catch their feet on the floor more often. The swing phase can be divided into three stages.

Acceleration   The force generated by the hip flexors, and to a lesser extent by the plantarflexors, accelerates the non-weight bearing limb forwards.

Mid swing   This corresponds with mid stance and it is at its shortest at the moment the swing phase limb passes the stance limb.

Deceleration   In this final stage of the swing phase, the lower limb muscles work to decelerate the swing limb in preparation for heel strike. The muscle action in this phase is usually eccentric and requires less energy than those times in the gait cycle when concentric activity is needed to accelerate a limb.

Other temporal and spatial components

Cadence   When considering pathological gait, a knowledge of the step rate is important and the term 'cadence' is used to indicate the number of steps taken per minute. The cadence mainly depends on the velocity of walking. In slow walking the cadence may be 40–50 steps per minute, whereas moderate walking will cause an increase in cadence to around 110 steps per

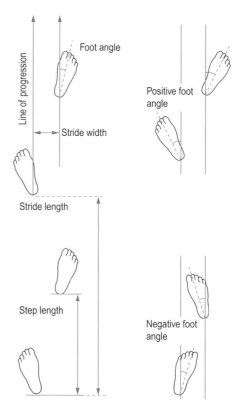

Figure 10.5   Characteristics of gait that can be measured from footprints.

minute and this figure will rise with increasing velocity until running occurs. If a patient has pain, joint stiffness, muscle weakness or poor balance, the cadence will be reduced. An increase in natural cadence is often taken to indicate an improvement in a patient's walking ability but it might be more appropriate to use the patient's ability to vary cadence as an indicator of walking skill.

The gait cycle contains a number of spatial components that are commonly measured as part of the analysis of gait (Fig. 10.5).

Stride length   This is the distance between successive foot-to-floor contacts with the same foot. For example, this might be the distance between the first point of contact of the right heel on the floor and the next point of contact of the right heel.

Step length   This is the distance between successive foot-to-floor contact with opposite feet. In this case, it could be the distance (in the line of progression) between the point of right heel strike and the point of left heel strike. There are two steps to every stride.

Step and stride length are dependent on several factors including the length of the lower limb, the age of the subject and the velocity of walking. Short lower limb length, increasing age and decreasing velocity will all reduce the step and stride length. Restriction in the range of hip flexion and/or extension is also a common reason for reduced step and stride length.

Foot angle   This is the degree of in-turning or out-turning of the foot: if the foot turns in there is said to be a negative foot angle; if the foot turns out, the angle is positive. The majority of the population walk with a positive foot angle of up to 30°. This angle is mainly associated with the degree of rotation at the hip joint and, to a lesser extent, the rotation between the tibia and the femur. In some cases tibial or femoral torsion will influence foot angle.

Stride or step width   This is the distance between the two feet and it is normally measured from the midpoint of the heels. This distance varies greatly between individuals and can vary between individual steps if the ground is uneven, but on average it is about 7 cm; however, when people have poor balance they tend to increase their stride width to give themselves a greater base of support. It is interesting to note that on slow walking the stride width tends to be greater than on rapid walking.

Joint and muscle activity in the stance phase

As shown in Figure 10.6, the pattern of joint movement is less complicated at the hip joint than the knee or ankle joints. Whilst the hip joint has only one phase of extension and one phase of flexion, the other two joints have two phases of each movement in each gait cycle. The range of movement at the hip and knee joints is more consistent between individuals but the movement at the ankle joint can be quite variable between one person and another.

Muscle activity, as indicated by electromyography, shows variability between subjects and also when different walking velocities are chosen. A guide to the common patterns of major muscle activity is given in Figure 10.7; the data for this were gathered from subjects walking at a moderate pace. It is interesting to note that in a substantial portion of the gait cycle there is little or no muscle activity occurring in the majority of the muscle groups. This supports the theory that gait is energy efficient.

Heel strike

At the instant of heel strike the hip joint is partially flexed and gluteus maximus and the hamstrings contract immediately to initiate hip extension. The knee joint will either be in full extension or flexed to about 5° and the quadriceps will be working eccentrically to control the knee flexion which follows immediately after heel strike. The ankle joint on heel strike is usually near the neutral position, though there can be a variation between individuals of up to 10° of dorsiflexion or plantarflexion. More than 10° of plantarflexion would be rare in a normal individual as it would render heel strike difficult and leave the toes vulnerable to stubbing on the floor. This position is produced prior to heel strike by concentric action of the dorsiflexor muscles and on heel strike there is an immediate change to eccentric activity to lower the forefoot to the floor. At the metatarsophalangeal joints there is a similar pattern of activity with the muscles positioning the joints in extension ready for heel strike and then lowering the toes into floor contact.

Foot flat

The hip joint is beginning to move into extension by concentric action of the hip extensors but the knee joint has flexed further in order to cushion the effect of heel strike and also to reduce the vertical displacement of the centre of gravity that would otherwise occur as the body passes over the stance limb. This knee flexion is controlled by eccentric work of the quadriceps group and measurements of knee movement taken in our laboratory show it can often be as great as 30°. At the ankle joint there is controlled plantarflexion to

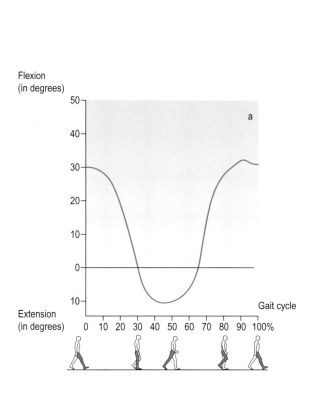

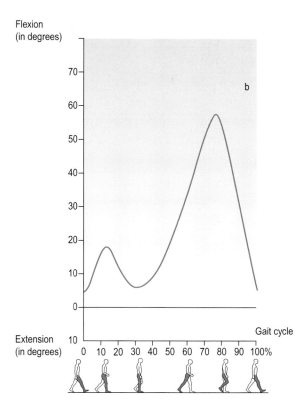

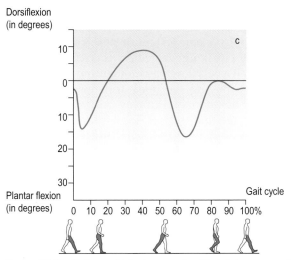

Figure 10.6   Pattern of hip, knee and ankle joint movement during a single gait cycle (walking velocity – 3.5 km/h). (a) Hip joint; (b) knee joint; (c) ankle joint.

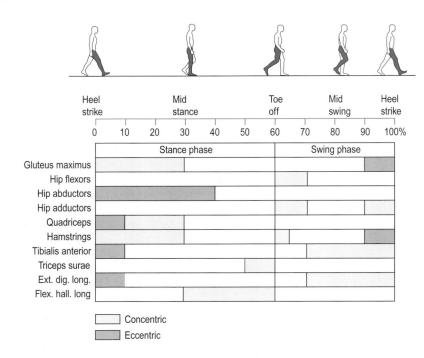

Heel strike | Mid stance | Toe off | Mid swing | Heel strike

0 10 20 30 40 50 60 70 80 90 100%

Stance phase | Swing phase

Gluteus maximus
Hip flexors
Hip abductors
Hip adductors
Quadriceps
Hamstrings
Tibialis anterior
Triceps surae
Ext. dig. long.
Flex. hall. long

☐ Concentric
▨ Eccentric

Figure 10.7 Muscle activity, as indicated by electromyography, is variable between subjects. It also varies with velocity and the faster the velocity, the more muscle input will be required. This figure shows the type and duration of muscle activity which might be expected in moderate velocity walking.

lower the foot to the floor which is undertaken by eccentric work of the dorsiflexors. Without controlled plantarflexion, the foot would 'slap' down uncomfortably and this can be heard in some patients. As the foot achieves good foot-to-floor contact there is a small amount of eversion to transfer the body weight across from the lateral border of the foot towards the great toe.

Mid stance

Hip extension continues but by now it is being produced by momentum and the muscles are no longer active. While the contralateral limb is in the swing phase, the pelvis is unsupported on that side and the hip abductors on the stance limb initially contract to control pelvic levels and lower the pelvis towards the swing side by eccentric muscle action. The knee joint remains in slight flexion. There is sometimes a minor burst of activity in the ankle dorsiflexors to pull the tibia forwards over the foot but once this movement has been initiated, momentum and gravity will take over. Depending on the velocity of the movement, the calf muscles may need to exert a slowing influence on the tibia through eccentric muscle action.

Heel–off, leading to push–off

At the beginning of this phase, the centre of gravity is in front of the stance foot so the force of gravity will increase the range of hip extension and ankle dorsiflexion. As full-range dorsiflexion is reached, the heel will rise off the floor and the plantarflexors will contract concentrically to provide the propulsive component of push-off. In slow to moderate walking velocities, this contraction is not usually very large as momentum is the major factor in moving the body forwards. In normal walking the hip extensors are only slightly active at this stage and, in fact, the hip and knee joints are usually starting to flex in preparation for the swing phase. At higher walking velocities the propulsion comes increasingly from the hip extensors, with the plantarflexors playing a major role in ankle stabilisation (Riley et al 2001).

Joint and muscle activity in the swing phase

Acceleration

Minor forces generated on push-off by the hip flexors and the plantarflexors accelerate the limb forwards in the swing phase assisted by momentum and gravity. The hip and knee joints are both flexing and there is a rapid movement towards dorsiflexion to ensure that the toes do not catch on the floor.

Mid swing

In mid-swing phase, flexion of the knee and hip joints continues to keep the foot sufficiently raised to avoid the toes catching on the floor. At this stage the foot may be lowered into slight plantarflexion.

Deceleration

The hip continues to flex, the movement being mainly produced by momentum and the hamstrings act eccentrically to slow down the movement at the hip joint. The knee joint moves from flexion to extension; it is interesting to note that the quadriceps play no part in this movement. The whole of the lower limb is being moved forwards by flexion of the hip and the resulting momentum causes knee joint extension. Towards the end of the deceleration phase, knee joint extension may have to be slowed down and this is achieved by eccentric action of the hamstrings. In preparation for heel strike, the dorsiflexors contract quite strongly to ensure that the foot is in the optimum position for heel strike.

Movement in the trunk, shoulder girdle and upper limbs

It is possible to walk with little movement of the trunk and no movement in the upper limbs but in these circumstances gait is awkward and tiring (Murray et al 1967). In the double-stance phase, when one hip is flexed and the other extended, the pelvis is rotated away from the lead limb. This causes some rotation of the lumbar spine towards the lead limb, which in turn leads to slight rotation of the thoracic and cervical spine in the opposite direction. The rotations in the spine are compensatory mechanisms designed to keep the head facing forwards. Stabilisation of head position in relation to the environment is an important factor in all lower limb activities. Normally the head is held in a fairly constant position in relation to the environment in order that visual information can be easily processed and balance maintained through unambiguous signals from the visual, vestibular and somatosensory receptors. If there is a functional need for the head to move excessively during gait then the head stabilisation mechanisms can be overridden but balance may be compromised (Mulavara et al 2002).

Reciprocal movements of the upper and lower limbs occur in unconstrained walking; for example, on heel strike the contralateral upper limb is in front of the body. Most movement occurs at the shoulder joint, with a lesser amount at the elbow, and normally the shoulder joint starts to flex or extend slightly before the same movement is seen in the elbow joint. The range of movement varies greatly between individuals and in the same individual it will vary according to the velocity of walking. Whereas the patterns of movement in the lower limb in the sagittal plane are very similar between individuals, they are more varied in the upper limb (Murray et al 1967). This is not surprising as the movement of the upper limb is not essential for the process of walking and the range of movement of upper limb joints is likely to be affected by the momentum imparted by the lower limbs and the degree of trunk rotation. There are several reasons why the upper limb moves during gait. It has been suggested that arm swing may impart momentum through the trunk to the lower limbs; subjective reports from fatigued walkers indicate that they have reduced the effort of walking by deliberately increasing their arm swing. It is also possible that arm swing acts to correct overrotation at the lumbar spine (Murray et al 1967).

Ground reaction forces in gait

Whenever the foot is in contact with the ground there will be vertical, anterior-posterior and mediolateral forces acting between the foot and the floor. Measurement of these forces using a force plate shows a consistent, intersubject pattern of vertical and anterior-posterior forces. The mediolateral forces are tiny and show much more variability between individuals (Fig. 10.8). At the beginning and end of the stance phase the vertical ground reaction forces are normally about 25%

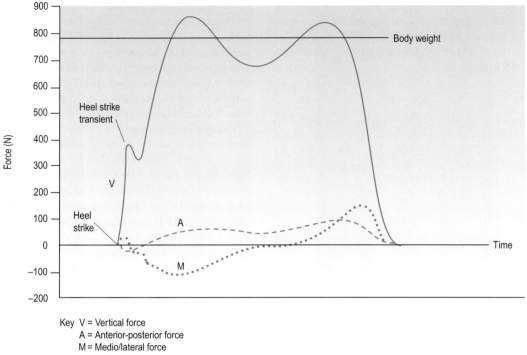

Key V = Vertical force
     A = Anterior-posterior force
     M = Medio/lateral force

Figure 10.8   Typical ground reaction force traces for an adult walking.

greater than body weight but much less than they would be in running. The anterior-posterior ground reaction forces are about 25% of body weight in each direction (Craik & Oatis 1995, Farley & Ferris 1998). With forces passing through the body on every step, there is the potential for injury. However, the relatively small forces involved, the structural mechanisms for shock absorption and the cushioning effect of knee flexion on initial foot–floor contact mean that repetitive strain injuries caused by ground reaction forces are rare in walking.

Energy expenditure and gait

The amount of energy required to walk at a comfortable pace is very small in comparison with other activities. Normal, easy walking on a firm surface requires about 0.080 kcal/min/kg. A gentle run requires 0.135 kcal/min/kg, swimming breast stroke requires 0.162 kcal/min/kg and playing squash 0.212 kcal/min/kg (McArdle et al 2001).

Task 10.5

This task will enable you to experience normal energy-efficient gait and compare it with disrupted gait where kinetic energy, potential energy and momentum are not used to their best effect.

Find somewhere where you can walk in a straight line for no less than 20 steps. Walk moderately quickly up and down your chosen area a few times, noting how much effort you need to complete this task. Now repeat the process but every third step you must stop completely and then restart at a quick pace. Make a comparison between the effort needed in the second task and that in the first task. If you walk far enough you may be able to measure differences in heart and respiratory rate between the two tasks.

Alterations in the normal structure of the human body or in the normal pattern of gait are likely to increase energy expenditure significantly. In normal gait, energy is conserved through the utilisation of momentum and kinetic and potential energy. There are rhythmical, vertical fluctuations of the centre of gravity in normal gait that produce similar fluctuations in kinetic energy and gravitational potential energy. In mid stance, when the centre of gravity is at its highest, gravitational potential energy is also at its highest and kinetic energy at its lowest. This situation is reversed during double stance and it is suggested that energy transfer mechanisms from the kinetic and potential energy contribute substantially to the overall energy requirements of gait (Farley & Ferris 1998). Figure 10.5 illustrates the vertical movements of the centre of gravity.

RUNNING

Running differs from walking in that there is no double-stance phase and there is a period when there is no foot-to-floor contact at all. In general terms, running and walking are very similar, though in running the movement is much quicker and the stride is lengthened. The vertical ground reaction forces generated are of the magnitude of 2.75–3.00 times body weight, which is considerably greater than walking, and heel strike may be replaced by toe strike (Farley & Ferris 1998). The trunk remains upright, although the line of gravity falls further outside the base than in walking. Movement of the upper limbs becomes essential and the elbows are more flexed than in walking.

10.2 Clinical considerations

Jogging is a common form of exercise and it can have a beneficial effect on joints. If a jogging style is adopted that encourages the hips and knees to move towards the limits of extension then it will stretch the flexor muscles and counteract the tendency of a sedentary life style to lead to slight hip and knee flexion contractures. Unfortunately many people choose to jog using relatively small steps that have no stretching effect at all. If you watch joggers you will see that the majority never fully extend the hips and knees.

WALKING BACKWARDS

Although it is uncommon for anyone to walk backwards for any great distance, it is necessary in everyday life to be able to take one or two steps in that direction. The pattern of joint movement is very similar to normal gait but the step length is reduced and heel strike is replaced by toe strike (Vilensky et al 1987).

WALKING UP AND DOWN STAIRS

This is a modified walking activity using similar patterns of joint movement and muscle action. There is a stance phase, a swing phase and a period of double support (Fig. 10.9). The activity is much more demanding than walking because the range of hip and knee joint movement is greater and there is considerable vertical translation of the centre of gravity (Andriacchi et al 1980, McFadyen & Winter 1988). The tibiofemoral forces, patellofemoral forces and anterior-posterior shear forces are considerably higher than in walking and therefore robust joint structures are needed if the activity is to be safely and painlessly performed (Costigan et al 2002). Stair ascent and descent have greater potential for falls than walking. In both these activities there is a single-stance phase when the body is in the most vulnerable position because the base of support is at its smallest. In stair activity, substantial vertical translation of the centre of gravity also occurs in single stance and this requires considerable muscular force. To achieve the single-stance component of stair activity requires good balance ability and for people whose balance is already challenged, they may be unable to go up and down stairs unless they have a banister for support.

When ascending stairs, the cycle is normally described as starting when the joints flex to place the foot on the step above. This is then followed by joint extension and the muscle activity is predominantly concentric. On stair descent the reverse pattern is seen. Most of the muscle activity is eccentric and the cycle is normally described as starting with the extended hip and knee positioning the foot on the step below, after which the joints move into flexion.

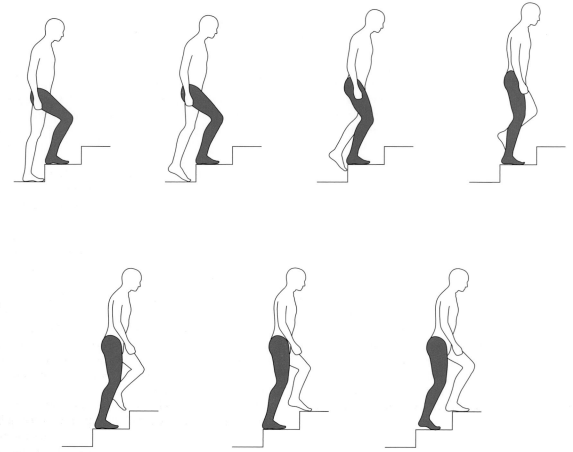

Figure 10.9   The pattern of movement in stair climbing.

Stance phase on ascent

This phase is sometimes referred to as 'pull-up' and it starts from the moment of foot contact on the step above. It is normally as long or longer than the stance phase in flat walking and has been reported at around 60% of the cycle (Riener et al 2002). In walking the first instance of foot-to-floor contact is through the heel but in stair ascent weight is initially taken on the anterior and middle third of the foot and then transferred to the remainder of the foot in readiness for full weight bearing.

On weight acceptance there is strong concentric contraction of the hip and knee extensors to extend the lead limb and raise the body up to and over the step. The forces generated are substantial. The quadriceps generate force at a level of around 1 Nm/kg/m, the greatest force occurring when the knee is flexed to about 60°. The vertical force through the tibia and also the compression force between the patella and the femur are estimated to be around three times body weight and may possibly be double that amount in some subjects (Costigan et al 2002). Gastrocnemius and soleus also work during the stance phase, moving the tibia posteriorly on the talus. As the single-support phase is entered, the hip abductors on the stance limb work strongly to prevent the pelvis dropping to the unsupported side and to pull the trunk laterally over the supporting limb.

In the latter part of the stance phase, when body weight is fully on the stance limb and the knee extended, the quadriceps work isometrically to maintain joint position while moving the centre of gravity in front of the stance foot. In some subjects the dorsiflexors undergo a low-magnitude contraction at this stage to facilitate the movement of the centre of gravity forwards.

In the final stages of the stance phase there is plantarflexion produced by strong contraction of gastrocnemius and soleus to accelerate the body forwards and upwards onto the new weight-bearing limb (Riener et al 2002). At this stage there is minimal activity in the knee and hip extensors (Andriacchi et al 1980, McFadyen & Winter 1988).

Swing phase on ascent

The swing limb must swing past the intermediate step and over the top step on which its stance will occur before the foot can be placed on that step. For this to occur, there has to be flexion of all the major lower limb joints, involving concentric work of the hip and knee flexors and the dorsiflexors. Early in the swing phase the hip joint flexes and the hamstrings flex the knee joint to pull the leg and foot posteriorly to achieve intermediate step clearance.

By mid swing the knee flexors are no longer contracting because the hip joint is sufficiently flexed to ensure intermediate step clearance. At this stage there may be some eccentric work of the quadriceps to control unwanted knee flexion.

In the later swing phase the hamstrings contract again to increase knee flexion so that the foot clears the top step, where it will eventually be placed. In order to avoid the foot catching on the top step, the amount of hip and knee flexion is quite extensive and this results in the foot being well above the step immediately before foot-to-step contact. To gain step contact the foot has to be lowered onto the step and this is achieved by slight hip extension controlled by eccentric activity of the hip flexors.

Through most of the swing phase, tibialis anterior works isometrically to hold the ankle joint in dorsiflexion so that the toe will not stub on the steps. Immediately before foot contact the dorsiflexors work eccentrically to lower the forefoot onto the step ready for weight acceptance on the forefoot (Andriacchi et al 1980, McFadyen & Winter 1988).

Stance phase on descent

The patterns of movement which occur when going downstairs are illustrated in Figure 10.10 and for convenience, they are subdivided into the weight acceptance phase and the lowering phase.

On weight acceptance, the initial foot contact is made with the anterior and lateral border of the foot. The ankle joint moves from the initial step-contact position of plantarflexion into a neutral or dorsiflexed position controlled by eccentric work of the calf muscles. The hip joints are in very slight flexion and the knee joint may flex up to 50° to cushion the instant of foot-to-step contact. This is controlled by eccentric work of the hip and knee extensors. The quadriceps then contract concentrically to extend the knee about 10° whilst the trunk moves horizontally to carry the centre of gravity over the stance limb. Tibialis anterior co-contracts with the calf muscles to control ankle position and to maintain weight bearing on the lateral border of the foot.

To lower the body weight (mid stance) to the next step entails controlled hip and knee joint flexion and ankle joint dorsiflexion. This mainly involves eccentric action of the quadriceps and, to a lesser degree, the calf muscles and hip extensors. The stance ankle is in maximum dorsiflexion with the body weight tending to force the movement further. To prevent over dorsiflexion at the joint, the plantarflexors may need to contract. Throughout this phase the hip abductors on the stance side maintain the level of the pelvis and pull the trunk over the stance limb.

Swing phase on descent

In the swing phase, the limb has to be raised off the higher step and swung forwards and downwards, clearing the intermediate step until it is in position to take weight at the start of the next cycle. The hip and knee flexors work concentrically to raise the foot off the top step and pull the limb forwards. Then the limb starts to extend ready for foot placement with eccentric work of

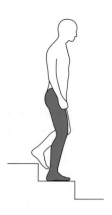 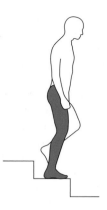 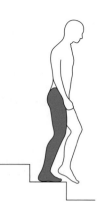

Figure 10.10 The pattern of movement in stair descent.

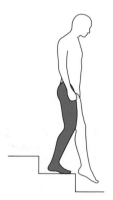 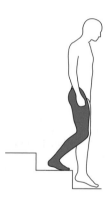 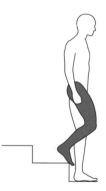

Task 10.6

Think about the ankle joint. Do you need the largest range of dorsiflexion when going up stairs or down stairs? Go up and down some stairs to see whether you have sufficient dorsiflexion to complete the task easily or whether you adopt a strategy to overcome lack of range. Talk to your friends because you may find a difference between individuals.

---

the hip flexors controlling hip extension and the hamstrings working eccentrically to decelerate the extension of the knee joint. The ankle joint drops into plantarflexion, controlled by eccentric work of the anterior tibial muscles which also maintain the foot in inversion in preparation for weight to be taken on the lateral border of the foot. The hip ipsilateral abductors contract just before the end of the swing phase in preparation for maintaining pelvic levels on weight acceptance (McFadyen & Winter 1988).

The amount of joint range needed for ascent and descent of stairs depends on the depth of tread. For standard-sized tread (16.5 cm), the hip joint must be able to move between full extension and about 60° of flexion, the range required at the knee joint is 0–100° of flexion and the ankle joint needs full dorsiflexion (McFadyen et al 1988, Tata et al 1983).

When going up stairs, the period of peak muscle torque and greatest instability occurs simulta-

10.3 Clinical considerations

You will be aware from your own personal experience that going up stairs requires much more energy than walking on the flat. The main problem is caused by the need to translate the centre of gravity vertically. In walking there are strategies to keep the vertical translation of the centre of gravity to a minimum but on stairs there is no choice because the centre of gravity must move through a substantial vertical distance. The largest amount of energy is expended on climbing stairs, although people will often feel that going down is the most difficult. Whilst stair descent uses less energy because the movement is in the direction of gravity and only requires control through eccentric muscle activity, it puts considerable strain on the knee joint. If people have problems with their patellofemoral joint then going down stairs becomes problematic. In addition going down stairs enables people to see how far the drop is and this can make frail or injured people feel vulnerable and inhibited.

neously at the start of the swing phase. The hip and knee joints of the stance limb are in considerable flexion and substantial effort is needed from the extensor muscles to raise the body; at the same time effort must also be directed to the maintenance of balance (Tata et al 1983).

When these facts are taken into consideration, it is no wonder that elderly and frail people find stair climbing difficult. To be able to use stairs safely it is necessary to have a wide range of movement at hip, knee and ankle joints, muscles capable of generating considerable force through a wide range, and a good sense of balance. Rehabilitation programmes for patients who have difficulties with stairs should always include activities which will increase joint range and the torque-generating capacity of muscle, and improve balance.

REFERENCES

Andriacchi T, Andersson G, Fermier R, Stern D, Galante J 1980 A study of lower limb mechanics during stair climbing. Journal of Bone and Joint Surgery 62A: 749–757

Arakawa K 1993 Hypertension and exercise. Clinical and Experimental Hypertension 15: 1171–1179

Baer GD, Ashburn AM 1995 Trunk movements in older subjects during sit to stand. Archives of Physical Medicine and Rehabilitation 76: 844–849

Costigan PA, Deluzio KJ, Wyss UP 2002 Knee and hip kinetics during normal stair climbing. Gait and Posture 16(1): 31–37

Craik RL, Oatis CA 1995 Gait analysis, theory and application. Mosby, St Louis, Missouri

Farley CT, Ferris DP 1998 Biomechanics of walking and running: centre of mass movements to muscle action. Exercise and Sport Sciences Reviews 26: 253–285

Hardman AE, Hudson A 1994 Brisk walking and serum lipid and lipoprotein variables in previously sedentary women: effect of 12 weeks of regular brisk walking followed by 12 weeks of detraining. British Journal of Sports Medicine 28: 261–266

Ikeda E, Schenkman M, Riley P, Hodge W 1991 Influence of age on dynamics of rising from a chair. Physical Therapy 71: 473–481

Janssen WGM, Bussmann HBJ, Stam HJ 2002 Determinants of the sit-to-stand movement: a review. Physical Therapy 82(9): 886–879

Kelly D, Dainis A, Wood G 1976 Mechanics and muscular dynamics of rising from a seated position. In: Komi P

(ed) Biomechanics. V B International Series on Biomechanics. University Park Press, Baltimore, Maryland

Kerr K, White J, Mollan R, Baird H 1991 Rising from a chair: a review of the literature. Physiotherapy 77: 15–19

Mak MKY, Levin O, Mizrahi J, Hui-Chan CWY 2003 Joint torques during sit-to-stand in healthy subjects and people with Parkinson's disease. Clinical Biomechanics 18(3): 197–206

McArdle WD, Katch FI, Katch VL 2001 Exercise physiology, energy, nutrition and human performance, 5th edn. Lea and Febiger, Philadelphia

McFadyen B, Winter D 1988 An integrated biomechanical analysis of normal stair ascent and descent. Journal of Biomechanics 21: 733–744

Mulavara AP, Verstraete MC, Bloomberg JJ 2002 Modulation of head movement control in humans during treadmill walking. Gait and Posture 16(3): 271–282

Murray MP 1967 Gait as a total pattern of movement. American Journal of Physical Medicine 46: 290–333

Murray MP, Drought AB, Kory RC 1964 Walking patterns of normal men. Journal of Bone and Joint Surgery 46A: 335–359

Murray MP, Sepic SB, Barnard EJ 1967 Patterns of sagittal rotation of the upper limbs in walking. Journal of the American Physical Therapy Association 47: 272–284

Pai YC , Rogers MW 1991 Speed variation and resultant joint torques during sit-to-stand. Archives of Physical Medicine and Rehabilitation 72: 881–885

Pereira MA, Kriska AM, Day RD, Cauley JA, LaPorte RE, Kuller LH 1998 A randomized walking trial in postmenopausal women: effects on physical activity and health 10 years later. Archives of Internal Medicine 158: 1695–1710

Riener R, Rabuffetti M, Frigo C 2002 Stair ascent and descent at different inclinations. Gait and Posture 15(1): 32–44

Riley PO, Schenkman M, Mann RW 1991 Mechanics of a constrained chair rise. Journal of Biomechanics 24: 77–85

Riley PO, Croce UD, Kerrigan DC 2001 Propulsive adaptation to changing gait speed. Journal of Biomechanics 34(2): 197–202

Schenkman M, Berger RS, Riley PO, Mann RW, Hodge WA 1990 Whole body movements during rising to standing from sitting. Physical Therapy 70(10): 638–652

Shepherd RB, Koh HP 1996 Some biomechanical consequences of varying foot placement in sit-to-stand in young women. Scandinavian Journal of Rehabilitation Medicine 28: 79–88

Smidt GL 1990 Gait in rehabilitation. Churchill Livingstone, New York

Tata J, Peat M, Grahame R, Quanbury A 1983 The normal peak of electromyographic activity of the quadriceps femoris muscle in the stair cycle. Anatomischer Anzeiger (Jena) 153: 175–188

Vilensky JA, Ganiewicz E, Gehlsen G 1987 A kinematic comparison of backward and forward walking in humans. Journal of Human Movement Studies 13: 29–50

Chapter 11

Function of the upper limb

Valerie Sparkes

CHAPTER CONTENTS

LEARNING OUTCOMES

At the end of this chapter you should be able to:

1. Discuss the factors that contribute to the
   function of the upper limb

2. Identify specific factors that affect the function
   of the individual sections of the upper limb

3. Discuss the function of the upper limb as part
   of the kinetic chain.

INTRODUCTION

This chapter, in outlining the function of the upper
limb, focuses on specific areas that contribute to
the upper limb and its role as part of the kinetic
chain. It will focus on some of the anatomical and
biomechanical aspects that are related to optimal
function. To answer the basic question 'What is
the function of the upper limb?' we need to look at
the activities of and demands on the upper limb
during daily life, including basic activities of daily
living and occupational and sporting demands.

When considering what anatomical and biomechanical features contribute to these functional
activities, we need to appraise the role of the bones,
muscles, ligaments, nerves, fascia, sensory receptors
and other soft tissues surrounding the joints, as
well as the central nervous system that controls
these systems (Terry et al 1991). For full appreciation

of the function of the upper limb, we need to consider it in relation to the other parts of the kinetic chain, including the trunk, pelvis and the lower limb.

FACTORS AFFECTING THE FUNCTION OF THE UPPER LIMB

The shoulder girdle

The primary function of the shoulder girdle is to allow freedom for the hands to function either alone or when using tools. The shoulder girdle is one part of the human body and can be viewed as one segment in a series of segments that are linked together. Body segments are sequentially activated to achieve functional or athletic tasks and the activation sequence is known as the *kinetic chain* (Kibler 1998, Kibler et al 2001). In assessing the performance of the shoulder girdle, it is essential to view it not in isolation but as a part of total kinetic chain activity (Kibler 1998, Kibler et al 2001). Any disturbance in function in any of the links in the kinetic chain can affect shoulder girdle function and any disturbance in shoulder girdle function can have an impact on the function of the other components of the kinetic chain (Kibler et al 2001). This will be further discussed at the end of the chapter.

The overriding feature of the glenohumeral joint is that although it is very mobile, it is one of the least stable joints of the skeleton. To achieve normal function, a balance between mobility and stability needs to be attained to avoid injury. Extensive range of movement and angulation is needed in the upper limb to achieve the variety of

---

Task 11.1

Imagine the scenarios listed below and think of the movements or positions that the lower limb, pelvis and trunk adopt during these activities:

- Reaching behind you to pull down the seat belt
- Performing a golf swing
- Lifting a large box
- Standing on tip toe to reach something from a high shelf.

---

tasks that daily life demands. However, due to the necessity of achieving the balance between mobility and stability, the humerus and scapula are constantly adapting their positions to maintain the optimum position for function (Moseley et al 1992). The term 'dynamic stability' is often used to describe this phenomenon, where structures such as muscles, tendons and ligaments are constantly adjusting to provide a stable base from which the limb can work and at the same time provide the power and coordination required for the task. However, the glenohumeral joint does not work in isolation. For a fully functioning upper limb, synchronised movement needs to occur in the glenohumeral, scapulothoracic, acromioclavicular and sternoclavicular joints, the elbow, wrist and hand and the surrounding musculature.

The scapula

The scapula functions primarily as a site for muscular attachments and forms the base from which the upper limb functions (Hadler et al 2000, Mottram 1997, Paine & Voight 1993). The achievement of normal positioning and control of the scapula is essential for optimal function (Mottram 1997). The scapula's concave surface sits on the convex rib cage and it is attached to the skeleton through the acromioclavicular joint and via the clavicle to the sternoclavicular joint.

The scapula is a very mobile structure and glides over and around the rib cage. It is primarily stabilised by muscles which attach to the spinous processes of the vertebrae and the ribs. These include trapezius, levator scapula, the rhomboids group, serratus anterior, serratus posterior inferior and superior and latissimus dorsi.

Role of the scapula

The scapula plays several roles to facilitate optimum functioning of the upper limb.

Normally it provides a stable base on which the upper limb functions. More specifically, in order to maintain dynamic stability of the glenohumeral joint, the musculature attached to and surrounding it must work in a coordinated fashion, exhibiting appropriate recruitment patterns (Mottram 1997, Voight & Thomson 2000). This is in order to maintain the correct alignment of the glenoid on which the humerus works (Kibler 1998). Optimal muscular activity is also facilitated by the maintenance of the normal length–tension relationship of the rotator cuff (Kamkar et al 1993).

The scapula must move in a controlled manner during movements of the upper limb and must accommodate the continual changing positions and functional demands of the limb (Moseley et al 1992). The scapula also acts as a base for muscle attachments, which provide both stability and movement to the upper limb. The muscles surrounding the scapula work as force couples in synergistic co-contraction to control the position of the scapula (Jobe & Pink 1993, Kibler 1998, Moseley et al 1992). The muscles responsible for controlling the scapula are all sections of trapezius, serratus anterior, rhomboids major and minor, levator scapula and pectoralis minor.

Pectoralis major and latissimus dorsi affect the scapula as they attach to the humerus. Other muscles which affect the scapula are deltoid, teres major, the rotator cuff muscles, subscapularis, supraspinatus, infraspinatus, teres minor, coracobrachialis, long head of triceps and the long and short heads of biceps.

The scapula needs to be able to protract, retract and rotate to allow the upper limb to be placed in the correct position for function. It needs to be able to retract to enable the cocking phase of throwing action, for example in the tennis serve, throwing a cricket ball and in the swimming recovery phase. Throwing activities involve a coordinated sequence of movements of the scapula and upper limb together with the appropriate trunk, pelvis and lower limb activity. The phases are:

- preparation or wind-up which begins with the start of motion
- cocking phase where the shoulder is abducted and externally rotated
- acceleration phase where the humerus internally rotates; this phase ends at ball release
- deceleration phase; the first one-third of the time from ball release to the end of the arm movement
- follow-through phase; the last two-thirds from ball release to the end of the arm movement (amended from Pink & Perry 1996).

Achievement of the cocking phase tensions the anterior chest musculature to prepare for the concentric phase of muscle action. The explosive phase of acceleration requires the scapula to protract in coordinated fashion. As the acceleration phase begins, smooth protraction and anterior glide of the scapula around the chest wall is required. This movement allows the glenoid to be maintained in the appropriate alignment with the head of the humerus. This movement of the scapula is mainly achieved by the eccentric contraction of predominantly rhomboids and middle trapezius. These muscles help dissipate some of the forces in the deceleration and follow-through phases (Pink & Perry 1996).

In overhead activities, such as throwing, the scapula has to rotate laterally to allow full abduction which is vital for full elevation. In most throwing activities the arm works at an angle between 85° and 100° of abduction so the muscles surrounding the scapula must draw the acromion away from the cuff to avoid compression (Fleisig et al 1994, Kamkar et al 1993, Kibler 1993, 1998). In all elevation movements it is necessary to clear the greater tubercle from the coracoacromial arch for the same reason.

Optimum scapula function is achieved not only by the muscles moving and controlling it but by movements at the acromioclavicular and sternoclavicular joints. As the shoulder abducts, the clavicle has to elevate, which requires a coordinated movement at the acromioclavicular and sternoclavicular joints.

11.1 Clinical considerations

If any of the muscles controlling the scapula do not function optimally there is the potential for compression of the structures underneath the acromion, including the subacromial bursae and the supraspinatus tendon. Other factors that can contribute to compression of these structures include dysfunction of the rotator cuff where the compressive force on the head of the humerus is lost, which results in an upward migration of the head of the humerus.

Scapulothoracic joint

Although not a classic bony articulation, the scapulothoracic joint is an important physiological joint that is vital to optimum function of the upper limb. The overall ratio of scapulothoracic to glenohumeral movement of 1:2 is achieved by movement of these two structures combined with rotation of the clavicle (Kumar 2002). Movement of the scapulothoracic joint is between two fascial planes and is controlled by the muscles surrounding it (Mottram 1997, Pratt 1994). The scapulothoracic joint and structures surrounding it are constantly seeking a position of stability in relation to the humerus so as to attain the optimum position of the glenoid.

Sternoclavicular joint

The sternoclavicular joint must be considered as an integral part of the upper limb as it links the shoulder girdle to the axial skeleton (Pratt 1994). The clavicle has been described as acting like a 'crankshaft' to allow elevation and rotation at the acromioclavicular end (Donatelli 1997, Pratt 1994). The clavicle acts as a strut to keep the lateral aspect of the scapula away from the chest wall. The disc between the sternum and clavicle, together with the ligaments, muscle and capsule surrounding the joint, facilitate movement of the clavicle on the sternum, allowing it to act like a hinge and so providing greater movement (Pratt 1994).

Acromioclavicular joint

Although supported by strong ligaments, the acromioclavicular joint is more lax than the sternoclavicular joint. It is supported by the conoid and trapezoid ligaments (coracoclavicular ligaments) and the acromioclavicular ligament. These ligaments are fundamental in controlling movements at this joint (Kumar 2002, Pratt 1994).

Scapular movements are translated to the clavicle through the coracoclavicular ligaments (Pratt 1994).

Subacromial space   The space between the acromion and the head of the humerus is critical to optimum function of the upper limb. This narrow space between the head of the humerus and the arch formed by the acromion, coracoid process and coracoacromial ligament facilitates general shoulder mobility but flexion and abduction in particular. In this small space are the subacromial bursae, supraspinatus muscle and its tendon, superior aspect of the joint capsule and the tendon of long head of biceps. Functionally, these structures are able to constantly move against each other within this small space without producing symptoms.

Glenohumeral joint

The glenohumeral joint is a highly mobile joint, capable of three degrees of freedom (Williams 1995), but also capable of remaining stable during a wide range of activities, for example supporting the weight of the limb during painting, reaching above the head and repetitive keyboard work. It has to be mobile and sufficiently powerful to support a wide variety of loads in varying positions, such as carrying bags of shopping or large boxes. The joint has to have the capacity to perform repetitive tasks of varying speeds and load, such as in packing boxes on a production line, playing squash, tennis and badminton. The extensive range of movement is achieved through a large humeral head moving on a relatively shallow glenoid fossa. Mobility is facilitated by a large capsule enveloping the joint, which is so lax that the bones can be distracted for 2–3 cm (Williams 1995). In normal functional movements the humerus must roll, spin and glide to keep in contact with the relatively small glenoid fossa.

Structures supporting the glenohumeral joint   As a highly mobile joint, the glenohumeral joint relies on the structures surrounding it for stability. The rotator cuff, which comprises the tendons of subscapularis, infraspinatus, teres minor and supraspinatus, is the major stabilising force of the glenohumeral joint and is known as a 'dynamic stabiliser' (Pink & Perry 1996). The rotator cuff together with the capsule and the glenohumeral ligaments play a pivotal role in controlling translation of the humeral head while it spins on the small glenoid surface (Pratt 1994). Ligaments, although contributing to the stability of the joint, only function as restraints at the extremes of movement. The rotator cuff can be viewed as the structure that steers the head of the humerus during upper limb movements, providing dynamic stability. Translation of the humeral head during elevation will also be reduced if the muscles surrounding the shoulder function in a coordinated manner, which requires pre-programming of muscle activation. In centering the head of the humerus, the rotator cuff maintains joint stability during function, especially within mid range when the ligaments and capsule are lax (Doukas & Speer 2001). The rotator cuff is attached close to the axis of rotation and adds to dynamic joint compression of the humerus into the socket, thus enhancing joint stability.

All muscles generate forces which are translated to the bones they attach to. The muscle system is constantly striving to maintain a balance of forces between muscle groups to produce optimum function. Dynamic stability is achieved through certain muscles and tendons controlling shear and translational forces generated by the prime movers of the shoulder, which include deltoid, triceps, biceps and latissimus dorsi, whilst still allowing movement to occur. This is essential for the appropriate spinning and gliding of the humerus within the glenoid to occur. The deltoid muscle mass makes up 41% of the scapulohumeral muscle mass and as well as being a prime mover of the glenohumeral joint, it contributes to its stability (Michiels & Bodem 1992). Being multipennate, it is fatigue resistant and its mechanical advantage is enhanced by its distal insertion on the humerus. During the initial phase of elevation in the glenohumeral joint, deltoid is active and produces a large degree of torque within the joint with the effect of producing a minimal superior glide of the head of the humerus. This is counteracted by the rotator cuff, which provides a firm fulcrum on which the deltoid is able to work (Jobe et al 1996). The force exerted by deltoid is at its maximum at 60° of elevation (Sarrafian 1983). Early rises in tension of supraspinatus during abduction have been noted which appear to facilitate centering the head of the humerus (Poppen & Walker 1976). Subscapularis, as a major depressor of the head of humerus, counteracts the upward shear of the deltoid muscle during upper limb function (Kabada et al 1992).

Although the precise role in terms of stability of the long head of biceps is not fully understood, through its tendinous attachments to the supraglenoid tubercle, the long head of biceps may influence the position of the head of the humerus within the glenoid by preventing anterior translation of the humerus (Doukas & Speer 2001, Kumar et al 1989). Both the long head and the short head appear to reinforce the glenohumeral joint anteriorly (Itoi et al 1993).

The kinematics of the joint will determine the extent to which muscle force results in a degree of stability (Herzog et al 1991). Rotator cuff function, and hence stability of the glenohumeral joint, is influenced by the angle of the glenoid, which in turn is dictated by the function of the muscles that control the scapula (van der Helm 1994). Terry et al (1991) found that the retroversion and posterior tilt of the head of the humerus and glenoid contributed to the joint stability.

Stability is further enhanced by the labrum, a fibrocartilaginous rim around the glenoid cavity (Williams 1995). The labrum deepens the cavity and facilitates the centring of the head of the humerus. It may also protect the bone and assist lubrication (Pink & Perry 1996). The negative intra-articular pressure within the glenohumeral joint may have a contribution to the stability of the joint (Pink & Perry 1996). It has been found that the negative intra-articular pressure increases when a downward load is applied to the dependent arm. This increase may prevent further downward glide of the humeral head (Kumar & Balasubramaniam 1985). When the arm is abducted the negative pressure may provide inferior stability to the humeral head (Weber & Caspari 1989).

Muscles acting on the pectoral girdle

Many of the muscles that provide stability to the glenohumeral joint also act as movers of the joint. There are many muscles that have an influence on the scapula and the glenohumeral joint.

The term 'scapulohumeral rhythm' has been coined to describe the combined coordinated activity of the scapula muscles and the rotator cuff muscles as they work together with deltoid and latissimus dorsi (Poppen & Walker 1976). As noted in Chapter 2, muscles work both concentrically

---

Task 11.2

Name the muscles whose tendons make up the rotator cuff.

Name the muscles that have attachments to the humerus and the spine.

Name the muscles that attach on the humerus and the scapula.

(shortening) and eccentrically (lengthening). In certain activities muscles may need to work eccentrically to decelerate a limb to produce a controlled movement to add precision to the task, for example performing a chip shot in golf.

In many throwing tasks where the glenohumeral joint is placed in external rotation, subscapularis, in working eccentrically, might slow down the action, producing control and absorbing energy. Therefore this action places less force on the ligaments and to some extent may protect them (Speer & Garrett 1993).

Properties of muscle affecting function of the upper limb

The term 'stiffness' refers to the ability of the muscle to provide resistance to deformation and provide support to the bones and joints (see Ch. 3). Muscle stiffness is determined by the intrinsic properties of muscle and neuromuscular control from the central nervous system. It is important to remember that muscles do not work in isolation. Coordinated muscular activity with appropriate timing is the key optimum function. In the upper limb, as in other areas of the human body, a system of force couples acts as the basis for motor control.

At the higher centres there is integration of visual, auditory and kinaesthetic information and

---

Task 11.3

Think of the action of reaching forwards to pick up a cup. Which joints and muscles are involved at the shoulder?

---

information regarding the demand of the task which produces a highly coordinated movement. (For further information see Chapter 4.) As well as stiffness, muscle length also contributes to joint function. In this highly mobile joint, muscles affecting both the scapula and the glenohumeral joint must have the appropriate extensibility to allow full movement to occur. In the final phase of glenohumeral elevation, muscles including latissimus dorsi, pectoralis major and minor, teres major and minor, infraspinatus and subscapularis must have sufficient extensibility to allow this to be achieved.

Neural tissue

For the upper limb to function optimally, it is vital to consider the function and properties of the nerves in that region. Properties of nerves include the ability to conduct information and to move and glide within the constraints of the surrounding anatomic structures which include soft tissues and bone. From wrist extension to flexion, the median nerve will slide nearly 2 cm at the wrist (Wright et al 1996). Some branches of the cervical plexus, for example the supraclavicular nerves (C3, C4), supply areas of the shoulder, with many of the branches running through muscles and close to joints (Williams 1995). The brachial plexus (C4–T2) is intimately entwined in the structures of the upper limb after emerging from the cervical spine. In certain areas of the upper limb there are tension points at which the nerves are relatively fixed or sit in a narrow channel and are therefore potentially prone to compression; for example, the ulnar nerve at the elbow sits in a groove on the dorsum of the epicondyle and the median nerve at the wrist lies between the retinaculum and tendons in the carpal tunnel.

Movement of the shoulder into functional positions can put nerves on tension. In normal circumstances nerves and surrounding structures glide on and between each other. As the anatomy suggests, there is a connection between cervical spine and upper limb movements.

Proprioception

Sensory feedback about the limb's position and direction is vital to allow modification of muscle activity to achieve optimum performance (Warner

---

Task 11.4

Try bending your head to the left side (cervical left side flexion). What do you feel? Now abduct your right arm with your elbow straight, to 90°. What do you feel? Now extend your wrist. What do you feel? Now finally extend your fingers. What do you feel?

Try the same with your left upper limb; does it feel the same or different?

---

et al 1996). Proprioception refers to afferent information received by higher centres from receptors in articular, muscle and cutaneous structures and is vital for coordinated function. Specialised nerve endings that have proprioceptive mechanisms, including Pacinian corpuscles, Ruffini endings and Golgi tendon organs, are found in capsules and ligaments of all joints. Although proprioceptors are a feature of all joints, most of the research in the upper limb has focused on the glenohumeral joint.

Neuroafferents have been noted within the capsulotendinous junction in the glenohumeral joint which will give feedback on shoulder position (Grigg 1993).

This input from receptors gives information about the position of the joint during all stages of functional activity and is vital for feedback during the task. Proprioceptive information is vital for programming movements and reflex muscular contractions, especially from the rotator cuff, to enhance stability of the glenohumeral joint (Warner et al 1996).

All tasks rely on pre-programming with information prior to and during the task as adjustments may need to be made during task performance (see Ch. 4). Any coordinated and skilled upper limb activity requires continual feedback from the sensory systems. Receptors must provide spatial and temporal information so that the task can be completed with optimum skill and efficiency.

This is particularly pertinent in the minimally restrained glenohumeral joint where coordinated activity of all the contractile tissue is essential for efficient control. In a reaching task, such as painting a picture or drawing, the neuromuscular system controlling the arm must integrate information such as limb position and force required

together with information from the eye to produce a smooth and controlled action. Where afferent information is diminished, due to injury for instance, the task may still be completed but often fine control and precision are lacking. In normal shoulders, there appears to be no difference in proprioception between the dominant and non-dominant hands and between males and females (Jerosch et al 1996, Warner et al 1996).

The elbow and forearm

These two regions will be considered together as their function is interlinked. The elbow functions in combination with the movements of the superior and inferior radioulnar joints. The elbow consists of two articulations, the humeroulnar and the humeroradial. The superior radioulnar joint consists of the head of the radius articulating with the ulna and the inferior radioulnar joint where the distal ends of the ulna and radius articulate with the carpus. The elbow is a stable joint when compared to the glenohumeral joint due to the shape of the proximal ulna (Guerra & Timmerman 1996), the radial head (Morrey et al 1983), the collateral ligaments and the aconeous muscle.

Elbow function

The elbow is an integral part of the upper limb as the link in the chain that can position the hand, adjust the length and height of the limb and transfer loads to the hand (Guerra & Timmerman 1996). Elbow function is vital to the basic task of bringing the hand to the mouth for eating, where the elbow flexors and supinators of the forearm work together. Flexion and extension of the elbow are accompanied by some degree of rotation of the ulna (Williams 1995). Pronation and supination that occur at the radioulnar joints place the hand in the most effective functional position. Pronation and supination allow the hand to be turned through 140–150° and in extension this can increase to nearly 360° with rotation of the humerus and the scapula (Williams 1995). The elbow often functions as a hinge, producing flexion and extension during activities such as sawing wood or hitting nails with a hammer and lifting objects up and down, for example.

Task 11.5

Think of different tasks that:

- use the elbow as a hinge in a flexion/extension movement
- put a compressive force through the elbow.

Task 11.6

Think of using a fork while eating. Consider the movements of all the joints involved in bringing the food on your fork to your mouth.

Task 11.7

Think of other tasks or athletic activities that load the elbow joint.

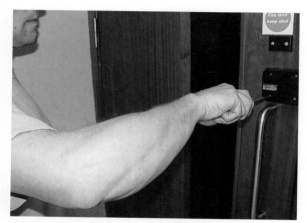

Figure 11.1   The action of using a screwdriver.

The forearm can exert a greater pressure in a supinated position than in pronation. This governs many power activities such as screwing nuts, turning handles or lifting heavy weights, where the most efficient position is one of forearm supination and elbow flexion.

Biceps brachii is utilised in all activities involving supination, such as turning a key or screwdriver (Fig. 11.1), as well as flexing the forearm to the upper arm. In demanding power activities, strength may be applied by grasp from the hand but considerable forces are applied through the forearm, the arm and the body. The mid-prone position is a strong functional position as can be seen when hammering and lifting boxes. Many functional activities involve a combination of elbow flexion in the mid-prone position with shoulder flexion. In a simple task like eating, there is a complex sequence of movements and positioning to bring the food to the mouth.

Muscles surrounding the elbow and forearm work in an integrated fashion, functioning as phasic agonists as well as antagonists. As well as producing fine controlled movements, the elbow has to absorb forces in heavy or athletic tasks. When the upper limb lifts heavy loads, triceps will recruit aconeous to stabilise the joint. Forces through the elbow during baseball pitching have been studied as many elbow injuries occur in this sport. The baseball pitch is divided into six phases: wind-up, stride, arm cocking, arm acceleration, arm deceleration and follow-through. Low muscle activity and low elbow joint forces have been noted during the wind-up and stride phases which are preparatory phases for dynamic muscle activity. High muscle activity and elbow forces were noted during arm cocking, arm acceleration and deceleration phases (Fleisig & Escamilla 1996).

Hand

The hand is a very specialised and versatile unit which has the potential for fine discrimination, coordination and dexterity as well as a powerful grip. The functional hand works as part of the coordinated unit of the upper limb. Development of hand skills is critical to performance of activities of daily living and to function throughout life. The hand can be used alone or with tools. It can act as a lever, where the hand can be fixed with the arm whilst the trunk moves. It can act as a base for support and balance and as a communicator.

Manipulation of objects by the hand is a fine and complex task, relying on an intact central nervous system to deliver the appropriate responses in terms of coordination and timing of activation, as in the need for the correct pressure to hold an object and the correct timing to release an object. Fine motor skills are essential to the manipulation of objects where there is a need for a coordination between mobility and balance, for instance in writing, where the hand needs to be able to perform the pinch grip and control the paper. As well as fine control manipulation, the hand has to be capable of holding tools and large objects.

The hands as a specialised sensory unit

One of the most important functions of the hand is the ability to perceive sensation (Mackel 1996). The hand is an active sensory organ, richly innervated with sensory receptors, and has a large representation area in the somatosensory cortex. The hand is capable of detecting objects even when there is no visual input, for example searching in a pocket or a bag, and is able to perceive different sizes, shapes and textures. The ability to use the hand has developed to its highest level in the adult human due to the presence of a specialised central nervous system.

Anatomy

The arrangement of the bones of the hand and the accompanying soft tissues allows for a diverse range of movements and tasks (Moran 1989, Strickland 1995). The skin covering the hand on the dorsum and the volar aspect plays a major role in the function of the hand as a tactile and discriminatory unit. The skin of the hand, especially on the volar aspect, is richly supplied with sensory nerve endings which aid discrimination of different sensations (Moran 1989). The skin also aids function, in particular gripping. The skin on the dorsum is mobile and aids flexion of the fingers whereas the volar skin is less flexible but has many creases in it which follow the lines of stresses imposed on it during function (Caillett 1994, Moran 1989).

Bones and soft tissues   The shape of the 29 bones in the hand and the neuromuscular system that controls it allow the hand to achieve a wide range of functions. Movements of the hand are produced by the coordinated effect of intrinsic and extrinsic muscle action as well as a balance between flexors and extensors. For example, complex movements such as writing require flexion at the metacarpophalangeal (MCP) joints and extension at the interphalangeal (IP) joints. During grip activities the intrinsic muscles, as well as the ligaments, ensure joint stability whilst the long flexors provide most of the force needed (Palmer 1991). Biomechanical studies have shown that the intrinsic muscles can exert a strong force of more than a third of the long flexors in the gripping action (Palmer 1991). The lumbricals contract during both MCP flexion and MCP extension. When the MCP joints extend, the lumbricals appear to be important in extension of the IP joints (Palmer 1991). Connective tissues of the hand, for example the flexor retinaculum, palmar aponuerosis and dorsal digital expansion, protect and bind groups of muscles to allow smooth movement. To reduce friction around tension points, each flexor tendon is contained in a sheath which contains a lubricating fluid, to aid smooth movement.

Some muscles that influence hand function do not directly insert into the hand. For example, brachioradialis inserts onto the base of the styloid process after crossing the cubital fossa. It flexes the elbow when the forearm is in mid pronation and supination which is essential in eating and drinking tasks.

The *thumb* is a vital functional unit of the hand as the carpometacarpal joint, together with a loose capsule, allows for a wide range of motion. This joint arrangement facilitates gripping and mani-

---

Task 11.8

Think of a task that requires the hand to be used for:

* a fine motor skill
* a power activity
* leverage of the body.

Task 11.9

Without you seeing them, get a friend to choose five household items of different textures that can be manipulated by the hand. Keeping your eyes closed, feel the objects and see how long it takes you to identify what they are.

pulation through a wide arc. The combined movements of flexion, medial rotation and adduction mean the thumb can be taken across the palm of the hand into 'opposition'. In opening the hand, the thumb is extended and abducted.

Wrist and hand movements

The optimum functional position of the hand is in the mid pronation position, with the wrist in extension and the digits in a moderate degree of flexion. Most functional activities of daily living occur with the wrist in a position between 10° of flexion and 35° of extension. Wrist movements involving the long muscles of the forearm are the key to the manipulations of the digits (Strickland 1995), with maximum strength in the power grip being facilitated by extension of the wrist. In functional activities the carpus is able to transmit forces from the hand through the forearm, for example when we get up from a chair. Gliding movements of the carpals on the radius are facilitated by capsular and ligamentous laxity and the carpals move in the opposite direction to the movement of the hand. The ligaments also provide stability of the carpals with appropriate gliding whilst the wrist and fingers are mobile.

Development of gripping

For most of an infant's first year grasp development relates to feedback from objects via the palmar surface, with the grasp reflex predominating initially (Holle 1981). During the second year evolving skills are associated with increasing cognitive abilities and environmental influences. Coordinated movements are developed through sensory experience and feedback through the hand. When beginning to bear weight, the hands and arms are used to support the body, to balance,

---

Task 11.10

Think of the function of the muscles listed below and how they influence hand function:

- Pronator teres
- Supinator
- Biceps brachii.

---

to walk and to manipulate objects. In the young child, force coordination is poorly developed. At age 1 year children might crush a fragile object such as an ice cream cone or a paper model but between the ages of 2 and 4 years they develop the skills to manage and handle fragile objects (Eliasson 1995).

The crawling position, where the hand and upper limb are used for support and propulsion, allows children to creep and in turn strengthens the upper limb and neck musculature. Strengthening of arms and hands also occurs as children pull on objects such as furniture to stand and support themselves (Case-Smith 1995). The development of neck and shoulder musculature together with increasing postural stability are the prerequisites for the control of reach activities. The first two years of life see dramatic developments in the use of the hand in terms of function and skill. Basic grasp and release skills develop into mature complex coordinated movements in the early years of development (Case-Smith 1995). At 10–12 months a child can manipulate tools, for example a spoon to feed or pencil to scribble.

All basic hand manipulation skills and those involving stabilisation of the object in the hand are seen to be present in normal children by age 7 years (Exner 1990).

Development of all manipulation skills requires coordination of the neuromusculoskeletal system surrounding the neck, shoulder, elbow and wrist.

For details of timescales for development of skills relating to feeding, self-care, dressing and washing, see Chapter 15 or Henderson (1995) and Zivani (1995)

The *hook grip* is where all the fingers are flexed towards the palm, for example in lifting a heavy suitcase or briefcase (Fig. 11.2). The fingers are flexed around the handle but the thumb is not involved.

The *power grip* is where the thumb is strongly flexed, the fingers are flexed towards the thenar eminence and the ulna is deviated. The thumb and the ring and little fingers contribute most to the power grip and this grip is used in many activities where power and stability are required, for example using a hammer or doing a bench press.

When gripping a hammer there is maximum flexion at the little finger and least at the index. In hammering, maximum area of contact is required

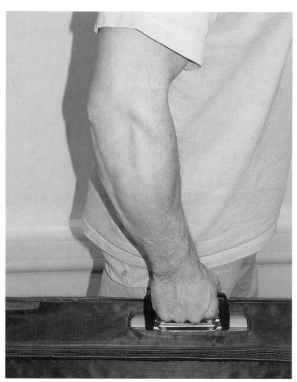

Figure 11.2 The hook grip and muscle work involved in carrying a suitcase.

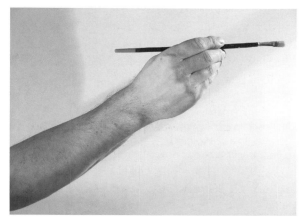

Figure 11.3 The fine control involved in using a paintbrush.

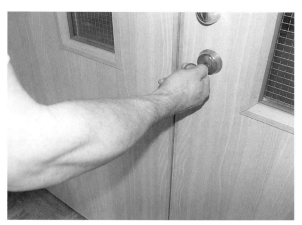

Figure 11.4 The use of the intrinsic muscles when turning a key.

to provide power with precision and control. In the power grip all the intrinsic and extrinsic muscles are used, with the hypothenar eminence muscles stabilising the medial aspect of the hand. The wrist extensors act as a stable base on which the power grip can function. Wrist extensors increase in activity, so as to direct the force onto the finger flexors so that they do not act on the wrist. Feedback from the sensory receptors in the hand is essential to exert exactly the right pressure required and coordinate the interaction of other muscles in the forearm to provide power. For example, in opening a heavy door the hand grips the handle and the forearm muscles provide the power.

The *precision or pinch grip* is used for fine manipulation and requires the thumb to be placed in contact with the finger tips (Fig. 11.3). To achieve this tip-to-tip approximation, the fingers must rotate and deviate in an ulnar direction. The precision grip utilises the coordinated action of the lumbricals and interossei to grip the object, with the hand being positioned by the wrist and forearm. The precision grip is more advanced than the power grip, appearing at around 9 months.

In the pinch grip, the MCP and proximal IP joints of the index are flexed while the distal IP joint can be flexed or extended. The opposed thumb pad meets the pad of the digit. This pad-to-pad grip is used, for instance, when holding a pen or sewing. In the *key grip* the extended thumb is held on the radial side of the index finger (Fig. 11.4).

Task 11.11

Pick some of the day-to-day activities listed below and look at the position of the wrist and forearm:

- The hand gripping a teapot
- Pouring tea
- Turning tap
- Holding a large glass
- Using a screw driver
- Carrying a bucket or a carrier bag
- Carrying a large box in front of you
- Writing
- Using a keyboard.

Task 11.12

Decide which grip is involved in the following activities:

- Playing tennis
- Playing chess
- Digging the garden with a spade
- Placing a full cup and saucer on the table
- Placing a letter into an envelope
- Lifting a heavy shopping bag
- Using a knife and fork.

The *lumbrical grip* is where the MCP joints are flexed across the palmar aspect, for example when holding a plate or something that needs to be kept horizontal.

Two-handed manipulative tasks are where both hands are involved in the task, playing the piano or guitar and working at a keyboard, for example. In some activities one hand can provide the stability whilst the other hand completes the task, such as peeling potatoes, sawing wood and unscrewing a jar lid.

THE UPPER LIMB AS PART OF THE KINETIC CHAIN

The kinetic chain refers to the relationship and interplay between each segment of the body. The upper limb is part of the kinetic chain linked to the other parts of the body. As discussed earlier, its

---

Task 11.13

Consider the attachment, origin and insertion of latissimus dorsi and list the segments of the body that it affects.

---

function relies on the optimum function of all the neurophysiological systems of the body and any rehabilitation programme must consider both open and closed chain activities as well as those to enhance dynamic stability (Wilk et al 1996). When considering the function of the upper limb, we need to think about the component parts of the trunk, including the cervical, thoracic and lumbar spine and pelvis, as the posture of the trunk can determine how effectively the upper limb functions (Crawford & Jull 1991, Lannerston & Harms-Ringdhal 1990). Full extensibility of the soft tissues related to the trunk, for example quadratus lumborum and latissimus dorsi, is essential for optimal upper limb function.

When power is required, for instance in a tennis serve, force generation and wind-up start with positioning of the feet. However, at the point of impact of the ball on the racket in a tennis serve, the feet may be off the ground. Individual body segments work together to position the upper limb in the correct functional position. For effective upper limb function there needs to be a transfer of forces from the proximal segments to the upper limb, which can be achieved through the stable but active upper limb base, the scapula. Up to 54% of the total force in a tennis serve will be generated from the lower legs, hips and trunk (Kibler 1995).

Proximal control

The function of the upper limb is primarily dependent on a stable base on which to work. The pelvis and more proximally the scapula can be viewed as the two interlinking platforms on which the upper limb functions. Function is also dependent on coordination between the scapular muscles and the muscles of the humerus, forearm, wrist and hand. Poor pelvic stability as a result of, for example, delayed muscle recruitment or atrophy of deep stability muscles (Hides et al 2001, Hodges & Richardson 1996) can lead to inefficient and uncoordinated activity of the upper limb. Hodges and Richardson (1996) have demonstrated that in rapid upper limb movements, transversus abdominis is activated prior to any arm movements. This pre-programmed activity of the transverse abdominal muscles ensures that the pelvis is stable prior to the upper limb moving. It has also been noted that the postural muscles of the lower limb are activated before the arm moves (Cordo & Nashner 1982), thus adding to the stable base on which the upper limb can function. This integrated action of postural activation in the pelvis and leg muscles, prior to arm movement, is an important prerequisite for the production of a coordinated action of the upper limb function. The importance of postural trunk control in the development of skills in children is demonstrated in the transition from the two-handed reach to a one-handed reach (Rochat 1992).

Open chain, closed chain

The upper limb works in both closed and open chain activities. Open chain activities include daily activities such as dressing and reaching up and sporting activities such as tennis and squash. Closed chain activities include rising from a chair or levering oneself out of the bath or up from the floor after a fall. In gymnastic activities these can include somersaults on the floor and the push-off from the vault and the beam. In studying closed chain activities such as press-ups and bench press, the highest EMG activity was noted in pectoralis minor in press-ups (Moseley et al 1992).

Many activities are a combination of open and closed chain activities such as using a walking stick, where the stick is planted on the ground, the arm is working in a closed chain pattern and the swing phase of the arm is open chain. In loading of the upper limb there is stimulation of all the upper limb muscles, including the scapular muscles, and proprioceptors within all the joints and ligaments. Weight-bearing activities can be used to promote stability within a notoriously mobile joint such as the glenohumeral joint by providing joint compression and muscular co-contraction which enhances dynamic stability

---

> ### Task 11.14
>
> Think of the role of the upper limb in the activities below:
>
> - A tightrope walker walking across a tightrope
> - A gymnast performing an exercise routine on the beam or a vault box
> - A patient with a plaster cast on his leg walking with crutches
> - A person with a stick who is unsteady
> - The rugby player who kicks a penalty or a conversion.

(Wilk & Arrigo 1993). The upper limb in a fixed position can also aid respiration. Patients will fix the humerus on a chair or bannister, for example, and pectoralis major can assist in pulling the sternum upwards and outwards to enlarge the thorax. This movement is assisted by serratus anterior and pectoralis minor.

The upper limb is used extensively to enhance balance and stability of the body in both closed and open chain situations. This may incorporate one or both upper limbs. In a situation where the lower limb musculature is weaker as a result of an injury, for example, the individual may increasingly rely on the upper limb for balance and stability during walking.

FUNCTION OF THE UPPER LIMB IN ACTIVITIES OF DAILY LIVING

Any simple movement, such as brushing your hair or cleaning your teeth, involves a series of complex and coordinated movements of the upper limb segments which is dependent on the coordinated activity of many muscles, nerves, ligaments and other soft tissues. Virtually any use of the hands involves movement of the scapula and the glenohumeral joint to position the hands in the appropriate functional position.

Many daily activities involve reaching and grasping an object and moving it, where the arm functions as one unit. The reach phase has been termed the 'transportation component' and the grasp the 'manipulation component' (Jeannerod

1984). In the phase of arm reaching, the proximal muscles and joints are used to place the limb in the appropriate position towards the object. The grasp phase starts whilst the limb is being moved towards the object and involves the activation of the intrinsic muscles of the hand (Jeannerod 1981). In the grasp phase the fingers have to anticipate the size and position of the object to attain a smooth and efficient action. This is achieved through information received through the visual senses. During any reaching task there is a phase of acceleration and deceleration of the limb with the muscles producing a combination of eccentric and concentric work. In activities such as eating there is a retrieval component where the hand is brought to the mouth.

The greater the speed of the reaching task, the less accurate the grasp activity may be. Visual feedback on the positioning of the hand is necessary for accuracy of the grasping task (Tillary et al 1991). However, even if the reaching movement is carried out without visual feedback, it can be achieved but may take more time or be less accurate. Rosbald (1995) indicates that the reaching task is probably pre-programmed prior to the task but adjustments can be made during the task if required.

CONCLUSION

This chapter has focused on the function of the upper limb, emphasising that all segments work in a coordinated fashion to achieve optimum function. In assessing the activity of the upper limb, we need to understand the function of each component part and its relationship to the other parts of the kinetic chain.

REFERENCES

Caillet R 1994 Hand pain and impairment, 4th edn. FA Davies, Philadelphia,

Case-Smith J 1995 Grasp release and bimanual skills in the first two years of life. In: Henderson A, Pehoski C (eds) Hand function in the child. Mosby, St Louis

Cordo PJ, Nashner LM 1982 Properties of postural adjustments associated with rapid arm movements. Journal of Neurophysiology 47:287–302

Crawford H, Jull G 1991 The influence of thoracic form and movement on ranges of shoulder flexion. MPPA proceedings, 7th Biennial Conference, Australia

Donatelli RA 1997 Functional anatomy and mechanics. In: Donatelli RA (ed) Physical therapy of the shoulder, 3rd edn. Churchill Livingstone, New York

Doukas WC, Speer KP 2001 Anatomy, pathophysiology, and biomechanics of shoulder instability. Orthopedic Clinics of North America 32(3):381–391

Eliasson AC 1995 Sensorimotor integration of normal and impaired development of precision movement of the hand. In: Henderson A, Pehoski C (eds) Hand function in the child. Mosby, St Louis

Exner CE 1990 In-hand manipulation skills in normal young children: a pilot study. Occupational Therapy Practice 1(4):63–72

Fleisig GS, Escamilla RF 1996 Biomechanics of the elbow in the throwing athlete. Operative Techniques in Sports Medicine 4(2):62–68

Fleisig GS, Dillman CJ, Andrews JR 1994 Biomechanics of the shoulder during throwing. In: Andrews JR, Wilk KE (eds) The athlete's shoulder. Churchill Livingstone, New York

Grigg P 1993 The role of capsular feedback and pattern generators in shoulder kinematics. In: Matsen FA, Fu FH, Hawkins RJ (eds) The shoulder: a balance of mobility and stability. American Academy of Orthopedic Surgeons, Rosemont, Illinois

Guerra JJ, Timmerman LA 1996 Clinical anatomy, histology and pathomechanics of the elbow in sports. Operative Techniques in Sports Medicine 4(2):69–76

Hadler AM, Itoi E, An K-N 2000 Anatomy and biomechanics of the shoulder. Orthopedic Clinics of North America 31(2):159–176

Henderson A 1995 Self-care and hand skill. In: Henderson A, Pehoski C (eds) Hand function in the child. Mosby, St Louis

Herzog W, Guimaraes AC, Anton MG et al 1991 Moment length relations of rectus femoris muscles of speed skaters/cyclists and runners. Medicine and Science in Sports and Exercise 23:1289–1296

Hides JA, Jull GA, Richardson CA 2001 Long term effects of specific stabilizing exercises for first episode low back pain. Spine 26:E243–248

Hodges P, Richardson CA 1996 Inefficient muscular stabilisation of the lumbar spine associated with low back pain: a motor control evaluation of transversus abdominis. Spine 21:2640–2650

Holle B 1981 Motor development in children. Blackwell Scientific Publications, Oxford

Itoi E, Kuechle DK, Newman SR et al 1993 Stabilising function of the biceps in stable and unstable shoulders. British Journal of Bone and Joint Surgery 75(4):546–550

Jeannerod M 1981 Intersegmental co-ordination during reaching at natural visual objects. In: Long L, Baddeley AD (eds) Attention and performance, vol 9. Lawrence Erlbaum, New Jersey

Jeannerod M 1984 The timing of natural prehension movements. Journal of Motor Behaviour 16:235–254

Jerosch J, Thorwesten L, Steinbech J et al 1996 Proprioceptive function of the shoulder girdle in healthy volunteers. Knee Surgery, Sports Traumatology and Arthroscopy 3(4):219–225

Jobe FW, Pink M 1993 Classification and treatment of shoulder dysfunction in the overhead athlete. Journal of Orthopaedic Sports Physical Therapy 18:427–432

Jobe CM, Pink M, Jobe FW et al 1996 Anterior shoulder instability, impingement and rotator cuff tears. In: Jobe FW (ed) Operative techniques in upper extremity sports injuries. Mosby, St Louis

Kabada MP, Cole MF, Wooten P et al 1992 Intramuscular wire electromyography of the subscapularis. Journal of Orthopedic Research 10(3):394–397

Kamkar A, Irrgang JJ, Whitney SL 1993 Nonoperative management of secondary shoulder impingement syndrome. Journal of Orthopaedic Sports Physical Therapy 17:212–224

Kibler WB 1993 Evaluation of sports demands as a diagnostic tool in shoulder disorders. In: Matsen FA, Fu F, Hawkins RJ (eds) The shoulder: a balance of mobility and stability. American Academy of Orthopedic Surgeons, Rosemont, Illinois

Kibler WB 1995 Biomechanical analysis of the shoulder during tennis activities. Clinics in Sports Medicine 14(1):79–85

Kibler WB 1998 The role of the scapula in athletic shoulder function. American Journal of Sports Medicine 26:325–337

Kibler WB, McMullen J, Uhl T 2001 Shoulder rehabilitation strategies, guidelines and practice. Orthopedic Clinics of North America 32(3):527–538

Kumar VP 2002 Biomechanics of the shoulder. Annals of the Academy of Medicine 31(5):590–592

Kumar VP, Balasubramaniam P 1985 The role of atmospheric pressure in stabilising the shoulder: an experimental study. Journal of Bone and Joint Surgery 67:719–721

Kumar VP, Satku K, Balasubramaniam P 1989 The role of the long head of biceps brachii in the stabilization of the head of the humerus. Clinical Orthopaedics 244:172–175

Lannerston L, Harms-Ringdahl K 1990 Neck and shoulder muscle activity during work with different cash register systems. Ergonomics 33(1):49–65

Mackel R 1996 The impact of injury and disease on the sensory function of the hand. Bulletin de la Societe Medecine 133(1):31–34

Michiels I, Bodem F 1992 The deltoid muscle: an electromyographical analysis of its activity in arm abduction in various body postures. International Orthopaedics 16:268–271

Moran CA 1989 Anatomy of the hand. Physical Therapy 69(2):1007–1013

Morrey BF, Tanaka S, An K-N 1983 Articular and ligamentous stability of the elbow joint. American Journal of Sports Medicine 11:315–319

Moseley JB, Jobe FW, Pink M et al 1992 EMG analysis of scapular muscles during a shoulder rehabilitation programme. American Journal of Sports Medicine 20(2):128–134

Mottram SL 1997 Dynamic stability of the scapula. Manual Therapy 2(3):123–131

Paine RM, Voight ML 1993 The role of the scapula. Journal of Orthopaedic Sports Physical Therapy 18:386–391

Palmer P 1991 Muscle function of the hand during resisted and non resisted activity. British Journal of Occupational Therapy 54(10):386–390

Pink M, Perry J 1996 Biomechanics. In: Jobe FW (ed) Operative techniques in upper extremity sports injuries. Mosby, St Louis

Poppen NK, Walker PS 1976 Normal and abnormal motion of the shoulder. Journal of Bone and Joint Surgery 58A:195–201

Pratt NE 1994 Anatomy and biomechanics of the shoulder. Journal of Hand Therapy 7(2):65–76

Rochat P 1992 Self sitting and reaching in 5 to 8 month old infants: the impact of posture and its development on hand eye coordination. Journal of Motor Behaviour 24(2):210–220

Rosbald B 1995 Reaching and hand eye co-ordination. In: Henderson A, Pehoski C (eds) Hand function in the child. Mosby, St Louis

Sarrafian SK 1983 Gross and functional anatomy of the shoulder. Clinical Orthopaedics and Related Research 173:11–19

Speer KP, Garrett WE 1993 Muscular control of motion and stability about the pectoral girdle. In: Matsen FA, Fu AH, Hawkins RJ (eds) The shoulder: a balance of mobility and stability. American Academy of Orthopedic Surgeons, Rosemont, Illinois

Strickland JW 1995 Anatomy and kinesiology of the hand. In: Henderson A, Pehoski C (eds) Hand function in the child. Mosby, St Louis

Terry GC, Hammon D, France P et al 1991 The stabilising function of passive shoulder restraints. American Journal of Sports Medicine 19:26–34

Tillary MI, Flanders M, Soechting JF 1991 A co-ordinated system for the synthesis of visual and kinaesthetic information. Journal of Neuroscience 11(3):770–778

Van der Helm FCT 1994 Analysis of the kinematic and dynamic behaviour of the shoulder mechanism. Journal of Biomechanics 27(5):527–550

Voight ML, Thomson BC 2000 The role of the scapula in the rehabilitation of shoulder injuries. Journal of Athletic Training 35(3):364–372

Warner JP, Lephart S, Fu FH 1996 Role of proprioception in pathoetiology of shoulder instability. Clinical Orthopaedics and Related Research 330:35–39

Weber SC, Caspari RB 1989 A biomechanical evaluation of the restraints to posterior shoulder dislocation. Arthroscopy 5:115–121

Wilk KE, Arrigo CA 1993 Current concepts in the rehabilitation of the athletic shoulder. Journal of Orthopaedic and Sports Physical Therapy 18(1):365–378

Wilk KE, Arrigo CA, Andrews JR 1996 Closed and open kinetic chain exercise for the upper extremity. Journal of Sport Rehabilitation 5(1):88–102

Williams PL 1995 Gray's anatomy, 38th edn. Churchill Livingstone, New York

Zivani J 1995 The development of graphomotor skills. In: Henderson A, Pehoski C (eds) Hand function in the child. Mosby, St Louis

Chapter 12

Function of the spine

Ann P. Moore   Nicola J. Petty

LEARNING OUTCOMES

When you have completed this chapter you should
be able to:

1. Describe how the spine functions to give
   support to the body during movement and
   weight-bearing activities

2. Discuss how the spine is able to give protection to soft tissues and vital organs during weight–bearing and physiological movements

3. Describe how the spine gives attachment for the muscles of the abdomen, thorax and upper and lower limbs

4. Explain how the spine allows movement of the human body

5. Explain how the spine contributes to the enhancement of movement of the upper and lower extremities

6. Describe how the spine is able to act as a shock absorber

7. Describe how the vertebral column gives shape to the human body in static and dynamic postures

8. Describe how the spine contributes to changes from static to dynamic postures.

INTRODUCTION

The spine is a complex, multisegmented structure which has many functions. It will be seen from this chapter that the spine is essential for weight bearing, protection and movement of the human body. A knowledge of the relationship of structure and function of the spine is of great importance to the clinician. When writing this chapter, the authors assumed that the reader has a knowledge of the basic structure of the spine.

The spine as a whole functions in a variety of ways. It gives support to the head, upper limbs and thoracic cage during movement and weight-bearing activities. It gives protection to the vital organs, such as the heart and lungs, and to soft tissues such as the spinal cord during physiological movements and weight-bearing activities. It provides attachment for the muscles of the abdomen and thorax and for some muscles of the upper and lower limbs. It allows movement to occur throughout its length and enhances movement of the upper and lower extremities. It enhances the visual and hearing fields. In addition, the spine gives shape to the human body in static and dynamic postures and facilitates changes from

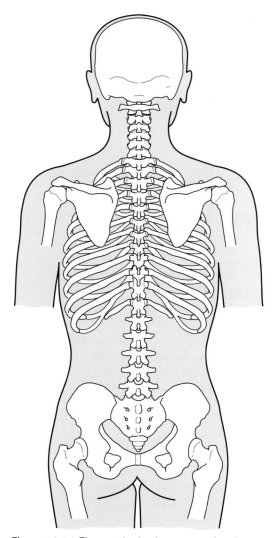

Figure 12.1 The vertebral column, posterior view (reproduced with permission from Kapandji 1974).

static to dynamic postures. Finally, it acts as a shock absorber. Each of these functions will now be considered in turn.

SUPPORT FOR THE HEAD, UPPER LIMBS AND THORACIC CAGE DURING MOVEMENT AND WEIGHT-BEARING ACTIVITIES

Normal movement can only take place if adequate support is available for the head, upper limbs and thoracic cage (Fig. 12.1). Such support is offered

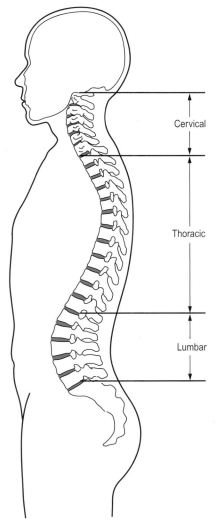

Figure 12.2 The vertebral column, lateral view indicating the spinal regions (reproduced with permission from Oliver & Middleditch 1991).

by the vertebral column and is discussed in this section.

The spine is composed of 33 vertebrae (Fig. 12.2), most of which consist of a vertebral body and a vertebral arch (Fig. 12.3). The vertebral bodies are, in the main, separated from each other in life by an intervertebral disc. The exceptions to this are found at the atlantooccipital joint and the atlanto-axial joint, where no such disc exists, and in the

sacrum, where the five sacral vertebrae are fused and do not contribute to spinal movement.

The atlantoaxial joint has a large range of rotation and the inclusion of an intervertebral disc at this level would severely limit this. It is also important that, in an area where the emerging brain stem is potentially vulnerable, this junction is well supported by ligamentous tissue. The union is therefore completed by the upward-projecting dens fitting into the osseofibrous ring rather than through a discal union. Similarly, at the atlanto-occipital joint a large range of flexion extension movement is permitted since there is no inter-vertebral disc restricting range of movement. The sacral vertebrae are fused in order to contribute to a solid and stable osseous pelvic ring which has to support the forces generated in weight bearing and locomotion.

The vertebral column is completed by the coccygeal region, which is composed of four vertebrae linked together by fibrous tissue: there is variable osteophytic union between either the first and second, second and third or third and fourth bones. The coccyx plays no supporting role in terms of spinal function but its movements are important in order to allow defaecation to occur.

Vertebral body support

The vertebral body consists of a cylinder of cancellous bone with trabeculae surrounded by a thin layer of cortical bone. The trabeculae act like struts, strengthening the vertebral body; the vertical trabeculae resist compressive forces and the horizontal trabeculae resist bowing of the struts and thus increase its strength (Bogduk 1997). This arrangement of the trabeculae can be seen in Figure 12.4. The vertebrae are thus able to resist the compressive and torsional stresses during movements of the spine and the tension caused by contraction of muscles which attach to it. The structure resembles a cardboard box which is full of packing material which prevents its collapse under compression during everyday movement. The compact bone represents the cardboard box and the trabeculae the packaging inside.

Vertebral bodies throughout the vertebral column vary in size and shape depending on their position in the column. The lumbar vertebrae are

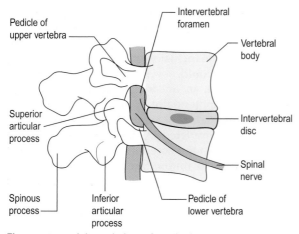

Figure 12.3 A lateral view of a spinal motion segment. The anterior weight-bearing part is shaded.

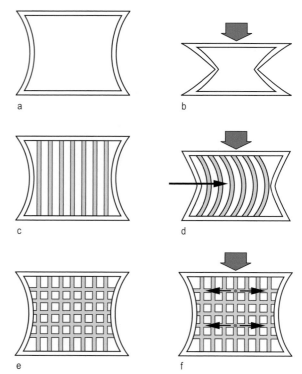

Figure 12.4 Reconstruction of the internal architecture of the vertebral body. (a) With just a shell of cortical bone, a vertebral body is like a box and collapses when a load is applied (b). (c) Internal vertical struts brace the box (d). (e) Transverse connections prevent the vertical struts from bowing and increase the load-bearing capacity of the box. Loads are resisted by tension in the transverse connections (f) (reproduced with permission from Bogduk 1997).

Task 12.1

Look at a skeleton of the spine or a model of the spine and study the spinal regions and their relative contours. Also note the position and angulation of the intervertebral discs.

---

larger and more heavily constructed than the thoracic vertebrae which, in turn, are more substantially built than the finer and more intricate cervical vertebral bodies (see Fig. 12.2). The size of the vertebra appears to be directly related to the amount of body weight that it must support. The cervical spine supports the head which accounts for approximately 10% of normal body weight; the thoracic spine supports the head and the weight of the upper limbs and thoracic organs; the lumbar spine supports the weight of the head, neck, thoracic cage and abdominal contents, and functions to transmit all this body weight through the sacroiliac joints via the sacrum to the pelvis and hence to the lower limbs in static and dynamic postures.

Intervertebral disc support

The intervertebral discs are interspersed between the vertebrae from the second cervical vertebra to

---

Task 12.2

Have a look at sagittal and coronal sections of a vertebral body and the distribution of the cancellous bone. Your educational establishment may have ready-prepared sections or alternatively you can obtain animal vertebrae from a butcher who will cut them into sections as needed. At first sight it might appear that the cancellous bone is randomly dispersed; in fact, it is distributed along the lines of weight bearing to enhance its strength. Look carefully at your sections and see if you can identify the way in which the trabeculae are organised.

the sacrum and constitute approximately one-fifth of the total length of the vertebral column. The shape of each disc corresponds to the shape of its adjacent vertebral body. The discs both allow and restrict movement between the vertebral bodies and transmit loads from one vertebral body to the next.

The discs vary in shape and size in the different regions of the spine. The discs are wedge shaped and thicker anteriorly than posteriorly in the cervical and lumbar spine, which contributes to lordosis in these regions. They are thinnest in the upper thoracic region and thickest in the lumbar region in order to bear a greater proportion of body weight. In proportion to the height of the vertebral body, the discs are thickest in the cervical region and this, in part, gives the cervical spine a greater range of physiological movement than the other regions of the spine. The discs form the main connection between adjacent vertebral bodies and are held in place around the periphery by Sharpey's fibres (Jackson 1966). The discs serve to keep the vertebral bodies apart during the maintenance of static and dynamic postures and therefore are well placed to contribute to the support mechanisms provided by the vertebral column.

The disc is composed of three parts:

- endplate
- annulus fibrosus
- nucleus pulposus.

The endplate is permeable and lies between the disc and vertebral body (Fig. 12.5). It is composed of hyaline cartilage (Ghosh 1990a). Water and nutrients pass between the nucleus and the cancellous bone of the vertebral body through the endplate.

The annulus fibrosus is a ring-shaped structure composed of concentric layers (or lamellae) of collagen fibres bound together and prevented from buckling by a matrix of proteoglycan gel. Approximately 70% of the annulus is composed of water, although this amount varies according to the load on the disc and its age. The inner annulus is attached above and below to the vertebral endplate and the outer part of the annulus is

---

Task 12.3

Look at a vertebral column and identify differences in the size and shape of the vertebral bodies in the five regions. See if you can suggest reasons for the features that you can see, noticing in particular the upward projections at the lateral aspects of the upper surfaces of the cervical bodies and the reciprocal bevelled surfaces of the lateral aspects of the lower surfaces of the cervical vertebrae. The upward projections are called uncinate processes and articulate with the vertebrae below at what is known as the uncovertebral joint (joints of von Luschka). These joints influence the degree and direction of movement and are thought to have a protective function for the lateral aspects of the intervertebral joints.

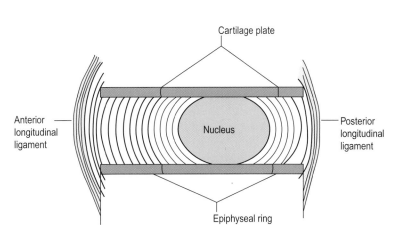

Cartilage plate

Anterior longitudinal ligament

Nucleus

Posterior longitudinal ligament

Epiphyseal ring

Figure 12.5   The cartilage endplate lies between the intervertebral disc and the vertebral body. The nucleus lies adjacent to the endplate. The anterior and posterior fibres of the annulus are attached to the anterior and posterior longitudinal ligaments respectively (reproduced from Macnab 1977).

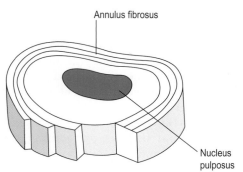

Figure 12.6 Horizontal section through a disc showing the layers of the annulus fibrosus (reproduced with permission from Oliver & Middleditch 1991).

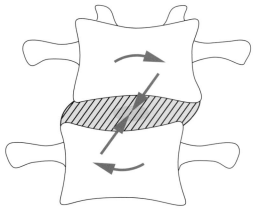

Figure 12.7 Anterior view of a spinal motion segment in the lumbar spine showing half the annular fibres stretched during rotation (reproduced with permission from Kapandji 1974).

attached to the periosteum and epiphyseal ring of the vertebral body and is strengthened by the anterior and posterior longitudinal ligaments.

The annular collagen fibres run parallel to each other and obliquely at between 40° and 70° to the horizontal, lying in opposite directions in adjacent layers, giving the annulus a lattice-like appearance (Fig. 12.6). The annulus contains both type I and type II collagen fibres (Ghosh 1988). Type I is found in tissues that are designed to resist tensile and compressive forces and type II is found in tissues designed to resist compressive forces (Bogduk 1997). The presence of type I and II fibres reflects the tensile and compressive loads applied to the annulus during static and dynamic postures. The lattice-like arrangement of the lamellae helps to limit movement between adjacent vertebrae. For example, during rotation half the fibres of the lamellae are stretched and the other half are relaxed (Fig. 12.7). On flexion, all the fibres posterior to the axis of movement are stretched and all the fibres anterior are relaxed. On extension, the anterior fibres are stretched and the posterior fibres are relaxed. On lateral flexion, the fibres ipsilateral to the direction of the motion are relaxed but on the contralateral side they are stretched.

The nucleus pulposus is a semifluid gel making up 40–60% of the disc and lies adjacent to the vertebral endplates of the vertebrae above and below. At its periphery the nucleus blends with the annulus in such a way that there is no distinct separation between the two components. The nucleus is made up of a loose network (not in layers like the annulus) of mainly type II collagen fibres (to resist compression) and a proteoglycan/water gel with some elastic fibres. Approximately 70–90% of the nucleus is composed of water.

The main property of proteoglycan gel is its water-absorbing capacity: by giving the disc a high osmotic pressure, water content is maintained even under the high compressive loads generated in normal weight-bearing postures and movement. The disc absorbs water and nutrients through the endplate from the vertebral body; the absorption of water creates a hydrostatic pressure within the disc which keeps the annulus under tension and helps to keep the vertebral bodies separated. The hydrostatic pressure varies according to the level of the disc, the posture adopted and any weights which are lifted. Nachemson (1976) measured intervertebral disc pressure in the lumbar spine during the maintenance of various postures and during various activities; the results can be seen in Figure 12.8.

A knowledge of how posture and load bearing can influence hydrostatic pressure within the disc is important to the clinician as it explains why, in some pathological states, some postures may be more painful and unachievable by the patient than others. For example, in a patient with an acute disc lesion, sitting is often very difficult to maintain for more than a minute: such a patient would prefer to lie in a weight-relieving posture in

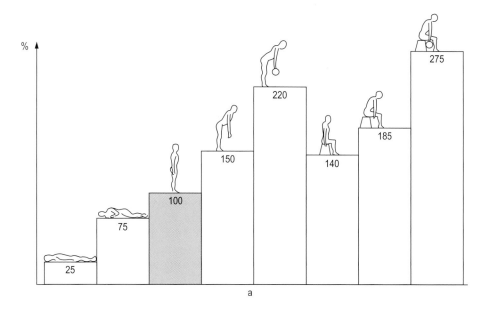

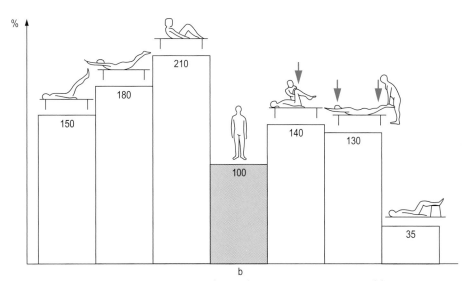

Figure 12.8 Relative change in pressure (or load) in the third lumbar disc: (a) in various positions; (b) in various muscle-strengthening exercises (reproduced by permission of Lippincott-Raven Publishers from Nachemson 1976).

order to minimise pain. Pain in this situation may be caused by a rise in hydrostatic pressure within the affected disc. Raised hydrostatic pressure may create or increase the symptoms arising from a disc lesion, the extruded disc material being brought into closer proximity with pain-sensitive structures and giving rise to local and referred pain.

The water content of the nucleus varies with age: at birth it is over 85% but drops to around

70% in the mature disc. The water content does not vary very much in the annulus and is about 70% throughout life. In humans, total body height reduces by approximately 19 mm (1% of stature) from the morning to the evening (Tyrell et al 1985) due to the loss of fluid from the discs on weight bearing and the absorption of fluid in non-weight bearing positions, particularly when recumbent.

Nutrition of the disc

The disc is avascular after the first decade of life so it then receives its nutrition mainly via tissue fluid exchange through the vertebral endplates and also from small blood vessels at the periphery of the annulus. The anterior annulus receives a better supply of nutrients than the posterior annulus. Fluid exchange is enhanced by movements of the spine, particularly movements in the sagittal plane (Adams & Hutton 1986), and reduced by static postures, particularly loading at end-range flexion or extension (Adams & Hutton 1985). If the nutrition of the disc is inadequate, disc degeneration may then occur (Ghosh 1990b). It is therefore vital to the health of the disc that the spine changes posture throughout the day and that prolonged static postures are avoided.

The intervertebral discs, together with the vertebral bodies and the supporting ligaments, particularly the anterior and posterior longitudinal ligaments, are well designed to support the body weight of the head and the upper limbs. The reader should note that this description is based on anatomical studies of the lumbar intervertebral disc. While a detailed description of the cervical disc is beyond the scope of this chapter, the reader should note that in the cervical spine the nucleus pulposus consists of fibrocartilage and the nucleus is not fully surrounded by the annulus fibrosus (Bland & Bushey 1990, Mercer 1995).

Vertebral arch support

The vertebral arch, lying behind the vertebral body, is made up of two pedicles and two laminae from which the spinous processes, two transverse processes, two inferior and two superior articular processes, project (see Fig. 12.3). The nature, shape and direction of these processes vary in different regions of the spine. The spinous processes and transverse processes function as points of attachment for supporting ligaments and muscles to increase their leverage. The articular processes bear an articular surface called an articular facet. The superior facet of one vertebra articulates with the inferior facet of the vertebra above, forming a zygapophyseal (apophyseal or facet) joint. These zygapophyseal joints are synovial joints and therefore have a synovial membrane lying deep to the fibrous capsule. The capsules which surround the joints are fairly lax to allow movement to occur.

Zygapophyseal joints are plane joints. When they are viewed in the dissected state, however, the articular surfaces are not completely flat – they undulate slightly and in life these undulations are evened out by the presence of small meniscoid inclusions. These inclusions are particularly well defined in the cervical and lumbar spines and are found in the superior and inferior recesses of each zygapophyseal joint. The role of the meniscoid inclusions is to increase surface area for distribution of loads acting through the joints and they may have a protective function for articular surfaces. They are composed of fatty cartilaginous and synovial tissue and are firmly attached to the fibrous capsule which surrounds the zygapophyseal joint.

The ligamentum flavum lies in close proximity to the joint, connecting the laminae of adjacent vertebrae and attaching to the anterior margin of the fibrous capsule. This highly elastic ligament is thought to assist the back extensor muscles to initiate restoration of the fully flexed spine to a more upright position. During this movement the elasticity of the ligament causes it to return to its normal length so that there is no buckling which could compromise the lumen of the vertebral canal. In addition, in the lumbar spine it protects the intervertebral disc by not allowing full flexion to be achieved too abruptly (Oliver & Middleditch 1991). Other supporting ligaments lie remote from these joints; they are the supraspinous, interspinous and intertransverse ligaments and can be seen in Figure 12.9.

The thoracic cage support

The thoracic cage forms a semi-rigid structure composed of 12 pairs of ribs which, apart from the

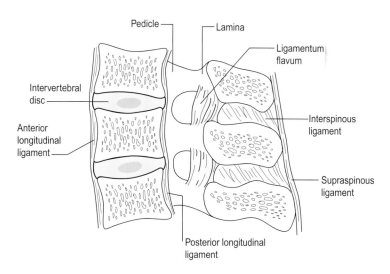

Pedicle

Lamina

Ligamentum flavum

Intervertebral disc

Anterior longitudinal ligament

Interspinous ligament

Supraspinous ligament

Posterior longitudinal ligament

Figure 12.9   Sagittal section of the lumbar spine showing supporting ligamentous structures (reproduced with permission from Oliver & Middleditch 1991).

two lower pairs of floating ribs, are united anteriorly by their costal cartilages to the sternum (see Fig. 12.1). The cage is completed posteriorly at the junction of the ribs with the vertebrae, the upper 10 ribs articulating with the vertebral bodies and the transverse processes of each of the upper 10 thoracic vertebrae. The thoracic cage forms the basis of attachment for muscles which link and give support to the upper limbs, via the shoulder girdle.

Due to its position relative to the spine and its relative inflexibility, the thoracic cage serves to restrict the physiological movements of flexion, extension and lateral flexion of the spine.

Movement of the thoracic cage occurs during respiration. Small movements of the ribs at the costovertebral joints produce large movements anteriorly of the sternum and laterally of the rib shafts. Because of the long leverage of the rib shafts and the direction and shape of the costotransverse joint surfaces, these changes in anteroposterior and transverse diameters of the thoracic cage increase its volume, reduce intrathoracic pressure and enable inspiration to occur.

The pelvic girdle support

The pelvic girdle comprises the two pelvic bones, the sacrum and the articulations between them (see Fig. 12.1). Posteriorly, the sacrum is wedged between the massive ilia of the pelvis and articulates with it via the two sacroiliac joints. The pelvic rim is completed anteriorly by the union of the two pubic bones at the symphysis pubis. The sacroiliac joints, which are synovial, are supported by some of the strongest ligaments in the body in order to maintain stability of the pelvic girdle. The symphysis pubis is a fibrous junction which is equally stable. Together, these articulations allow minimal movement during weight bearing and locomotion and maintain a solid base of support for the spine, head and upper extremities. The pelvic girdle is intimately linked with the lower extremities via the hip joints. Body weight is transmitted via the pelvis to the lower extremities; likewise impact from ground reaction forces during weight bearing and locomotion is transmitted via the lower extremities through the pelvis and on to the spine.

PROTECTION FOR SOFT TISSUE AND VITAL ORGANS DURING PHYSIOLOGICAL MOVEMENTS AND WEIGHT-BEARING ACTIVITIES

Vertebral canal structures

The vertebral canal serves to support and protect the spinal cord and cauda equina with its accompanying spinal meninges, blood vessels and

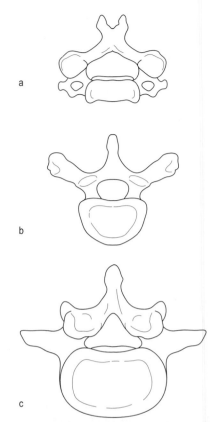

Figure 12.10 Segmental variations in the shape of the spinal canal: (a) cervical; (b) thoracic; (c) lumbar (reproduced with permission from Butler 1991).

lymphatic drainage vessels. During movement of the spine, the spinal cord, together with its meninges, undergoes changes in length, tension and position. From spinal extension to spinal flexion there is about 5–9 cm of elongation, with most of the movement occurring in the cervical and lumbar regions (Breig 1978, Louis 1981), and an increase in tension (Butler 1991). On flexion, the spinal cord and meninges elongate, become thinner and move anteriorly in the spinal canal. On extension, they become shorter and fatter and move posteriorly (Breig 1978). With right lateral flexion, the spinal cord shortens on the right and elongates on the left-hand side (Breig 1978).

Thus, with normal physiological movements, the space taken up by the spinal cord and nerve roots in the spinal canal will vary. If pathology causes any encroachment into the spinal canal, the spinal cord or nerve roots may be compromised and this may be accentuated by certain physiological movements. It must be remembered that any blood vessels accompanying the spinal cord and its meninges or the nerve roots and their dural sleeves may also be compromised by pathology. Limb movements can also affect the neural tissue in the spinal canal; for example, the straight leg raise (SLR) increases tension in the lumbar and sacral nerve roots and their meningeal covering.

The boundaries of the vertebral canal formed by the vertebral body anteriorly and the vertebral arch posteriorly are well adapted to protect the spinal cord and its meninges as they are made of compact bone which is very resistant to compressive forces.

The lumen of the vertebral canal varies in its shape in different parts of the spine depending upon the size of the neuromeningeal tissue passing through it. It is triangular and large in the cervical spine to allow for the enlarged spinal cord close to the brain stem; in the thoracic spine it is smaller and circular; and in the lumbar region the lumen widens and becomes more triangular in shape to accommodate the cauda equina (Fig. 12.10). Within the vertebral canal are small clusters of fat pads which fill in the recesses of the canal and act as cushions to the soft tissue structures during movements of the spine. This is a very important function during rapid spinal movement when the spinal cord moves forwards in the canal during flexion and backwards during extension and also when physiological movements are accompanied by compression, for example when jumping. The fat pads protect the sensitive neuromeningeal tissues from sudden impact.

The intervertebral foramen as a protective structure

The intervertebral foramina are gaps between the vertebrae and lie laterally (see Fig. 12.3). The posterior wall of an intervertebral foramen is formed by the zygapophyseal joint, the anterior wall by the vertebral bodies and intervening disc, and the superior and inferior walls by the pedicles of the vertebrae above and below, respectively.

Within each intervertebral foramen lies the spinal nerve, sinuvertebral nerve, adipose tissue, blood and lymphatic vessels. The adipose (fatty) tissue together with the osseous fibrous ring serves to protect the structures in the intervertebral foramen during physiological movements when the diameter of the intervertebral foramen is altered. The cross-sectional area alters significantly during flexion and extension; in the lumbar spine flexion increases the area by 30% and extension decreases the area by 20%, whereas rotation and lateral flexion reduce the area (on the side to which the movement is directed) by 2–4% (Panjabi et al 1983).

Normally the spinal and sinuvertebral nerves occupy one-third to one-half of the cross-sectional area of the foramen and in normal circumstances the alteration of the intervertebral foramen with movement does not adversely affect the enclosed tissues. However, certain individuals have transforaminal ligaments in the lumbar spine which are vestigial ligaments and have been described in detail by Golub and Silverman (1969). They span the intervertebral foramen and so reduce its vertical height and cross-sectional area. They occur quite naturally to a variable extent in some individuals but are absent in others. If they exist in association with minor pathology, the foraminal space, during physiological movements, may be significantly reduced and compression of the soft tissue structures may occur, leading to clinical signs and symptoms of a large space-occupying lesion. In other words, the presence of these ligaments may give a false impression to the diagnostician in terms of the true nature and size of the lesion. Transforaminal ligaments may also be present in

the thoracic and cervical spines but the evidence for this is not extensive at the present time.

In the thoracic cage, the vertebral column, which lies posteriorly, is perfectly positioned to offer protection to the vital organs and their protective membranes, i.e. lungs, pleura, heart and pericardium. In addition, the descending thoracic aorta is well protected from external trauma as it lies deep within the thorax on the anterior surface of the vertebral column.

In the cervical spine the transverse processes are punctuated by the foramina transversaria for the passage of the vertebral arteries. The vertebral arteries on the left and right join anterior to the brain stem to form the basilar artery and this feeds into the circle of Willis which supplies a large area of the brain (Fig. 12.11).

The foramina transversaria offer the two vertebral arteries protection from compression during physiological movements and external trauma. This protective device can, however, create some difficulty during physiological movements in the pathological state, when osteophytic growth from zygapophyseal joints can impinge on the vertebral artery, thus impeding blood flow and producing vertebrobasilar insufficiency. The most common symptom is dizziness; other symptoms which depend on the area of the brain stem affected can include 'drop attacks', visual disturbance, diplopia, nausea, disorientation, dysarthria, dysphagia, ataxia, impairment of trigeminal sensation, sympathoplegia, hemianaesthesia and hemiplegia (Bogduk 1994).

PROVISION OF ATTACHMENTS FOR THE MUSCLES OF THE ABDOMEN AND THORAX AND FOR SOME MUSCLES OF THE UPPER AND LOWER LIMBS

The spine via its many bony processes offers direct or indirect attachment to muscle structures which have one or more of the following functions:

- segmental stabilisation of the spine during movement and normal posture
- production of gross movement over a large number of segments
- stabilisation and physiological movement of the limbs relative to the trunk.

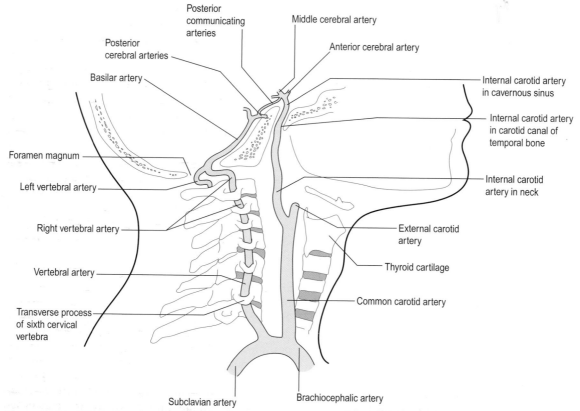

Figure 12.11   The pathway of the vertebral arteries through the cervical vertebrae to the brain stem (reproduced from Palastanga et al 1994).

Segmental stabilisation of the spine during movement and normal posture

Muscles whose function relates to segmental stabilisation and posture lie much closer to the vertebral column than muscles which produce gross movement. By virtue of the length of the vertebral processes, muscles increase their mechanical advantage because of the greater leverage that is available.

A spinal motion segment consists of two adjacent vertebrae with their intervening disc as shown previously (see Fig. 12.3). Each individual motion segment is potentially unstable without its supporting ligaments and muscles. The muscles which span the motion segment are very important in stabilising adjacent vertebrae during gross

movements of the spine which are produced by larger muscle groups. The concept of deep and superficial muscles functioning in different ways was first put forward by Bergmark (1989). In the lumbar spine the deep stabilising muscles include multifidus, rotatores, interspinales and intertransversarii. Multifidus spans between one and four vertebrae and the latter two muscles link adjacent vertebrae. The main action of multifidus is to produce posterior sagittal rotation of the vertebrae which occurs during extension, and to control this movement during flexion (Macintosh & Bogduk 1994). During rotation of the trunk the contraction of the prime movers, the oblique abdominal muscles, would tend to produce trunk flexion. Multifidus in the lumbar spine acts with erector spinae to oppose the flexion pull of the obliques, ensuring pure axial rotation (Macintosh & Bogduk 1986).

The rotatores, interspinales and intertransversarii muscles are thought to act as stabilisers. One suggestion is that they act as large proprioceptive transducers since they have been found to contain 2–6 times the density of muscle spindles found in the longer muscles (Bastide et al 1989, Nitz & Peck 1986, Peck et al 1984). They would thus provide feedback on spinal position and movement.

In standing, the spine is well stabilised by its joints and ligaments so that there is little back muscle activity; individuals vary, however, and there may be slight continuous activity, intermittent activity or no activity (Valencia & Munro 1985). Back muscle activity in sitting is similar to that in standing (Andersson et al 1975) but with the arms supported or with the backrest reclined, it is reduced (Andersson et al 1974).

The degree of lumbar lordosis and the position of the pelvis are interdependent and are to some degree controlled by the surrounding muscles. Contraction of the back extensors and hip flexors will tend to increase lumbar lordosis and cause an anterior pelvic tilt; contraction of the abdominals and hip extensors, on the other hand, will produce a flattening of the lumbar lordosis and posterior pelvic tilt. The balance of contraction of these muscle groups can be influenced by pathological processes of the spine (Aspinall 1993, Cooper et al 1993, Hides et al 1994, Jull & Janda 1987) and therefore assessment of muscle function is important in the examination of a patient with spinal pain (Richardson et al 1999).

In the cervical spine, joints and muscle systems are very closely associated with stabilisation movements of the head and eyes and the function of the body's vestibular system (important for balance activities) and also the proprioceptive system. The cervical spine then is essential for the general control of body posture and balance (Keshner 1990, Winters & Peles 1990). The cervical spine, like the lumbar spine, has superficial muscles spanning a number of cervical spine segments, i.e. multisegmental muscles, which have a role in the production of gross cervical spine movements, for example the upper fibres of trapezius, sternocleido-mastoid muscle and scalenus anterior, medius and posterior. These muscles are very important for gross cervical spine movements. The cervical spine also contains a deep intersegmental muscle system, for example longus colli and longus capitis which are responsible for controlling cervical spine movements produced by the 'global/superficial muscles'. These deep cervical muscles have, along with the deep lumbar muscles, been termed 'local muscle structures'. Much work has been carried out on the interaction between the deep and superficial cervical flexor muscles by Falla et al (2003) (much of Falla et al's interesting work is still in press at the time of writing).

Jull (2000) has demonstrated different activation patterns in deep and superficial cervical spine muscles in patients complaining of neck pain with overactivity occurring in the superficial muscles and loss of or reduction in the stability of the cervical spine occurring with underactivity of the deep cervical neck flexors.

Production of gross movement over a large number of segments

Muscles which produce this type of gross movement tend to be more remote from the vertebrae; for example, it is the more superficial members of the erector spinae group which are concerned with gross movement of the trunk. This is because these muscles span up to five or six vertebral segments and are thus able to produce more gross segmental movements. In the upright position, the trunk muscles, notably the abdominals and back extensors, initiate movements into flexion, extension and lateral flexion. Once the centre of gravity is displaced, the contralateral group will contract eccentrically to control the movement against gravity. For example, on spinal flexion, the trunk flexors will initially contract to displace the centre of gravity forwards, then the movement will be controlled by eccentric work of the back extensors which increases with increasing angles of flexion (Shultz et al 1982). It should be noted that because of the direction of the back extensor muscle fibres (being parallel to the spine), activity in these muscles causes a proportional increase in intradiscal pressure.

The abdominal muscles which lie some distance from the spine achieve the movements of physiological flexion, side flexion and rotation of the trunk in combination with other muscles of the trunk and in association with the deeper muscles of the back. None of the abdominal muscles are attached directly to the spine: however, transversus abdominis and the internal abdominal oblique muscles have attachments to the lower thoracic and lumbar spines via the thoracolumbar fascia. Together, these three abdominal muscles and their fascial attachments provide a complex bracing mechanism to protect the lumbar spine during flexion movements and lifting activities. The exact mechanism of lifting still remains unclear, despite much research in this area. A detailed discussion of the various mechanisms put forward is beyond the scope of this chapter.

Stabilisation and physiological movement of the limbs relative to the trunk

The spine gives attachment for levator scapulae, serratus anterior, latissimus dorsi, trapezius and rhomboids minor and major which are all important muscles for the production of shoulder girdle movement and for stabilisation of the scapula in order to facilitate movements of the upper limb. In addition, the spine affords attachment for psoas major and piriformis, muscles which have direct influence on the lower extremity during gait.

SPINAL MOVEMENT

Functionally, the spine is considered to consist of a large number of spine motion segments which contribute to overall spinal movement (see Fig. 12.3). The motion segment consists of the interbody joint which allows movement to occur under compression and the two zygapophyseal joints which are concerned with guiding the direction of the movement which takes place. We have considered these two joints earlier in the chapter. The motion segment is well developed to allow movement to occur between adjacent segments since the collagenous fibres of the annulus are compressible to a small extent, are capable of being torsioned and also of being stretched longitudinally. In addition, the nucleus pulposus acts rather like a water cushion stabilised

by the surrounding annulus and adjacent vertebral segments and is capable of deforming in response to changes of both static and dynamic postures (Fig. 12.12). The size of the intervertebral disc varies according to vertebral level. The discs are thickest in the most mobile segments of the vertebral column, i.e. in the lumbar and cervical spine, and thinnest in the thoracic spine. The two synovial zygapophyseal joints together complete the triad motion segment. Their structure has been described earlier in this chapter.

Note that in the cervical region (apart from C0–1 and C1–2), the inferior articular facets face downwards and forwards at an angle of approximately 45° (Fig. 12.13). The superior articular facets of the vertebra below lie in a complementary position, facing upwards and backwards. In the thoracic spine the zygapophyseal joints are orientated so that the inferior facets of the vertebra above face forwards and slightly medially, lying almost in a coronal plane, and therefore the superior facets of the vertebra below face backwards and laterally. By contrast, the facets of the lumbar spine are curved so that the inferior articular facets face both laterally and forwards while the superior facets face medially and backwards.

As segments are viewed progressively from C2 to the sacrum, it will be noted that the change in the direction of the articular facets is a gradual process. The inclination of zygapophyseal joints will affect the range and direction of the motion available at each segmental level as can be seen below (Figs 12.14, 12.15).

The upper cervical joints, the atlantooccipital (C0–1) and atlantoaxial (C1–2), are atypical motion segments since there is no intervertebral disc between these two junctions and the direction of the facets is quite different from the rest of the cervical spine. The C0–1 articulation is the only joint within the vertebral column which does not have a triad joint, there being only two articulations at this level which are synovial condylar joints. The superior facets of C1 are significantly expanded to enable the condyles of the occiput to be supported. They are elongated and cup shaped, facing slightly medially and in the anteroposterior direction lie at 45° to the sagittal plane. The configuration and direction of the joint surfaces facilitate anteroposterior sagittal rotation and

a   b

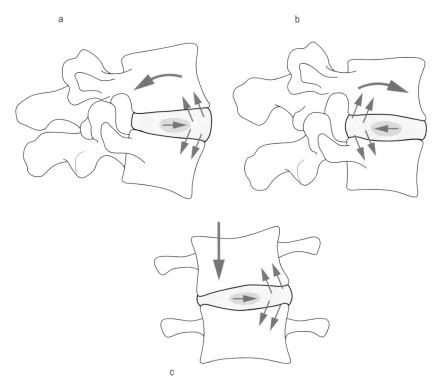

c

Figure 12.12   Effect of movement on deformation of the intervertebral disc. (a) Extension: the upper vertebra moves posteriorly, the nucleus moves anteriorly and the annulus is tensioned anteriorly. (b) Flexion: the upper vertebra moves anteriorly, the nucleus moves posteriorly and the annulus is tensioned anteriorly. (c) Lateral flexion: the upper vertebra tilts towards the side of flexion, the nucleus moves in the opposite direction, where the annulus is tensioned (reproduced with permission from Kapandji 1974).

translation of the occipital condyles on the superior articular facets of C1, allowing a large range of flexion and extension at this level. The C1–2 joint is formed by a pivot joint between the odontoid peg of the axis and the anterior arch of the atlas. This junction creates a very mobile joint in terms of physiological ranges of rotation, as can be seen from Figure 12.15.

There are six degrees of freedom at each spine motion segment: sagittal rotation and translation, coronal rotation and translation, horizontal rotation and translation (Fig. 12.16). Flexion consists of anterior sagittal rotation and anterior translation, extension consists of posterior sagittal rotation and posterior translation.

Atlantooccipital joint (C0–1)

Flexion and extension are the largest ranges available at this segment, with slight lateral flexion also possible. During flexion of the head on the neck, the occipital condyles roll on the lateral masses of C1 and also translate forwards. The

atlas translates backwards and tilts upwards and posteriorly. In extension the reverse movements occur.

Atlantoaxial joint (C1–2)

Rotation is the largest range available. During rotation to the left, the right inferior facet of C1 moves forwards and slightly upwards on the superior facet of C2 and the left inferior facet of C1 moves backwards and slightly downwards. The forward and backward movements constitute rotation and the upward and downward movements constitute lateral flexion, therefore rotation is accompanied by some lateral flexion movement. Some flexion, extension and lateral flexion movements are also available at this level (see Figs 12.14 and 12.15).

Lower cervical region (C2–6)

Flexion and extension, lateral flexion and rotation are all possible at these levels. During flexion the

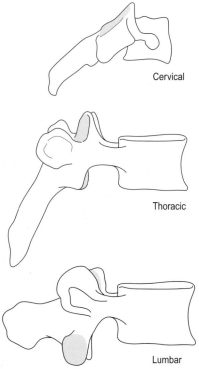

Figure 12.13 Orientation of the articular facets (shaded) in the cervical, thoracic and lumbar regions (reproduced from Palastanga et al 1994).

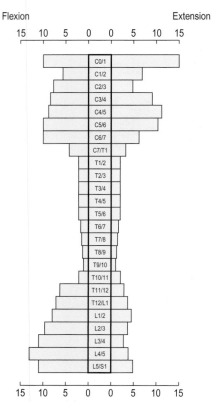

Figure 12.14 Average ranges of spinal segmental movement (flexion and extension) (reproduced with permission from Oliver & Middleditch 1991).

Task 12.5

Look at the vertebral column and notice the changes in the direction of the articular surfaces in each region of the spine.

---

vertebrae undergo anterior sagittal rotation and anterior translation. The intervertebral foramen increases in size during this movement. During extension the vertebrae undergo posterior sagittal rotation and posterior translation. The intervertebral foramina decrease in size during this movement.

Rotation is coupled with lateral flexion to the same side. For example, with rotation to the right, the left inferior articular facet of the upper vertebra glides superiorly, anteriorly and laterally on the superior articular facet of the vertebra below; the right inferior articular facet of the upper vertebra glides inferiorly, posteriorly and medially on the superior articular facet of the vertebra below. The anterior, posterior, medial and lateral movements constitute rotation movements and the inferior and superior movements constitute lateral flexion.

In the same way lateral flexion is accompanied by rotation. With lateral flexion to the right, the left and right inferior articular facets of the upper vertebrae glide in a similar way as in right rotation. The inferior and superior glides produce the lateral flexion, the anterior, posterior, medial and lateral movements produce the rotation.

Cervicothoracic junction (C6–T2)

Similar movements occur in this region as above.

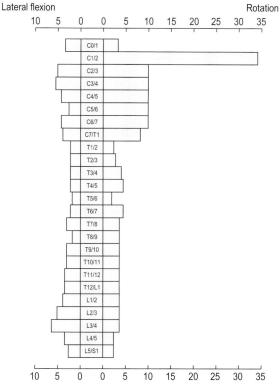

Figure 12.15   Average ranges of spinal segmental movement (values given to one side) for lateral flexion and rotation (reproduced with permission from Oliver & Middleditch 1991).

Thoracic region (T3–10)

This is the least mobile area of the spine. During flexion the inferior articular facets of the superior vertebra slide superiorly with a small amount of forward translation. In extension the reverse movements occur. Rotation is always coupled with lateral flexion as the zygapophyseal joints slide relative to each other. In lateral flexion to the left, the inferior facets of the superior vertebra on the right glide superiorly and translate slightly forwards and, on the left side, slide inferiorly and translate slightly backwards.

Lumbar region

Flexion is the freest movement. In the lumbar spine there are around 10° of anterior sagittal rotation and 2 mm of anterior translation during flexion

and around 3° of posterior sagittal rotation and 1 mm of posterior translation on extension (Pearcy et al 1984). Movements during lateral flexion and rotation are less clear.

Lateral flexion is always accompanied by a degree of rotation. Lateral flexion to the left, for example, is accompanied by axial rotation to the opposite side at the upper lumbar levels. At the two lower levels, lateral flexion to the left is accompanied by rotation to the left (Pearcy & Trebewal 1984). Figure 12.17 depicts the overall pattern of movement of the lumbar spine during the active physiological movement of lateral flexion in standing of a young asymptomatic male subject. It can be seen that lateral flexion to the left is accompanied by rotation to the left and with lateral flexion to the right, there is rotation to the right. The lateral flexion movement in this case is accompanied by flexion; however, in other subjects lateral flexion may be accompanied by extension.

It should be noted that range of movement is not static; there is a reduction in range with increasing age. The lumbar spine, for example, has a reduced range of movement, in both males and females, with increasing age (Leighton 1966). This is due to an increase in stiffness of the intervertebral disc (Twomey & Taylor 1983). Range of spinal movement also varies between males and females, although there is conflicting evidence from the literature. One study found that up to the age of 65, men had a greater sagittal mobility than females but the reverse was true after 65 (Sturrock et al 1973).

Sacroiliac joints

Movement of the sacroiliac joints occurs during flexion and extension movements of the trunk. Anterior rotation of the base of the sacrum with posterior rotation of the apex is termed 'nutation'. The reverse movement is known as 'counternutation'. There is approximately 1° of nutation during flexion and 1° of counternutation during extension of the lumbar spine in standing (Jacob & Kissling 1995). The direction of the movement varies between individuals; in some flexion is accompanied by nutation and in others by counternutation.

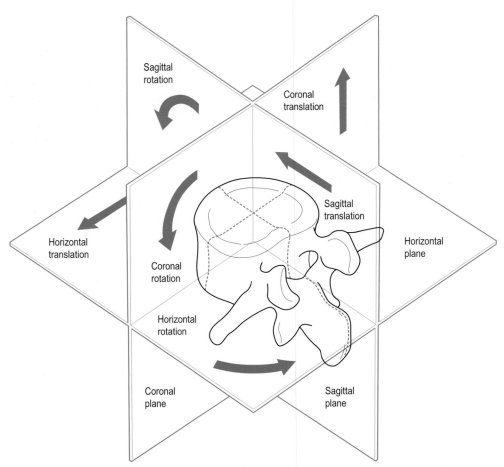

Figure 12.16 Planes and directions of motion showing the six degrees of freedom at a spinal motion segment (reproduced with permission from Bogduk 1997).

Task 12.6

Palpating the external occipital protuberance and the spinous process of C2, nod your head into flexion and extension and feel how much movement is available.

Task 12.7

Feeling the spinous process of C2, rotate your head from right to left and back again and see how much rotation movement is available at the C1–2 region. The movement takes place further down the cervical spine when the spinous process of C2 begins to move under your finger.

Task 12.8

Sitting in front of a mirror and palpating the spinous processes of two or three of your own mid-cervical vertebrae, look at the range of flexion and extension, lateral flexion to the right and the left and rotation to the right and left that occurs when you move and feel what happens to the vertebrae as these movements take place. Be aware that movements occurring in the spine are rarely 'pure' movements and you will feel, for example, that rotation is accompanied by slight side flexion.

Task 12.9

Ask a colleague to sit with the neck exposed and then flex the cervical spine from fully extended to fully flexed. Notice the quality of the movement that takes place when viewing your colleague from behind. Ask several other colleagues to do the same. See if you can detect any differences in the range of movement occurring at different levels between different individuals and see if you can decide why these differences occur. You may, for example, notice that one individual appears to have tighter musculature posteriorly which may limit range of movement.

Task 12.10

With two or three colleagues in a sitting position, ask each of them to cross their arms over the front of their chests and ask them then to move first from a neutral position into flexion then extension, then second, into lateral flexion and then third, into rotation. See if you can pinpoint where the movement occurs within the thoracic spine and how much range there is at one or more segments and how this may vary between individuals.

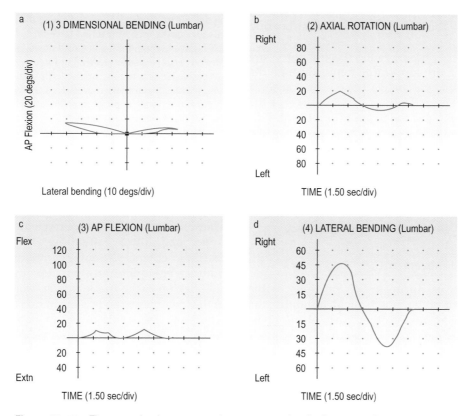

Figure 12.17   These graphs demonstrate the accompanying flexion, extension and rotation movements which occur during lateral flexion movement of an asymptomatic subject: (d) shows lateral flexion (the primary movement); (a) shows the overall movement as if looking from above; (c) shows accompanying flexion and extension movement; (b) shows accompanying rotation to the left and right. The CA-6000 Spine Motion Analyser is able to measure three-dimensional spinal movement in real time (reproduced with permission from Orthopedic Systems Inc., Hayward, California, 1993).

This movement does not occur as a result of muscle activity but as a result of mechanical forces placed upon the base of the sacrum during load bearing through the lumbar spine. The movement is restricted by the sacrotuberous and sacrospinous ligaments and also by the interosseous ligaments which bind the sacrum together with the iliac. These nutation and counternutation movements occur readily during gait and weight-bearing activities.

During stance phase, ground reaction forces are transmitted via the supporting femur through the hip to the ipsilateral pelvic bone. This causes a tendency for shear (sliding) to take place at the symphysis pubis and the SI joint (Fig. 12.18). This shearing force is enhanced by the weight of the dependent leg on the contralateral side. Also during gait, anterior and posterior rotation of the pelvis relative to the sacrum occurs. It should be noted, however, that due to the very strong ligaments supporting the sacroiliac joints, the range of movement is extremely small.

General spinal movement

The spine moves during most functions of the body as a result of the muscles which stabilise the trunk for movements of other parts of the body. For example, when one is sitting and lifting one's hand to one's mouth as in eating or drinking, the trunk will often move forwards into flexion. The pelvis tilts forward and the trunk flexes, initiated by the trunk flexors and controlled by the trunk extensors working eccentrically. This activity allows the body and hence the mouth to come closer to the food which is to be eaten. In drinking, the trunk is stabilised and the head and neck extend to enable liquid to be taken into the mouth and the neck is then brought back into the neutral position in order for swallowing to be facilitated.

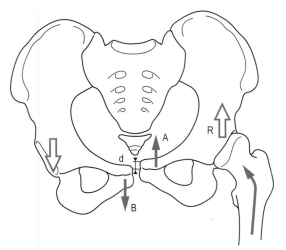

Figure 12.18   The forces around the pelvis when standing on the left leg (stance phase) and taking the right leg forward in walking. The ground reaction force (arrow R) elevates the left hip while the right hip is pulled down by the weight of the free leg. This causes a shearing force at the pubic symphysis tending to raise on the left (A) and lower on the right (B) (d is the distance moved due to this shear force). The forces will be in the opposite direction at the sacroiliac joints, the left ilia will tend to lower and the right ilia will tend to be raised (reproduced with permission from Kapandji 1974).

Enhancement of movement of upper and lower extremities and enhancement of visual and hearing fields

The spine serves to enhance movement of both the upper and lower extremities: for example, in reaching activities the range of motion of the upper limb can be significantly enhanced by rotation and side flexion of the trunk, and an example relating to the lower limb can be seen in hurdling activities where the trunk side flexes above the flexed hip and knee in order to gain clearance of the hurdle.

The trunk also serves to increase the field of vision. This is accomplished by rotatory movements of the head on the neck or of the trunk as a whole, allowing the eyes to be brought into a more optimum position for viewing the targeted object. Trunk movements can also enhance hearing fields in the same way.

Movements of the spine generally aid maintenance of balance by allowing the subject's centre of gravity to be brought over the base of support; for example, in one-leg standing, the trunk will side flex, rotate, flex and extend in whatever sequence is necessary to maintain the upright posture.

In the car, drivers will frequently rotate their head on their neck and their neck on their thorax and even sometimes the upper part of the thorax in an attempt to enhance the visual fields in order to perform safe driving activities, for example when reversing.

In addition, one can often see people who are listening intently to another's conversation rotate their neck and slightly side flex their head in order to bring one of their ears into closer proximity with the person who is speaking.

THE SPINE AS A SHOCK ABSORBER

Impact forces, e.g. during running and jumping, are transmitted upwards to the spine through the lower limbs and pelvis. Downward forces due to body weight are transmitted through the spine to the pelvis; these are reduced significantly by the presence of the spinal curvatures which help to stagger the transmission of these forces. These forces are absorbed to a degree by the trabeculae of the cancellous bone and the cartilaginous components of the intervertebral discs.

GIVING SHAPE TO THE BODY IN STATIC AND DYNAMIC POSTURES

The spine in normal subjects takes on a characteristic appearance in both dynamic and static postures. If spinal contours are enhanced or lost, it can be a manifestation of poor postural control, muscle weakness or imbalance, bony deformity or bony and/or ligamentous pathology. It can also relate to habitual postural stances, which can be related to work or leisure pursuits, or these habitual postures can be a manifestation of a psychological disturbance. For example, in depression the upper cervical spine is often extended so that the chin is poked forward, the lower cervical spine and the thoracic spine are flexed, the lumbar spine is flexed, producing a flattened lordosis, and there is some flexion of the hips and knees and the patient walks with a shuffling gait. A change in the contours of one region will often be accompanied by compensatory changes in other regions.

The spine also moves in a characteristic way. Analysis of spinal movement is important for the clinician in order to assess the presence of pathology or spinal dysfunction. It is important that contributions by all segments of the spine are monitored in terms of a total regional/spinal movement. If one spine motion segment is blocked (hypomobile), movement of the whole spinal region may be affected, causing limited or abnormal movement and this is sometimes compensated for by the development of hypermobility in adjacent segments.

THE SPINE FACILITATING CHANGES FROM STATIC TO DYNAMIC POSTURES

The spine serves a useful function when the body requires movement from a static to a dynamic posture or from one static posture to another static posture. The mobility in the spine allows the subject's centre of gravity to be brought over the base of support; for example, when getting up from a chair the thorax and trunk are flexed forwards over the pelvis, towards the knees, so that the lower limbs can raise the trunk from the chair, whilst the trunk remains in a stable posture.

Spinal movements are integral to a number of everyday movement changes which take place between static postures, for example rolling from supine to side lying, attaining an upright sitting position from side lying, changing position from sitting to standing, moving from standing into a stepping position. In addition, the spine moves fluidly during walking, running and jumping activities. Complex spinal movements also occur during hopping, going up and down stairs, standing on one leg and standing on tip-toe.

It is likely that the trunk can be used to produce deceleration of a moving body in conjunction with the lower limbs; for example, in running the trunk flexes slightly over the lower limbs. When the runner decelerates, the trunk is brought into a more upright, slightly extended position which increases air resistance by increasing turbulence and also moves the centre of gravity posteriorly. This in itself retards motion.

In most circumstances the trunk, head and neck can initiate gross movements of the body, e.g. in

---

Task 12.12

You have now become used to looking at spinal movements in your colleagues. Now ask a colleague with the spine suitably exposed (so that you will be able to see the cervical, thoracic and lumbar regions) to carry out some generalised body movements so that you can observe what happens to the spine. Ask your colleague to lie first of all on a plinth in supine lying. Then ask your colleague to do the following:

- roll from supine lying into side lying and back again
- from side lying get into an upright sitting position
- from the upright sitting position with feet on the floor move from sitting to standing
- in standing, take a step forward and then a step backwards
- walk forwards while you view the spine from the posterior aspect
- jump with both feet together on a number of occasions
- stand on one leg so you can view what happens in the thoracic, lumbar and cervical spines as weight is taken on the leg

- close both eyes while standing on one leg so that you can see what happens to the spine in that situation.

During all these activities ascertain which areas of the spine are moving and which movements are occurring in these areas of the spine, and what other movements are occurring in either the upper or lower limbs or both at the same time.

By completing this last activity, you will have put into practice many of the theoretical concepts addressed in this chapter. It is important that you use your observation skills very carefully during this last exercise and having successfully completed it with one individual, try it on a number of other individuals. You may be surprised at the differences which occur between individuals in terms of the contribution that each area of the spine makes in these very fundamental movements of the human body.

---

rolling where either the head and neck or the pelvis can initiate the movement followed by the upper or lower extremity.

Since the early American Association booklets on joint motion published in 1965, there have been various developments and innovations in spinal motion analysis. The last decade has seen an upsurge in production of three-dimensional real-time instrumentation (for example, the CA 6000 Spine Motion Analyser, Isotrak, Coda, Vicon and Spinatrak) which will in the future revolutionise our understanding of spinal motion. More recently, various researchers (Dopf et al 1994, Dvorak et al 1995, McGregor et al 1995, Troke et al 2000, Van Herp et al 2000) have been involved in testing the reliability and validity of these instruments, analysing spinal motion and in some cases producing normative databases (mainly in the lumbar spine).

REFERENCES

Adams MA, Hutton WC 1985 Gradual disc prolapse. Spine 10: 524–531

Adams MA, Hutton WC 1986 The effects of posture on diffusion into the lumbar intervertebral discs. Journal of Anatomy 147: 121–134

Andersson BJG, Jonsson B, Ortengren R 1974 Myoelectric activity in individual lumbar erector spinae muscles in sitting: a study with surface and wire electrodes. Scandinavian Journal of Rehabilitation Medicine 3(suppl): 91–108

Andersson BJG, Ortengren R, Nachemson AL et al 1975 The sitting posture: an electromyographic and discometric study. Orthopedic Clinics of North America 6: 105–120

Aspinall W 1993 Clinical implications of iliopsoas dysfunction. Journal of Manual and Manipulative Therapy 1: 41–46

Bastide G, Zadeh J, Lefebvre D 1989 Are the 'little muscles' what we think they are? Surgical and Radiological Anatomy 11: 255–256

Bergmark A 1989 Stability of the lumbar spine: a study in mechanical engineering. Acta Orthopaedica Scandinavica 230(suppl): 20–24

Bland J, Bushey DR 1990 Anatomy and physiology of the cervical spine. Seminars in Arthritis and Rheumatism 20: 1–20

Bogduk N 1994 Cervical causes of headaches and dizziness. In: Boyling JD, Palastanga N (eds) Grieve's modern manual therapy, 2nd edn. Churchill Livingstone, Edinburgh

Bogduk N 1997 Clinical anatomy of the lumbar spine, 3rd edn. Churchill Livingstone, Edinburgh

Breig A 1978 Adverse mechanical tension in the central nervous system. Almqvist and Wiksell, Stockholm

Butler DS 1991 Mobilisation of the nervous system. Churchill Livingstone, Edinburgh

Cooper RG, Stokes MJ, Sweet C, Taylor RJ, Jayson MIV 1993 Increased central drive during fatiguing contractions of the paraspinal muscles in patients with chronic low back pain. Spine 18: 610–616

Dopf CA, Schlomo SM, Geiger DF, Mayer PJ 1994 Analysis of spine motion variability using a computerised goniometer compared to physical examination. Spine 19: 586–595

Dvorak J, Vajda EG, Grob D, Panjabi MM 1995 Normal motion of the lumbar spine as related to age and gender. European Spine Journal 4: 18–23

Falla D, Jull G, Hodges P 2003 Neck pain patients demonstrate reduced activation of the deep cervical flexor muscles during performance of cranio-cervical flexion test. World Physical Therapy, 14th International WCPT Congress, Barcelona, Spain

Ghosh P 1988 The biology of the intervertebral disc, vol 1. CRC Press, Boca Raton, Florida

Ghosh P l990a Basic biochemistry of the intervertebral disc and its variation with ageing and degeneration. Journal of Manual Medicine 5: 48–51

Ghosh P l990b The role of mechanical and genetic factors in degeneration of the disc. Journal of Manual Medicine 5: 62–65

Golub BS, Silverman B 1969 Transforaminal ligaments of the lumbar spine. Journal of Bone and Joint Surgery 51A: 947–956

Hides JA, Stokes MJ, Saide M, Jull GA, Cooper DH 1994 Evidence of lumbar multifidus muscle wasting ipsilateral to symptoms in patients with acute/subacute low back pain. Spine 19: 165–172

Jackson R 1966 The cervical syndrome. Charles C Thomas, Springfield, Illinois

Jacob HAC, Kissling RO 1995 The mobility of the sacroiliac joints in healthy volunteers between 20 and 50 years of age. Clinical Biomechanics 10: 352–361

Jull GA 2000 Deep cervical neck flexor dysfunction in whiplash. Journal of Musculoskeletal Pain 8(1-2): 143–154

Jull GA, Janda V 1987 Muscles and motor control in low back pain: assessment and management. In: Twomey LT, Taylor JR (eds) Physical therapy of the low back. Churchill Livingstone, Edinburgh

Kapandji IA 1974 The physiology of the joints, vol 3: the trunk and the vertebral column. Churchill Livingstone, Edinburgh

Keshner EA 1990 Controlling stability of a complex movement system. Physical Therapy 70: 844–854

Leighton JR 1966 The Leighton flexometer and flexibility test. Journal of the Association for Physical and Mental Rehabilitation 20: 86–93

Louis R 1981 Vertebroradicular and vertebromedullar dynamics. Anatomica Clinica 3: 1–11

Macintosh JE, Bogduk N 1986 The biomechanics of the lumbar multifidus. Clinical Biomechanics 1: 205–213

Macintosh JE, Bogduk N 1994 The anatomy and function of the lumbar back muscles. In: Boyling JD, Palastanga N (eds) Grieve's modern manual therapy, 2nd edn. Churchill Livingstone, Edinburgh

Macnab I 1977 Backache. Williams and Wilkins, London

McGregor AH, McCarthy ID, Hughes SP 1995 Motion characteristics of the lumbar spine in the normal population. Spine 20: 2421–2428

Mercer SR 1995 Clinical anatomy of cervical disc instability. Proceedings of the Manipulative Physiotherapists Association of Australia 9th Biennial Conference, Gold Coast, Australia, p 101–103

Nachemson AL 1976 The lumbar spine: an orthopaedic challenge. Spine 1: 59–71

Nitz AJ, Peck D 1986 Comparison of muscle spindle concentrations in large and small human epaxial muscles acting in parallel combinations. American Surgeon 52: 273–277

Oliver J, Middleditch A 1991 Functional anatomy of the spine. Butterworth-Heinemann, Oxford

Palastanga N, Field D, Soames R 1994 Anatomy and human movement, structure and function, 2nd edn. Butterworth-Heinemann, Oxford

Panjabi MM, Takata K, Goel VK 1983 Kinematics of lumbar intervertebral foramen. Spine 8: 348–357

Pearcy M, Trebewal SB 1984 Axial rotation and lateral bending in the normal lumbar spine measured by three-dimensional radiography. Spine 9: 582–587

Pearcy M, Portek I, Shepherd J 1984 Three dimensional X-ray analysis of normal movement in the lumbar spine. Spine 9: 294–297

Peck D, Buxton DF, Nitz A 1984 A comparison of spindle concentrations in large and small muscles acting in parallel combinations. Journal of Morphology 180: 243–252

Richardson C, Jull G, Hodges P, Hides J 1999 Therapeutic exercise for spinal stabilization in low back pain. Churchill Livingstone, Edinburgh

Shultz A, Andersson GBJ, Ortengren R et al 1982 Analysis and quantitative myoelectric measurements of loads on the lumbar spine when holding weights in standing postures. Spine 7: 390–397

Sturrock RD, Wojtulewski JA, Dudley Hart F 1973 Spondylometry in a normal population and in ankylosing spondylitis. Rheumatology and Rehabilitation 12: 135–142

Troke M, Moore AP, Maillardet FJ, Hough A, Cheek E 2001 A new, comprehensive normative database of lumbar spine ranges of motion. Clinical Rehabilitation 15: 371–379

Twomey LT, Taylor JR 1983 Sagittal movements of the human lumbar vertebral column: a quantitative study of the role of the posterior vertebral elements. Archives of Physical Medicine and Rehabilitation 64: 322–325

Tyrell AR, Reilly T, Troup JDG 1985 Circadian variation, stature and the effects of spinal loading. Spine 10: 161–164

Valencia FP, Munro RR 1985 An electromyographic study of the lumbar multifidus in man. Electromyography and Clinical Neurophysiology 25: 205–221

Van Herp G, Rowe PJ, Salter PM 2000 Range of motion in the lumbar spine and the effects of age and gender. Physiotherapy 86: 42

Winters JM, Peles JD 1990 Neck muscle activity and 3D head kinematics during quasi/static and dynamic tracking movements in multiple muscle systems. In: Winters J M, Woo S (eds) Biomechanics and movement organisation. Springer Verlag, New York

Chapter 13

Posture and balance

Clare Kell   Robert W.M. van Deursen

LEARNING OUTCOMES

When you have completed this chapter you will be
able to:

1. Discuss an evolutionary approach to posture and
   balance

2. Describe the ideal postures and the adaptations
   necessary for the journey through life

3. Discuss the mechanisms for maintaining a
   functional posture

4. Discuss the interdependence of control
   mechanisms during the maintenance of balance
   when performing everyday activities

5. Discuss the therapeutic relevance of regaining
   altered posture and balance.

INTRODUCTION

Posture is variously defined as an attitude or
position of the body (Cech & Martin 2002); the
maintenance for a period of time of a position in
space as a prelude or background to movement
(Bray et al 1999); the intrinsic mechanisms of the
human body that counteract gravity (Basmajian
1964); or the position ordinarily held when locomotion ceases but distinct from positions of rest,
feeding or other incidental poses (Morton 1929), to
mention but a few. In some cases, while it is not

stated in the same sentence as the definition, authors proceed to discuss the position of upright stance, giving the misleading impression that definitions apply and are of interest to this position only.

In this chapter the term 'posture' refers to the alignment of body segments such that the position of the body is ready for engagement in functional activity and responsive to both anticipated and unexpected perturbations or disturbances in balance. Such a definition acknowledges the active nature of posture and its maintenance which, while essentially operated at a subconscious level, is a prerequisite to an efficient, effective, task-orientated existence.

After briefly reviewing the evolution of man's bipedal posture, the chapter will consider the body's segmental alignment in the positions of upright stance, unsupported sitting and prone lying. We shall then challenge the reader to consider the relevance of these 'standards' in the reality of human movement and function across life and work spans. The chapter will conclude with an in-depth discussion about the intrinsic and extrinsic requirements and systems essential for the maintenance of posture and postural control.

EVOLUTIONARY THEORY

Evolution of the human bipedal posture

For generations scientists have argued about the origins of the human upright posture: did we 'come up' from all-fours (a quadruped existence) or did we 'come down' from the trees (a brachial existence)? In 1929 Dudley Morton, an American surgeon and natural history researcher, proposed a theory suggesting that our ancestry lay with the tree-dwellers. Concerned with postural evolution, Morton described the move of life from sea to land as the first time that organisms began to feel the full force of gravity on their structural being. On the land, to maintain postural stability, it became essential for animals to orientate their centre of gravity (COG) within their base of support. Morton regarded the posture of any animal as the result of the force interactions it experienced, e.g. internal muscle forces versus the external forces of pressure, gravity, etc. Dependent upon the **su**m of the current

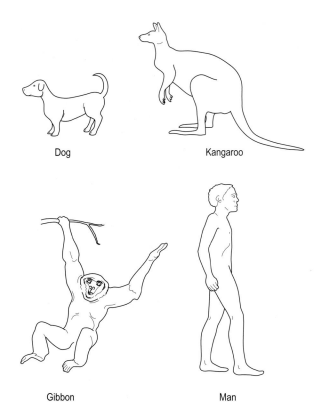

Figure 13.1   Various postures of land-dwelling mammals.

Dog

Kangaroo

Gibbon

Man

Task 13.1

Look at the pictures in Figure 13.1. Try to locate the BOS, COG and LOG in each case. What do you notice? Now think about the functional abilities of each of the animals. Is there a link between standing posture and function?

---

forces experienced, an animal's posture would be susceptible to ongoing change and development.

A common evolutionary trait was to have a spine linking four limbs held at 90° and in contact with the ground. Some animals evolved through this posture to standing on two hind limbs only. Morton suggested that a classic form of this evolutionary development is the modern kangaroo that maintains an essentially bipedal stance with a heavy tail counteracting the raised COG (Fig. 13.1). What is noticeable, however, is the kangaroo's saltatory or jumping gait pattern – the only form of fast locomotion for hind legs maintaining the primitive hip angle. It is the biomechanics of the hind leg angle that Morton felt precluded this evolutionary path for the human erect posture. Morton's theory suggested that elongating the structures about the hip would have required such large forces that lumbar spine involvement would have been unavoidable. Since the lumbar spine is more mobile than the hips, Morton proposed that lumbar spine hyperlordosis (overarching) would have resulted before the hips themselves were stressed.

However, brachiation, with the animal suspended from trees using its upper limbs, would have facilitated the gravitational interaction of elongating the trunk and extending the hips as seen in the modern gibbon. Morton's theory suggests that, with the exception of the gibbon, which remains primitive in primate evolution, primates have continued to adapt to the arboreal environment by developing powerful shoulders and longer arms and reducing strength and length in the lower limbs. While essential for efficient and effective tree existence, this segmental relationship has had the effect of raising the primate's COG and weakening its hips – a condition of secondary reversion to quadrupedalism (Morton 1929, p. 156). At some stage between the primitive gibbon and the modern primate, man must have explored life on the ground; we possess the primate's grasping hand, long arms and mobile shoulders but the gibbon's erect posture. Our keen sense of equilibrium is said to be a feature essential for our ancestral tree-dwelling habitat.

The spine and its role in the development of bipedalism

The adoption of the erect posture gave the human speed and agility but at the price of reduced stability resulting from the now raised COG and reduced base of support (BOS: outlined by the outer edges of the feet) through which the line of gravity could act during balanced functional activities (see Ch. 3). With the body's weight now being transmitted to the supporting surface (through the spine, hind limbs and feet) from a significant height, the human needed a system for transmitting the load.

The human spine is an amazing, biomechanically efficient structure designed as an 'S' shape (Fig. 13.2) so that the curves can support the column while simultaneously offering a spring-like response to the loading. This elastic rod with its combination of curves and arches spreads the body's weight while offering both support and flexibility to the body as a whole (Hamill & Knutzen 1995). The load-bearing segments at the neck, hips, knees and ankles are balanced on and under the spine by the activity of sets of antagonist muscles that cross the joints 'like the springs of an anglepoise lamp' (Rothwell 1994, page 259). But such a many-linked chain produces its own problem: how are all the segments going to stay on top of each other as we move? We shall return to this issue later in the chapter.

Evolution of man's foot

As man's contact point with his supporting surface while in upright stance, the foot is important in any discussion about human posture and a basic knowledge of its anatomy and biomechanics is essential. The developing erect posture and bipedal locomotion changed the function of human hind legs. If we agree with Morton's theory of postural evolution, we can see that, no longer needing a mobile grasping foot, humans required a structure

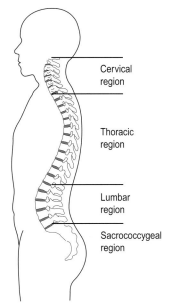

Figure 13.2 The curves of the vertebral column.

Cervical region

Thoracic region

Lumbar region

Sacrococcygeal region

that could both offer a relative rigidity to support the weight of an upright posture against the force of gravity on a small base and be capable of propulsion. To this end, the human is the only primate to have developed a foot characterised by a permanent arch (Reeser et al 1983).

As with the spine, the arch of the foot combines great strength with flexibility. Supported in quiet stance by the local bones and ligaments, the longitudinal arch offers stability and surface area contact, dissipating the weight-bearing load. System flexibility is provided by a mobile forefoot that is under intrinsic muscle control. This mobility permits weight distribution during gait with the musculature becoming very active to support the arch when it is under most strain (when rising onto toes) so that it is still present as the gait cycle proceeds (Hicks 1955, cited in Reeser et al 1983).

THE MODERN HUMAN POSTURES

In this section attention is turned to the reality of the upright posture in the modern human. The theories of force interaction on postural development (Basmajian 1964) will be applied across the life span and then extended to discuss the self-imposed influences of our habits and environments.

Development of the 'S'-shaped spine across the life span

Cech and Martin (2002) described postural and functional development throughout life, the salient points of which are summarised below.

At birth the newborn infant spine is characterised by two concave forward-facing curves in the thoracic and pelvic regions. The latter curve is facilitated by the sacrum being composed of individual sacral bones at this stage. At about 3–4 months of age, as the infant tries to raise its head from the prone lying position, gravitational interaction causes the convex forward development of the cervical spine. The final curve, the convex forward lumbar curve, begins to form as the baby sits up. Standing and walking increase the lumbar lordosis so that the COG lies over the pelvis in standing. At this stage the child's feet are still flat. The location of COG differs from adult-

hood, being higher (around T12) and anterior in the trunk in response to the baby's proportionately larger head and liver. A relatively high COG challenges stability, which is commonly countered in toddlerhood by a wide base of support (Fig. 13.3).

Cech and Martin suggest that foot arches and spinal curves approach adult form by the age of 6 years. It must be remembered, however, that the child has many more years of growth in front of it when the spine formation can be challenged and adapted in response to environmental stressors. Nissinen et al (1993) emphasise the specific vulnerability of the spine to formation stressors for the duration of puberty when growth occurs as a spurt, leaving supporting structures temporarily challenged. These spinal structure-related-to-function issues are essential to both postural assessment and management and will be dealt with specifically later in the chapter.

By the age of 22 years, when growth has stopped (Nissinen et al 2000), the spinal curves and the position of the body's COG within it will have matured. Ignoring for the moment all the factors that can influence individual posture, the position of upright stance will remain unchanged until a point in later life when ageing results in a changing interaction between physical ability and gravitational pull. As physical strength and mobility decline, gravity exerts its influence to change the ageing stance posture, drawing it into

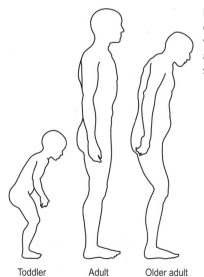

Figure 13.3 The curves of the vertebral column across the life span.

Toddler   Adult   Older adult

flexion (lowering the COG) and reversing those curves developed during infancy (Cech & Martin 2002). As a consequence, there is a tendency for the ageing population to display a posture of upright stance with a reduced cervical spine curve (see Fig. 13.3), a flattened lumbar lordosis and lowered and biomechanically inefficient longitudinal arches in their feet.

The ideal alignment of segments

An ideal posture is one that aligns the body segments so that the torques and stresses generated by gravity are minimised at each point in the chain (Pearsall & Reid 1992). Such a posture would require the least internal expenditure of energy to maintain; the forces of gravity would be neutralised by minimal internally generated counterforces (active muscle work) (Basmajian 1964).

What must be remembered, however, is that there is no uniform ideal. One person's posture is not identical to another's; each is responding in a unique way to their gravitational environment given their unique combination of physical, muscular and soft tissue characteristics. As a result care should be taken when labelling posture as 'poor' or 'non-ideal'. Until a careful history and examination is made of the patient and the environment within which they exist, it would be quite wrong to start adjusting to the consensus ideal promoted by researchers in their investigations. Woodhull et al (1985) and Pearsall and Reid (1992) concluded that the most striking finding from their work was the postural variability between subjects. Pearsall and Reid suggested that each subject was displaying a posture that optimally compensated for their specific anthropometric differences (p. 84). Woodhull et al cautioned that, while some subjects' postures are probably biomechanically 'better' than others, there is no reason to assume that the average is better than any one example (p. 115).

Upright stance

The location of the line of gravity (LOG; see Ch. 3) through the human body in upright stance has been investigated using various methodologies including X-ray analysis, force platform analysis and staged immersion in water. The consensus is that, for the normal adult, the line of gravity ideally intersects the sagittal plane through the following points:

- the mastoid process or tragus of the ear
- just anterior to the shoulder joint
- just posterior to the hip joint
- just anterior to the knee joint
- just anterior to the ankle joint (Pearsall & Reid 1992, Woodhull et al 1985).

Woodhull et al (1985) tried to locate the passage of the LOG about the hips and knees and found that the line passes 1–2 cm behind the centre of the hip joint and 1–2 cm in front of the lateral epicondyle of the knee. The research suggested that this position of gravity generates torques (turning forces) that tend to keep both joints in slight extension while standing.

So, what does the ideal upright stance posture look like if it adopts this segmental alignment in response to gravity? The most striking thing about truly ideal posture would be the left-to-right symmetry of the stacked segments with no single muscle group seen to be heavily active except the erector spinae (Hamill & Knutzen 1995). Viewing the posture from behind (posterior view), the observer would expect to see the following anatomical landmarks symmetrically aligned with the horizontal: ear lobes, breadth of shoulders, scapulae, waist creases, posterior iliac spines (dimples), buttock creases and knee creases (Fig. 13.4a). With the bare feet anteriorly placed and approximately 8 cm (hip distance) apart, the tendo calcanei would follow a perpendicular line to the floor. The spinous processes would follow a direct line from head to floor with no deviation to left or right (scoliosis).

A front or anterior view (Fig. 13.4b) is good for noting central alignment, for example centrality of the chin above the sternum, a central and relaxed umbilicus, upward-facing anterior iliac spines, anterior-facing patellae. The observer would also notice a symmetrical distribution of weight through the feet: if you ran your hands around the edge of the feet you would feel that they were equally accepting their base of support, rocking neither inwards nor outwards, and the longitudinal arches would be identical and run in line with the floor.

a Posterior view

b Anterior view

c Lateral view

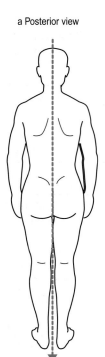
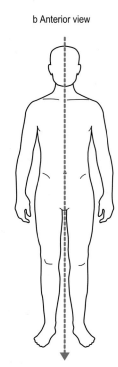
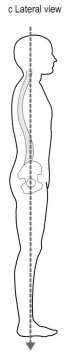

Figure 13.4 The 'ideal' alignment of segments in standing. (a) Posterior view; (b) anterior view; (c) lateral view.

Observing the ideal upright stance posture from either side (lateral view) would show the head balanced on the neck with no excessive chin protrusion or retraction. The spinal curves would demonstrate an open 'S' shape such that the rib cage was facing anteriorly and the abdomen would be flat but relaxed. A side view would show only one cheekbone, one shoulder, one scapula, one nipple, one buttock and one knee (Fig. 13.4c); if two of anything can be seen, segmental rotation is occurring. To clearly assess segmental rotation, the posture should be observed from both sides.

Sitting

When sitting, the height of the COG drops in relation to space but rises within the body (see Ch. 3) and the BOS is increased with less load being placed on the lower extremities. In general terms, this posture requires less energy to maintain than that of upright stance, being inherently more stable. What has changed, however, is the angle of the pelvis on the lumbar spine as the former is tilted backwards to allow the ischial tuberosities to be the focus of weight transference to the base (Hamill & Knutzen 1995). The resulting flattening of the lumbar spine leads to significant loading on the intervertebral discs and stretching of the posterior structures of that vertebral segment. Prolonged unsupported sitting can therefore have a detrimental effect on the lumbar spine. Supporting the lumbar spine with an appropriately measured and placed chair rest will dramatically reduce lumbar vertebral loading.

Ideally, therefore, the sitting posture should be supported by a chair whose backrest is high enough to support the upper thoracic spine (Fig. 13.5) and which inclines slightly backwards so that the lumbar spine is encouraged to stay in slight flexion (Kisner & Colby 1996). The person's bottom should be placed to the back of the seat with up to two-thirds of their thighs supported on the chair base to avoid compression of the posterior knee structures. Ideally the chair height should be adaptable so that the knees and ankles can be at right angles as the feet are placed hip distance apart on the floor.

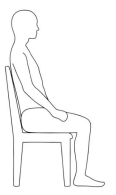

Figure 13.5 The 'ideal' alignment of segments in sitting.

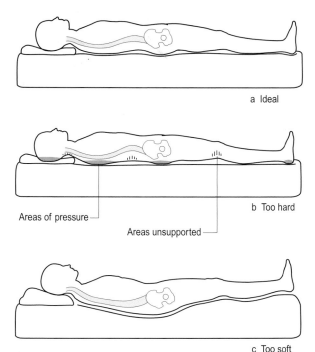

a Ideal

Areas of pressure

b Too hard

Areas unsupported

c Too soft

Figure 13.6 Possible mattress influences on segmental alignment in supine lying. (a) The 'ideal' alignment; (b) the possible effects of a very firm mattress; (c) the possible effects of a very soft mattress.

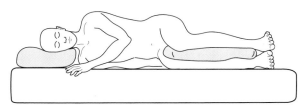

Figure 13.7 The 'ideal' alignment of segments in side lying.

Task 13.2

Observe your colleagues or people around you. How are they sitting? What factors could you change? How are you sitting at the moment? How long can you remain in this position? What is making you feel the need for change?

Lying

Lying is a posture of great stability with both a low COG and a very large BOS. In this position we can achieve equilibrium with gravity with little if any energy expenditure (Basmajian 1964). Basmajian stated that it is in lying that we spend most of our first year and about half of our lives thereafter! So it is important that we understand what is happening to the alignment of our segments in this position.

First, we must remember that the lying position is composed of three distinct segmental orientations relating to the postures of supine (face up), prone (face down) and side lying. Each posture offers different contact points to the supporting surface and therefore exposes different areas to gravitational influence. The ideal supine position is one that mirrors the segmental alignment of upright stance (Basmajian 1964). This position can only be achieved when the supporting surface is adaptable enough to permit indentation of the backward-protruding structures, e.g. the occiput, scapulae, thoracic spinous processes, sacral spines, ischial tuberosities and heels (Fig. 13.6a). Too hard a surface will lead to these areas succumbing to pressure injuries (Fig. 13.6b) and too soft a support

will result in mass spinal flexion (Fig. 13.6c). Pillows should be kept to a minimum (unless required for medical reasons) to avoid malaligning adjacent segments in the chain.

Due to the necessity to maximally rotate the cervical spine in order to breathe, and the accompanying hyperextension of the lumbar spine, the prone position is not advised for long periods.

The ideal side-lying posture again aims to mimic upright stance alignment. The influence of gravity in this position, however, necessitates support from external structures, most commonly pillows (Fig. 13.7). For the reasons outlined above, the supporting surface should allow indentation of prominent bony structures but not be too soft to encourage side flexion. In side lying the cervical and lumbar curves require support due to their 'hanging free' between the wider head and pelvis. As with supine lying, however, the use of external support must be targeted to the individual, supporting but not exaggerating existing curves. If a pillow under the head is required, it should be accompanied by or include an extra support for the neck. The best option is to place a roll to support the neck; the worst is to use a man-made fibre pillow that forces the head into side flexion and by morning supports only the ear! Similarly, a small roll may be needed to support the lumbar spine at the waist. Finally, in the side-lying position, gravity draws the top leg towards the bottom and the ideal hip distance separation of the lower limbs is lost, with resulting rotation of the lumbar spine towards the lower side. To counteract this rotation, it is advisable to lie with a pillow positioned between the knees.

The above description provides the ideal posture for segmental alignment and reduction of stressful torque. While seemingly 'overpadded', this support is used widely throughout patient care environments.

Summary

This section has reviewed the 'ideal' segmental alignment in three frequently described resting postures. The reader is urged to remember that the 'ideal' is used as a frame of reference for postural assessment purposes and not as a guide to therapeutic outcome; the latter depends upon an individual's functional environment. Postural analysis should be conducted in *each* position listed above as poor alignments will emerge or become unmasked when gravitational and stability influences are changed. The most obvious change is seen when moving from standing to sitting when trunk rotation disappears as legs of different length are removed from the supporting chain.

Requirements for achieving the ideal posture

A quick observation of our fellow humans will show us that very few people demonstrate an

---

Task 13.3
For each of the 'postural requirements' listed, note down a patient problem that may result in their not fulfilling that requirement. How long is your list? How many people do you think have some form of postural deviation from the 'ideal'?

ideal posture. Why is this? Why do some people develop 'problem/symptomatic' postures and not others?

If we accept that our posture results from the interaction between our physical status and gravity then, as gravity remains essentially static, the changes must be happening to us physically. This observation requires some expansion. The maintenance of any posture requires the following: a integrated system for detecting the posture, checking whether it is really what was wanted, and then bringing about any necessary change; effective and efficient muscles that can be appropriately recruited and then maintain the activity required; soft tissue structures of the appropriate length and flexibility to restrain and permit movement as designed; a psychological state that is motivated to engage with postural control; an environment that permits postural alteration, e.g. there will be problems trying to stand upright with high-heeled shoes and short, tight skirts! The influence of the key factors will be considered below but for now we shall focus on things that can influence muscle strength, soft tissue flexibility and therefore segmental alignment across the life and work spans.

Several detailed studies have observed childhood postures in upright stance and followed those children until growth has stopped. Of interest to our discussion is the percentage of children who, while completely asymptomatic, display asymmetrical spinal postures. Juskeliene et al (1996) found asymmetry in 46.9% of 6–7 year olds while Nissinen et al (1989) reported spinal asymmetry in 21% of 10 year olds. At 13 years old, the Nissinen population exhibited all sorts of postural combinations that were more common in girls than boys (Nissinen et al 1993), but when growth had stopped (age 22 years), equal numbers of boys and girls had asymptomatic, asymmetrical postures with the most common presentation being a right scoliosis (Nissinen et al 2000). So what sort of things could be causing these asymmetries?

Factors influencing segmental alignment

In childhood

Juskeliene et al (1996) reported that increased rates of asymmetry were found in two groups of children: those who had frequent childhood illnesses (defined in this study as having four or more acute illnesses in a year) and those who undertook low physical activity. The least asymmetry was found in the most active children. The researchers concluded by stressing the importance of muscle health and strength in the development of growing spinal alignment.

Following their sample over a long period of time allowed Nissinen et al to make the following observations: left-handedness is a powerful determinant of hyperkyphosis (too much of a thoracic curve), probably resulting from working at desks designed for right-handed students (Nissinen et al 1995); puberty is a very 'dangerous' time for spinal development because of the imbalance of bone growth spurt and delayed growth and development of supporting and controlling soft tissue structures; post puberty, twice as many girls as boys had developed a scoliosis because their sitting height (height while sitting at a desk) had grown faster than the boys' and at a younger age – and they were still all using the same, standard class desks (Nissinen et al 1993). The message from this sample appears to be a concern for the environments in which children spend a considerable part of their day.

Gillespie (2002) reviewed the impact on spinal development of the current use in childhood of computers (desk- and laptops) and electronic games (hand-held and computer or screen based). While reporting staggering numbers of hours spent by children and young people in these activities (note the observation about physical activity above), Gillespie made the following observation: 'Children and adolescents are increasingly engaged in activities that simulate work demands known to cause repetitive strain injury in working adults' (p. 249).

She goes on to explain how children spend long periods of time in deep concentration while adopting postures that are not suited to their needs. Specifically, Gillespie (2002) talks about school desk and chair heights and their fixity (see above), the tendency for sharing computers at school but with only one mouse and keyboard, the tendency for children to use desktop computers at home set up for their parents (although she does make the astute observation that many units are not in fact set up appropriately for the adults using them either!) and the use of Game Boys® and laptops on any surface that will take them. Although not seeking to correlate her findings to specific postural developments, the article alerts interested parties to the normal daily routines and spinal stresses of many of today's young people. As explained in the following section, habitual adoption of awkward positions can easily lead to asymmetrical development and subsequent problems stacking and aligning segments needed as a basis for widespread, adaptive functional activity.

Gillespie concluded on a positive note by observing that, unlike adults, children, when uncomfortable, are happy to climb onto tables, chairs, lie on the floor, etc. and in so doing may be reducing the actual negative influence that they experience; she suggests that perhaps adults could learn from the unselfconscious attitudes of children (p. 256)! Figure 13.8 depicts the 'ideal' computer station posture with the screen height and angle adjusted so that a comfortable head position is maintained.

In adulthood

Maintaining a fixed posture So, if reduced physical activity and the adoption of awkward, sustained postures are risk factors for children, what factors influence adult posture? Grieco (1986) considered this issue while reviewing the likely impact on spinal evolution of taking millions of years to become 'homo erectus' and the relatively recent enforcement of 'homo sedens' in the execution of many of today's employment tasks (p. 347). Grieco reviewed the positions and ergonomics of work stations and working patterns and made the following observations:

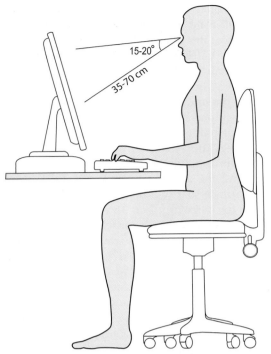

15-20°

35-70 cm

Figure 13.8 The 'ideal' computer-station posture.

- Enforced posture should be considered as a risk factor (to soft tissue and spinal injury) on the same level as the lifting of weights and vibration.
- Ischaemia in the paravertebral muscles occurs from prolonged isometric contraction as seen in the maintenance of unsupported postures (and that can be any posture: sitting, standing, etc.).
- The problem, in terms of spinal injury, is one of postural fixity rather than the loading of the spine at any one time; vertebral disc nourishment occurs via a pump or sponge mechanism, i.e. due to changing pressure resulting from change in posture.
- Ergonomic chairs may decrease the loading on the spine in general but because occupiers are more comfortable, they do not move around and then postural fixity becomes a problem.
- People who are uncomfortable move around.
- All employees should be educated in the use of their ergonomically sound devices and have 10-minute 'postural pauses' (p. 359) built into their work pattern at least every 50 minutes.

In conclusion, Grieco (1986) suggested that adults are susceptible to the same environmental stressors as children but now in the pursuit of employment. Postural education is a key factor in his argument.

Other causes of fixed postures We must not forget that there are many adults in our population who, for reasons of poor stimulation, loneliness, weakness, illness, etc., remain static or confined to one posture for substantial periods of time. Prolonged sitting for whatever reason will lead to the functional adaptation of a reduced lumbar spine lordosis, an increased thoracic kyphosis and reduced range of movement at the hips and knees into extension (Cech & Martin 2002). As the ideal thoracic alignment is designed to encourage maximal efficiency of lung function, people with static postures, especially a thoracic hyperkyphosis, are at risk of developing pathologies associated with poor ventilation, e.g. reduced lung capacity and tidal volumes leading to chest infections and reduced efficiency of the thoracic venous pump, causing problems for lower limb venous return and fluid distribution (Bray et al 1999). These problems are compounded if people are elderly and therefore their soft tissues are already reducing in flexibility and strength.

Hormone–related changes Cutler et al (1993) analysed the postures of 136 healthy women who were pre- and postmenopausal to see if there was a relationship between hormonal levels and postural hyperkyphosis (the so-called 'dowager's hump' attributed to postmenopausal osteoporotic women). The results suggested that there was no link between degree of kyphosis and age, hormone levels or calcium intake. Again, there appeared to be a weak link with exercise levels; while many women displayed a kyphosis, the more active women were better able to straighten out of the kyphosis at will.

Temporary influences on postural alignment The classic, temporary influences on posture include situations where weight distribution alters, as in pregnancy, and where pain and/or pathological processes alter mood, tolerance levels and general engagement with the environment (Clancy & McVicar 2002). If the underlying cause of these postures is rectified promptly no lasting adaptation to the new posture should occur, as a return to functional activity will restrengthen supporting muscles and soft tissues.

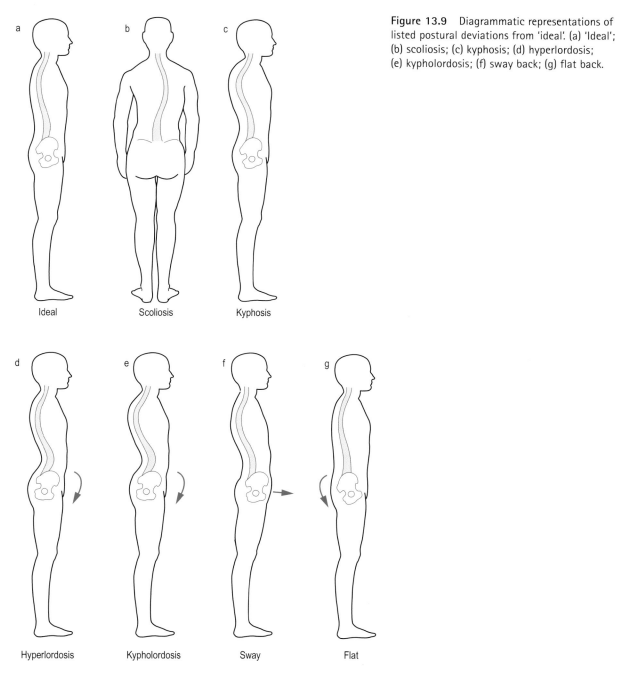

Figure 13.9 Diagrammatic representations of listed postural deviations from 'ideal'. (a) 'Ideal'; (b) scoliosis; (c) kyphosis; (d) hyperlordosis; (e) kypholordosis; (f) sway back; (g) flat back.

Ideal   Scoliosis   Kyphosis

Hyperlordosis   Kypholordosis   Sway   Flat

Defined postural deviations from the ideal

Classical postural analysis has characterised non-ideal postures into six categories: scoliosis, kyphosis, hyperlordosis/hollow back, a combined kypholordotic posture, sway-back and flat-back postures (Fig. 13.9). Nominally (by title), all refer to deviations from the spinal ideal. Readers should note that this naming system rarely indicates that the defined deviation originated within the spine itself.

The following section will briefly describe each of these postural 'types' and discuss how the spinal deviation impacts on the segmental align-ment of the whole body. A malalignment in one part of the body will have to be compensated for in another in order to keep the line of gravity falling within the base of support. Compensations seen will depend on the patient and context but could include structural realignment and/or increased muscle work in adjoining segments.

Scoliosis

- A static (fixed) or mobile (correctable) lateral curve usually seen in the thoracic and lumbar spinal regions.
- Soft tissues and muscles on the side of the concavity will be shortened and strong while those on the convex side will be longer and weaker.
- Depending on the severity of the scoliosis, a compensatory side flexion may be seen further up the segmental chain.
- If the deviation is due to a problem lower down the chain, the scoliosis may itself be the compensation.

Kyphosis

- Again can be static or mobile. Many people adopt short-term slouched postures with no lasting effect.
- Always refers to an increased anterior curvature of the thoracic spine.
- A common posture in the older population.
- An increased kyphosis affects the higher seg-ments such that the eyes focus on the ground unless the cervical spine compensates by in-creasing its lordosis, a position likely to cause muscle tension and joint compressions. Common symptoms of this effect are pain and headaches, as the neck is not biomechanically designed to adapt to this position.
- A long-standing kyphotic posture will result in shortening all musculature on the anterior chest wall, e.g. pectoral muscles, and the lengthening of the erector spinae to compensate.
- Severe kyphosis may result in impaired lung function due to altered biomechanics for thoracic expansion.
- Occasionally a kyphosis is the result of a compensation for shortened hip flexors.

Hyperlordosis

- A situation where, in upright stance, the pelvis is held in anterior tilt.
- Classically seen after pregnancy and when abdominal musculature is weak.
- This position leads to an increased lumbar lordosis that shortens both the spinal extensors and the anterior muscles controlling the pelvis – iliopsoas, rectus femoris and tensor fasciae latae (Palastanga et al 2002).
- The drawing forward of the pelvis will lengthen and weaken the glutei and abdominal muscles.
- The posture is called 'kypholordotic' when combined with a compensatory increased thoracic kyphosis.

Sway back

- Also known as 'relaxed', the characteristic profile of this posture is the slouch.
- Adopting this posture uses the least amount of active muscle work as the posture is generally maintained by soft tissue and ligament length, e.g. pushing the pelvis forwards so that the hips go into extension allows the pelvis to hang on the anterior ligaments of the hip.
- This posture is commonly adopted by boys with Duchenne muscular dystrophy, for example.
- Working back up the segments, this anterior pelvic shift will need to be compensated for by an increased lumbar lordosis and thoracic kyphosis. The head will usually be held forward of 'ideal'.
- Depending upon the extent of the pelvic shift, the knees may be locked into extension so that stance is maintained via bony approximation.
- A really mixed picture of altered joint and muscle biomechanics is presented by this posture, each deviation requiring careful assessment and consideration of the cause/compensation conundrum.

Flat back

- The key feature of this posture is a posterior tilting pelvis, which reduces the lumbar lordosis and gives the back its characteristic 'flat' appearance.
- People adopting long-term slouched sitting positions commonly develop this posture.

- A posterior tilting pelvis may result in the person standing in hyperextension at both hips and knees with lengthened hip flexors.
- Abdominal muscles are likely to be tight and strong with the erector spinae reciprocally weak and long.
- Further up the segmental chain, the loss of lumbar lordosis will be compensated by an anteriorly positioned head, which in turn may be compensated by a slightly increased thoracic kyphosis.

Summary

This section has outlined the common features of a number of classically described postural deviations from the ideal. The reader should remember, however, that owning one of these postures does not automatically give the bearer pain, discomfort or any other problem. Kisner and Colby (1996) give detailed examples of where problems may arise for each postural type but note that most people are symptom free. It is also important to note at this stage that the existence of a pure 'flat back', for example, is as rare as the 'ideal' alignment. As we know, each person's posture is the result of their interaction with their environment. While the given labels are useful for initial consideration, postural assessment and intervention can only occur on a case-by-case basis.

MAINTAINING A FUNCTIONAL POSTURE

Introduction

Now that normal posture has been defined and the influences that affect segmental alignment have been described, the chapter will consider the concept of balance or postural control.

How do we use posture to frame purposeful movement? Despite the potential instability of a relatively high COG above a small BOS, humans are able to maintain their posture and control the alignment of all segments so that purposeful movements occur about a stable base. In a nut-shell, human postural control requires information from and integration between the systems responsible for visual, vestibular and somato-sensory input and motor output. Despite the size of the task, we are only fleetingly aware of the systems' ongoing efforts to move and support our body in relation to gravity. Lackner and DiZio (2000) describe the perception of effortless ability to stand on one foot, our bodies seemingly unaware of the huge forces that are being transmitted through our supporting segments – it is only when we are ill or fatigued that we feel every gramme of load!

This section of the chapter will review the components of the postural control system and discuss how they are integrated to produce the background for functional activity. We adopt the 'systems theory' approach to motor control described by Shumway-Cook and Woollacott (2001) and will conclude with a discussion about the factors that influence normal postural control and consideration of the impact of abnormal control on effective and efficient movement.

Some definitions

To facilitate clear discussion, we will begin by explaining how we intend to use certain terms.

Lee (1988) and Williams et al (1994) describe a 'system' as a device or set of elements that transforms input into a single or a selection of desired outputs. To function, a system requires inputs, outputs and a means for the two to communicate together. In this context, the term 'control system' refers to an ability of the system to set and then achieve its output; for example, when reaching for an object our postural control system is able to decide and then execute the correct amount of compensatory postural reaction (outputs) to maintain balance (centre of gravity over base of support).

Regulation refers, in this instance, to the ability of the system to do more than simply control for an output in a given situation (Lee 1988). Regulation is the ability of the system to maintain the control-desired output but responsively, i.e. in response to feedback gained from what is actually happening. Therefore, to carry our example further, we can reach for an object successfully despite internal changes (e.g. we sneeze) or external challenges (someone knocks into us). It is this ability of the postural control system to regulate and react responsively to its environment that gives the human an exceptional array of highly skilled functional activities.

How does postural control work?

To answer this question, this section will consider each 'step' in the postural control cycle: sensory information input, integration and effector result.

Input requirements

For any system to produce an effective product, it must receive good, up-to-date and relevant input data. Such is the intensity and diversity of the information required to frame functional movement that three input systems are used: the vestibular system, the visual system and the somatosensory system.

The vestibular system Located in the inner ear are two sensory systems that send information down the 8th cranial nerve, the vestibulocochlear nerve. The cochlear portion of the cranial nerve carries information from the cochlear portion of the inner ear concerned with auditory stimulation – we hear with this part. Although not directly related to balance, over- or unexpected stimulation of this system can affect postural control, as we shall see later. The vestibular system comprises the other part of the inner ear complex and is responsible for our awareness of head orientation with respect to gravity and the head's linear and angular acceleration, i.e. any change in velocity and direction.

While this is not the place for detailed physiological discussion, it is important at this point to note that the sensory receptors of the vestibular system are constantly firing and that it is the change in firing rate and pattern that is detected and interpreted by the interpretation centre for this system - the vestibular nuclei of the brain stem.

The visual system The eyes provide the sense of sight but also play an essential role in giving us information about where our bodies are in space. This latter sense is sometimes called visual proprioception (Shumway-Cook & Woollacott 2001). Visual proprioception informs the brain about body position in space, the relationship between one body part and another and the motion of our body. This latter sense is the eyes' ability to distinguish the site of viewed movement: is it the object I am watching, is it my eye in my head or is it my head itself moving? It is suggested that information from the eyes passes to the superior colliculi (roof of the midbrain) where sensory maps compute how close to the body, and how close to the midline of the body, the movement is occurring (Shumway-Cook & Woollacott 2001).

The somatosensory system The awareness of joint position is provided by a complex interpretation of information collected from the unmyelinated Ruffini fibres in the joints themselves, the muscle spindles of those muscles passing over the joints and the effector motor command signals (Lackner & DiZio 2000). In the hand, where precise joint proprioception is crucial, a fourth input, from the cutaneous mechanoreceptors in the hand itself, adds to the information pool. In a similar way the mechanoreceptors in the feet provide important information about the distribution of pressure through different areas of the soles of the feet.

While we are able to think about the position of our limbs, proprioception is an essentially subconscious sense. It is thought that information from the somatosensory receptors listed here passes directly to the motor neurones controlling postural stability at spinal level. In this way, sensory information can modulate movement that results from commands originating in higher centres of the nervous system (Shumway-Cook & Woollacott 2001, p. 66).

What sort of input information do we require?

Lee (1988) offered a detailed review of the types of information needed by the postural control system. A summary of some key points is made here.

In order to form an output, it is important to know where you are at the start; therefore input data must describe the *initial conditions*. We learn these patterns of setting up a move (the postural reference) and can be 'caught out' when something changes, e.g. we have a leg in plaster. To avoid frequent falls every time something changes, information is also needed about alterations to both the internal and external environments that would challenge our balance. These *challenges to*

Task 13.4

Why do we need to know all this information? Think about the perturbations you might experience when walking along a crowded pavement. How do you cope with postural challenges you can see coming? What happens if someone runs into you from behind? Why is there a difference?

balance are also called perturbations and are described as being mechanical in origin if they occur as a result of external or self-generated forces or sensory if they are the result of an unexpected sensory input, e.g. an object moves quickly into our visual field or a loud crash occurs. Such is the complexity of the information received that the brain is able to determine the strength, duration, frequency and direction of the perturbation.

Integration and action

Now the postural control system sensors have provided the system with the information it requires, it is time to act. Shumway-Cook and Woollacott (2001) suggested the following routes for system output to achieve the intended outcome.

Information from the superior colliculi (visual system) passes to three main regions:

1. regions of the brain stem that control eye movements
2. the tectospinal tract that helps control neck and head movement
3. the tectopontine tract that, through connections with the cerebellum, processes eye–head control.

In this way the visual system is controlling output so that the postural control system can be sure about head position and movement in space.

The vestibular system uses the various vestibular nuclei in the brain stem to output to different sites. The vestibular nuclei collect and redistribute information to other interpretation centres, e.g. the cerebellum, reticular formation, the thalamus and the cerebral cortex, but can also affect system output directly. Collectively the nuclei will influence the antigravity muscles of the neck, trunk and limbs via the vestibuloocular and vestibulospinal tracts.

As mentioned earlier, information from the somatosensory system is able to influence motor output at spinal level. Such a direct communication system allows for quick response times and is used to good effect where the sensors detect the likelihood of a fall. For example, if a person is standing, the pressure receptors in the feet will detect the perturbation and respond by effecting actions to either widen the BOS (induce a stepping reaction) and/or lower the COG. We use this response every time we shift our COG over one leg (as in walking); detecting increased pressure under one foot, the somatosensory system responds by increasing extensor motor tone on the supporting side and simultaneously increasing flexor tone on the opposite side. Both these actions working together have the effect of transferring the COG over the new BOS (the supporting limb; Rothwell 1994).

Rothwell (1994) suggested that the visual, vestibular and proprioceptive subsystems respond to slightly different disturbances in balance. The visuospinal system controls slow shifts in balance, the vestibulospinal system controls both static and faster inputs with the proprioceptive system also sensitive to faster stimuli. However, Lee (1988) warned the therapist that, while some overlap of system sensitivity does exist, it is not complete. For example, if you close your eyes you will sway more in standing because the vestibular and proprioceptive subsystems are unable to completely correct for slow error (p. 298). Information from the subsystems may not be equally weighted or important, i.e. one type of sensory input may be dominant and therefore have the most influence in determining postural response. In most contexts it is the vestibular inputs that are critical in deciding what is actually going on in both the internal and external environments (Cech & Martin 2002, Lee 1988). Rothwell (1994) concluded that, despite the subsystem integration, only one (any one) of the three main sources of afferent input is required for effective balance to exist (p. 262).

Are things going as we planned? Regulation

Once a movement has begun, the sensory systems cannot relax. The postural control system requires ongoing information about the effect of the planned response; this is called *feedback*. Again, Lee (1988) provides a very interesting discussion about feedback, defining the process as an active method for controlling error. Sensory inputs inform higher centres about the achieved or expected output and then an error signal, representing the difference between actual and desired output, is detected. The response is a modification of signal output. We are normally unaware of this process as feedback involving all the subsystems occurs at an automatic level.

Of course, no system is perfect and relying on a feedback system has its problems. The process just described has many 'steps' to produce a movement and for feedback to be effective, the whole process has to be completed repeatedly as the movement/correction continues. 'Loop delay', or the time it takes to make a correction, is one of the big problems with feedback systems (Lee 1988, p. 297). Additional conduction problems or difficulties with central processing will adversely delay anticipatory and feed-forward information. Some patients will therefore move with a high risk of error and thus have difficulty producing efficient and effective movement control.

To combat some of these problems, we have another mechanism for making adjustments: the feed-forward or anticipatory control loop (Massion 1992, Rothwell 1994). Feed-forward is a process where, in a known or commonly experienced situation (where the likely perturbations have been learnt), signals for postural compensation and modification are sent before (in anticipation of) receipt of sensory information that the intervention is actually required. Anticipatory control occurs during most of our regular daily activities, e.g. writing, stepping, etc., reducing movement execution times considerably and therefore increasing the efficiency of the task. Problems arise when the environment changes and the system is already executing the now wrong modification!

Of course, one of the ways to counter these problems is to start thinking about what you are doing – how you are positioned and your segments aligned – before you execute a movement. This conscious preparation for activity, preparing a posture suitable for the intended task, is essential and recommended by many therapists (Butler & Major 1992, Lee 1988, Williams et al 1994). Problems

arise, however, when the adjustments during activity become conscious. Think about the following situation. You are walking down the stairs in a busy building, holding your books in front of you (so you can't see your feet) and chatting to your companions; all is fine and you arrive safely at the bottom. How does the difficulty of the activity (walking down the stairs) change when you start to worry about where your feet are? Now what is going on? Several things are happening here. First, you are adding in extra communication loops and increasing the time delay from sensory input to motor output but second, in order to see your feet, you are probably going to have to lean forwards to see the steps. What does this do to your COG?

Task 13.5

Take the situation given above. What do you think is happening in your vestibular system when you look down at the step? How does your visual system cope with sensing the height you could fall? What happens if a step is suddenly a different height from the rest?

Is it a good idea to make patients' postural control responses conscious? Or should we try and build up segmental, automatic control by staging the complexity and difficulty (in terms of segments needing to be controlled against gravity) of the activities we ask them to practise (Butler & Major 1992)?

Summary

This section has reviewed some basic physiology and discussed the systems used to maintain balance while the body is performing functional activities. We have seen that movement requires the dynamic and ongoing interplay of vision, proprioception, contact cues, efferent control and internal (learnt) models. Such multisensory input is essential for body orientation, the apparent stability of our surroundings and ultimately for movement control (Lackner & DiZio 2000, p. 286). Finally, it must be acknowledged that not all postural control occurs at a purely subconscious level. In their research, Schlesinger et al (1998) suggested that increasing attention is needed to maintain balance when postural tasks and/or coexisting secondary tasks increase in complexity. The effect of 'multi-tasking' on postural control is considered later in this chapter.

Simplifying the postural control responses in standing

Small perturbations to stable postures, such as upright, quiet standing, can be accommodated without any central control due to the intrinsic elastic properties of muscle (Rothwell 1994). Together with reflex loop innervation, muscles are provided with a stiffness similar to that of a spring. During small perturbations muscle acts as a stretching spring, resisting the disturbance. In upright standing, with the COG projected anterior to the ankle joints, it is the calf muscle that is thought to play an important role in accommodating small perturbations.

When in upright stance, the body employs three main strategies to combat further threats to balance and stability (Nashner 1990, cited in Shumway-Cook & Woollacott 2001). The process is subconscious and reduces response times by treating effector muscles as groups or 'muscle synergies'. A synergy describes the functional coupling of groups of muscles that are constrained to work together (Shumway-Cook & Woollacott 2001). Sending one signal to a synergy will therefore get a wide-ranging, set response – cutting out 'the middle-man' and therefore reducing response times and increasing efficiency.

Nashner (1990, cited in Shumway-Cook & Woollacott 2001) reports three main synergies that form the basis of the subsequent named movement strategies.

The ankle strategy

The ankle strategy is used when the foot is fully supported on the contact surface so that the dorsiflexors and plantarflexors about the ankle joint can exert their influence through 'reverse action', i.e. if we sway backwards the anterior tibialis muscles will contract to bring us back to the midline, pulling the body over the foot. Similarly a forwards sway will cause gastrocnemius to become active (as the perturbation is now greater than can be accommodated by intrinsic properties

alone) and draw the COG forwards over the BOS (Cech & Martin 2002). The ankle strategy (also known as the 'inverted pendulum'; Popov et al 1999, Rothwell 1994) is effective for correcting small perturbations when standing on a firm surface (so active when you stand quietly) and obviously requires intact joint range and muscle strength about the ankle (Shumway-Cook & Woollacott 2001).

Of course, humans can make the task of balancing in upright stance hard for themselves and many people choose to do this by the footwear they use! Basmajian (1964) described the results of an EMG study into the resting activity of lower limb muscles while wearing different footwear. As early as 1956 it was known that high heels increase the resting activity of the calf muscles because the COG is shifted forwards (Fig. 13.10). It appears that high-heeled shoe wearers partially compensate for the threat to balance by combining this increased muscle work with a simultaneous increase in lumbar lordosis.

The hip strategy

When the perturbations are greater than a small sway, when the disturbance is quickly applied or when the foot is on a small contact surface the body uses the hip strategy. Using the large muscles of the hip and knee together, the hip strategy is better able to control the COG and prevent a fall (Shumway-Cook & Woollacott 2001). Cech & Martin (2002) cited a study by Allum et al (1998) who report that the hip strategy is evoked in preference to the ankle strategy for all perturbations that come from a mediolateral direction. Whatever the size of the perturbation, the study concluded that mediolateral forces activate muscle synergies in a proximal-to-distal order.

The stepping strategy

The stepping strategy has been referred to above and is evoked when the perturbation is strong enough to really threaten stability. In this instance a gross movement, i.e. a step, hop, etc., is required to widen the BOS so that the COG can fall within it and balance be regained.

Figure 13.11 summarises the boundaries to stability in upright stance and the sequence of strategy adoption.

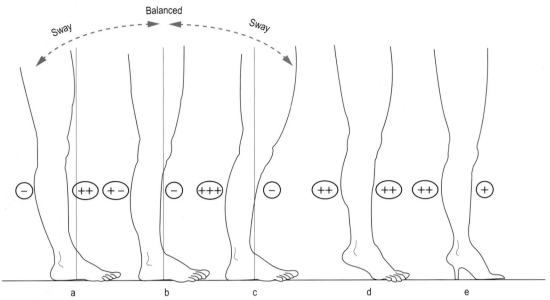

Figure 13.10 Muscular activity in leg muscles.

Task 13.6

Think about the posture of high-heeled shoe wearers (Fig. 13.10). Refer back to sections describing 'ideal' posture and 'classic deviations'. Describe the likely 'label' and compensations further up the body if the posture of the high-heeled shoe wearer is held and/or becomes the norm.

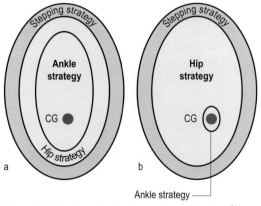

Figure 13.11 Boundaries for motor strategies. (Reproduced with kind permission from SERDI Paris.)

Summary

This section has reviewed the postural control system and will conclude with a summary of the body systems and structures identified as essential for functional postural control (readers requiring more detailed information are encouraged to consult the original texts referred to above).

Requirements for an integrated postural control response

- Intact sensory system: sensors, nerves, communication pathways.

- Intact central nervous system: conduction pathways, internal communication networks, framework for pattern reference/learnt response patterns relevant to individual shape and body symmetry/alignment.

- Intact muscloskeletal system: effector pathways including nerves, neuromuscular junctions, strength and endurance of muscles, range of movement about effector joints.

- Psychological engagement with surroundings: remember that the reticular formation is responsible for coordinating postural muscle tone activity in response to levels of higher centre arousal.
- An external environment that allows accurate postural changes to be made when perturbations occur.

Task 13.7

How does your posture change when you are tired or in pain? What will be your response to perturbations in these conditions?

Factors that affect postural control

Obviously anything that impairs the function of the systems listed above will affect postural control responses, but there are some common situations that will challenge balance responses.

The effects of ageing

The effects of the ageing process on the postural control systems of healthy people can be summarised thus:

- Body sway increases with age. Only a small proportion (c30–37%) of elderly people are able to maintain balance using the ankle strategy.
- The function of the sensory systems declines as part of the ageing process but the visual system becomes increasingly important as sensation and muscle strength reduce in the lower limbs and vestibular system function also declines.
- Both nerve conduction and central processing in the brain stem slow with age (Kristindottir et al 2001, Lord et al 1991, Perrin et al 1997, Woollacott & Shumway-Cook 1990).

The effects of coexisting multisystem activity

Many interesting studies have been conducted to look at the effects of adding activities ('multi-tasking') to people trying to maintain increasingly difficult postures. As balance regulation requires

---

Task 13.8

How do you think the changes seen with ageing will be noticed in terms of postural control? If these changes occur in the healthy elderly population, how will coexisting multi-pathology, cataracts, etc. compound their postural control problems?

---

increasing amounts of information-processing capacity (attention), greater demand is made on the available higher centre resources, in turn reducing the capacity for coexisting activity (Lajoie et al 1993), e.g. memory and comprehension activities. Schlesinger et al (1998) reported that the effect is compounded if the person is deprived of sleep, a potential cause for concern if someone is a shift-worker.

Hodges et al (2002) and Dault et al (2003) have investigated the effects of changing patterns of respiration and the muscle work of articulation on postural control. Both groups of researchers reported that these everyday activities have demonstrable effects on postural control. Hodges et al suggested that the perturbations of respiration cause measurable counterbalancing activity in the trunk and lower limb muscles – a highly coordinated control system requiring multisegment synergies.

The effects of high or low levels of exercise

Prolonged exercise (e.g. a 25 km run) has been shown to reduce postural control. Leper et al (1997) suggested that this is due to the system's sensory receptors readjusting their levels of sensitivity in response to the hyperstimulation experienced during exercise. Speers et al (1998) also found that system recalibration occurred when they tested postural control responses in a sample of astronauts before and after space flight. The authors suggested that, in this instance, the recalibration was due to hypostimulation experienced during weightlessness. Interestingly, when their sample of astronauts returned to land they were using hip correction strategies far more frequently than ankle strategies.

One of the effects of prolonged low activity levels may be an increase in body weight. The effect of obesity on postural control has stimulated

---

Task 13.9

Why do you think astronauts demonstrate this postural control adaptation in the weightless environment?

---

much research activity with results suggesting that obesity negatively affects postural responses, especially if perturbations come from mediolateral directions (Goulding et al 2003, McGraw et al 2002). While not ignoring the influence of probable coexisting poor muscle endurance, both studies suggested that obese people have intact proprioceptive and sensory systems. Postural control could be challenged because of an altered muscle:body weight ratio increasing body inertia so that more force generation is required for both the perturbation and the appropriate correction to occur. The cost of postural control is therefore high.

Summary

In this section we have thought about the systems required to make postural control efficient and effective and discussed some normal conditions under which predicted responses are challenged. Obviously, however, there are innumerable instances when internal and/or external events can unexpectedly prevent normal balance responses occurring, e.g. a limb amputation, lesions of the central nervous system, etc.

RELEVANCE TO THERAPEUTIC PRACTICE

This final section relates the given theoretical understanding to current therapeutic practice. We shall review the possible precursors to abnormal, symptomatic posture and postural control and offer some examples of therapeutic options. Our goal is to facilitate understanding so that therapists consider some general routes to help manage and improve patients' safety and functional activity.

Symptomatic postural alignment

Identifying causes for symptomatic postures

Earlier in this chapter we described the ongoing interaction between the internal muscle and soft tissue forces and the external forces of gravity, friction and inertia. At any time different force 'balance' will affect postural change. The task for the therapist is to identify the symptom's primary source and discuss with the patient the likely cause(s). We have discussed the importance of taking the patient through a detailed postural assessment in, and between, each of the three main resting postures to note how the patient's current posture deviates from the stated 'ideal'. Causes of postural deviation may include muscles that are too weak, soft tissues that are too tight or long, or joint movements impeded by swelling or hampered by actual or anticipated pain.

Relieving the symptoms and preventing recurrence

It is essential that people suffering with symptomatic postures are given the opportunity to rest in positions of ease, where their postures are supported, reducing the effort needed for their maintenance. Readers are referred back to the sections describing supported sitting and lying postures. Secondary intervention will manage symptom control and recurrence prevention through detailed ergonomic review, appropriate muscle strengthening and joint realignment disciplines. Postural rehabilitation is a long-duration activity requiring high patient motivation and patient–therapist interaction and support. At all times therapists must be aware of the individual needs of their patient and the context/environment in which that patient operates, helping to make therapeutic intervention relevant wherever possible.

Problems with postural control: balance re-education

Identifying the causes

If a patient with a recent amputation or spinal cord injury is referred for balance re-education then the reasons for balance problems may seem apparent, but therapists must also consider the impact of coexisting pathology, e.g. vision, vestibular processing, general system ageing, etc. Whatever the cause of the balance problem, it is likely that the patient's soft tissues will have adapted quickly to the new environment and stimuli. It is essential that the musculoskeletal system is prepared so that it is in the 'best condition' possible to respond to demands made upon it by the central nervous system. For example, sensory endings cannot provide adequate information when surrounded by oedema nor can the muscle function as required if its connective tissue has shortened or adhered.

When muscles, soft tissues, etc. have been prepared for action, it is important to help the patient integrate the changes made into functional activities. Remember that there are essentially two ways in which the postural control system operates: it is able to maintain our segmental alignment in quiet postures where no or minimal perturbations are expected; and it maintains balance when perturbations are great, e.g. while performing multitask or functional activities. This knowledge can be used to help stage patients' rehabilitation. Reflecting upon the needs of a functional postural control system allows us to develop a tailored rehabilitation programme. The points below reflect the range of questions that should be considered by the therapist when developing such a programme.

Some questions to ask

- Is there a need to try and increase existing sensory stimulation levels? Could we use a mirror or approximate the joints to increase mechano-receptor input? Is the department too noisy?
- How good is the patient's segmental control? Should we reduce the difficulty of the starting position by lowering the COG and increasing the BOS?
- Is the patient's problem with segmental or inter-segmental control? Should we work to achieve subconscious control segment by segment or does the patient have problems initiating or controlling the muscle synergies?
- So, should the patient be fairly static or is he ready to have his balance challenged by expected and unexpected perturbations? Remember the existence of the feedback and feed-forward systems: it is normal to have difficulty responding to perturbations from behind and those that come at high frequency – patients are not necessarily responding abnormally if they have problems with these!

Task 13.10

You have two referrals, one for an elderly lady with a history of frequent falls and the other for an elderly lady who has recently fractured an ankle. Would you consider balance rehabilitation for both patients? What would be the focus of your rehabilitation in each case? Note down a brief management plan for each – consider if and how they differ. What are your thoughts?

- The patient is thinking very hard about his balance reactions but is this a problem? As we have seen, patients can be encouraged to think about preparing their segmental alignment for functional activity. Directly thinking about postural control during simple functional activities can cause more problems but is essential during advanced, difficult postural conditions and when performing multiple tasks simultaneously.

This list is incomplete but is intended to help readers consider the issues that may be impacting on their patients' functional activity efficiency and effectiveness. The key is adequate musculoskeletal preparation followed immediately by integration into controlled functional activity. The nervous system is continually adapting and we need to ensure that the components of the postural control system are challenged in such a way that compensations occur towards the normal.

CONCLUSION

This chapter has explored the origins and norms of the upright human posture and the demands that are placed on whole body systems in order to produce effective functional activities. We have described the 'ideal' postural alignment and discussed the real-life influences that make segmental alignment unique to the individual. We have acknowledged the complexity of postural control, the multisystem integration needed and the frequency of balance problems in the patient and general populations. An understanding of posture and its control is essential for all involved in the rehabilitation of human movement.

REFERENCES

Basmajian JV 1964 Man's posture. Archives of Physical Medicine and Rehabilitation 45: 26–36

Bray JJ, MacKnight ADC, Mills RG 1999 Lecture notes on human physiology, 4th edn. Blackwell Science, Oxford

Butler PB, Major RE 1992 Biomechanics of postural control and derived management principles. Physiotherapy Theory and Practice 8: 183–184

Cech DJ, Martin S 2002 Functional movement development across the life span, 2nd edn. W B Saunders, Philadelphia

Clancy J, McVicar AJ 2002 Physiology and anatomy: a homeostatic approach, 2nd edn. Arnold, London

Cutler WB, Friedmann E, Genovese-Stone E 1993 Prevalence of kyphosis in a healthy sample of pre- and postmenopausal women. American Journal of Physical and Medical Rehabilitation 72: 219–225

Dault MC, Yardley L, Frank JS 2003 Does articulation contribute to modifications of postural control during dual-task paradigms? Cognitive Brain Research 16: 434–440

Gillespie RM 2002 The physical impact of computers and electronic game use on children and adolescents: a review of current literature. Work 18: 249–259

Goulding A, Jones IE, Taylor RW, Piggot JM, Taylor D 2003 Dynamic and static tests of balance and postural sway in boys: effects of previous wrist bone fractures and high adiposity. Gait and Posture 17: 136–141

Grieco A 1986 Sitting posture: an old problem and a new one. Ergonomics 29: 345–362

Hamill J, Knutzen KM 1995 Biomechanical basis of human movement. Lippincott, Williams and Wilkins, Philadelphia

Hodges PW, Gurfinkel VS, Brumagne S, Smith TC, Cordo PC 2002 Coexistence of stability and mobility in postural control: evinced from postural compensation for respiration. Experimental Brain Research 144: 293–302

Juskeliene V, Magnus P, Bakketteig LS, Dailidiene N, Jurkuvenas V 1996 Prevalence and risk factors for asymmetric posture in preschool children aged 6-7 years. International Journal of Epidemiology 25: 1053–1059

Kisner C, Colby LA 1996 Therapeutic exercise: foundations and techniques, 3rd edn. F A Davis, Philadelphia

Kristinsdottir EK, Fransson P-A, Magnusson M 2001 Changes in postural control in healthy elderly subjects are related to vibration sensation, vision and vestibular asymmetry. Acta Otolaryngologica 121: 700–706

Lackner JR, DiZio PA 2000 Aspects of body self-calibration. Trends in Cognitive Sciences 4: 279–288

Lafont C, Boroni A, Allard M et al (eds) 1992 Falls, gait and balance disorders in the elderly. Elsevier, Paris

Lajoie Y, Teasdale N, Bard C, Fleury M 1993 Attentional demands for static and dynamic equilibrium. Experimental Brain Research 97: 139–144

Lee WA 1988 A control systems framework for understanding normal and abnormal posture. American Journal of Occupational Therapy 43: 291–301

Leper R, Bigard AX, Diard J-P, Couteyron J-F, Guezennec CY 1997 Posture control after prolonged exercise. European Journal of Applied Physiology 76: 55–61

Lord SR, Clark RD, Webster IW 1991 Postural stability and associated physiological factors in a population of aged persons. Journal of Gerontology 46: 69–76

Massion J 1992 Movement, posture and equilibrium: interaction and coordination. Progress in Neurobiology 38: 35–56

McGraw B, McClenaghan BA, Williams HG, Dickerson J 2000 Gait and postural stability in obese and nonobese prepubertal boys. Archives of Physical and Medical Rehabilitation 81: 484–489

Morton DJ 1929 Evolution of man's erect posture. Journal of Morphology and Physiology 43:147–179

Nissinen M, Heliovaara M, Seitsamo J, Poussa M 1989 Trunk asymmetry and scoliosis. Anthropometric measurements in prepubertal school children. Acta Paediatrica Scandinavica 78: 747–753

Nissinen M, Heliovaara M, Seitsamo J, Poussa M 1993 Trunk asymmetry, posture, growth and risk of scoliosis. Spine 18: 8–13

Nissinen M, Heliovaara M, Seitsamo J, Poussa M 1995 Left handedness and risk of thoracic hyperkyphosis in prepubertal schoolchildren. International Journal of Epidemiology 24: 1178–1181

Nissinen M, Heliovaara M, Seitsamo J, Kononen MH, Hurmerinta KA, Poussa M 2000 Development of trunk asymmetry in a cohort of children ages 11 to 22 years. Spine 25: 570–574

Palastanga N, Field D, Soames R 2002 Anatomy and human movement: structure and function, 4th edn. Butterworth-Heinemann, Oxford

Pearsall DJ, Reid JG 1992 Line of gravity relative to upright vertebral posture. Clinical Biomechanics 7: 80–86

Perrin PP, Jeandel C, Perrin CA, Bene MC 1997 Influence of visual control, conduction and central integration on static and dynamic balance in healthy older adults. Gerontology 43: 223–231

Popov KE, Kozhina GV, Smetanin BN, Shlikov VY 1999 Postural responses to combined vestibular and hip proprioceptive stimulation in man. European Journal of Neuroscience 11: 3307–3311

Reeser LA, Susman RL, Stern JT 1983 Electromyographic studies of the human foot: experimental approaches to hominid evolution. Foot and Ankle 3: 391–407

Rothwell J 1994 Control of human voluntary movement. Chapman and Hall, London

Schlesinger A, Redfern MS, Dahl RE, Jennings JR 1998 Postural control, attention and sleep deprivation. NeuroReport 9: 49–52

Shumway-Cook A, Woollacott M 2001 Motor control: theory and practical applications, 2nd edn. Lippincott, Williams and Wilkins, Baltimore

Speers RA, Paloski WH, Kuo AD 1998 Multivariate changes in coordination of postural control following spaceflight. Journal of Biomechanics 31: 883–889

Williams LRT, Caswell P, Wagner I, Walmsley A, Handcock PJ 1994 Regulation of standing posture. New Zealand Journal of Physiotherapy 22: 15–18

Woodhull AM, Maltrud K, Mello BL 1985 Alignment of the human body in standing. European Journal of Applied Physiology 54: 109–115

Woollacott MH, Shumway-Cook A 1990 Changes in posture control across the life span - a systems approach. Physical Therapy 70: 799–807

Chapter 14

Tension and relaxation

Marion Trew

CHAPTER CONTENTS

LEARNING OUTCOMES

When you have completed this chapter you should be able to:

1. Understand the difference between positive and negative stress

2. Understand the basic physiological changes in tension and relaxation

3. Recognise the common changes in movement patterns or posture that occur in situations of tension

4. Describe several different methods of inducing relaxation.

INTRODUCTION

Often minor degrees of stress or tension can affect normal posture and patterns of movement and where levels of tension are very high, human movement will be noticeably disrupted. Tension that leads to abnormal posture and movement may also lead to muscular and joint pain and a tension spiral is produced where tension leads to pain and the pain leads to more tension (Fig. 14. 1). This chapter considers stress or tension in general terms and how it may affect movement. The chapter concludes by considering several different relaxation techniques and emphasises the importance of the individual taking 'ownership'

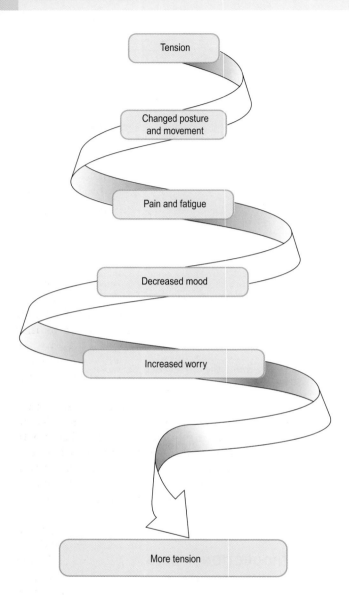

Figure 14.1   The tension spiral.

of the relaxation process rather than being a passive participant.

Though the general population is familiar with the words 'tension' and 'relaxation', a surprisingly large number of people are unable to recognise these two states in themselves. This may be because a well-developed sense of physical self-awareness is not common, probably because there is a tendency to regard the body as something to be accepted until it starts to go noticeably wrong. It may also be because concepts like stress, tension and relaxation are not easy to define precisely (Table 14.1). Despite this, everyone has the potential to know what tension and relaxation are, though

Table 14.1   Definitions of stress, tension and relaxation

Stress	Tension	Relaxation
Strain	Strain	Loosen
Pressure	Rigidity	Less close
Force	Barely suppressed emotion	Less rigid
Response to adverse stimulus	Conflict	Passive
Constraining influence	Anxiety	Being at rest
Disruption of homeostasis	Tautness	Diminished awareness
Demand exceeding ability		Emotionally at ease
Physical and emotional wear and tear		

some people may need guidance to recognise these states in themselves. When people are able to monitor their own levels of tension and relaxation, they have taken the first step in being able to control and modify their reactions to stress.

NORMAL LEVELS OF AROUSAL

It is quite normal to vary between periods of stress when arousal is high and periods of low arousal and relaxation. In fact, these differences in the level of arousal are essential for efficient activity. When action is needed, the arousal level is high, the level of muscle tone is raised and non-essential systems become relatively inactive. When there is no call for high levels of mental and physical activity, then it is appropriate for the general level of arousal to be reduced so that energy may be conserved and depleted energy stores may be replenished.

In addition, all individuals have natural periods of greater or lesser mental and physical arousal throughout each day. The most obvious example is the wake/sleep cycle. At a more detailed level this basic rhythm is also evident in the various functions of the body: the rhythmical contraction and relaxation of the heart, the inspiratory and expiratory phases of the breathing cycle and in movement, where one muscle group contracts whilst the antagonists relax to allow the movement to take place. These alternating rhythms can be speeded up or slowed down in response to

both internal and external stimuli, depending on the needs and demands of the particular situation.

Relaxation requires a de-emphasis of arousal states and, in particular, a reduction in muscular activity but because the mind and body are inextricably linked, there may also be a reduction in mental activity. Mental activity such as anxiety, emotional tension and fear can all have a deleterious effect on tension and when considering relaxation it is not possible to divorce emotional states from physical states (Elton 1993). The body-mind effect reflects the links between the autonomic nervous system and the cerebral cortex of the brain and when trying to induce relaxation, it is essential to be aware of this association.

When the natural balance between tension and relaxation is disrupted it can lead to an excessively high level of mental and physical arousal during which the muscular, respiratory and cardiovascular systems start to exhibit inappropriate activity. This is variously described as stress, tension, anxiety or an inability to relax and it leads to feelings of mental and physical tiredness, headaches, abnormal joint postures and a loss of the fine control of movement (Basmajian & Wolf 1990). In severe cases, other systemic manifestations such as dizziness, dysfunction of the digestive system, shortness of breath and disruption of the immunological response may occur (Baker 1987). Stress is defined by Selye (1984) as the non-specific result of any demand upon the body. This result can be mental, somatic or both. The physiological responses to stress are controlled by the autonomic nervous system and the psychological responses are thought to be controlled from the hypothalamus and the limbic lobe of the cerebral cortex.

PHYSIOLOGY OF STRESS AND RELAXATION

The autonomic nervous system is divided into two separate systems, the sympathetic and the parasympathetic, and they control the viscera. Afferent impulses from the viscera are integrated either at spinal level or within the reticular formation of the pons, medulla and midbrain. The two systems frequently act in a complementary manner affected by the quantity and type of synapse transmitter. The sympathetic system releases noradrenaline and the parasympathetic nerve endings release acetylcholine. Noradrenaline is also released as a hormone by the adrenal gland, thus enhancing the effect of the sympathetic system.

The cardiovascular centres of the pons are responsible for the regulation of blood pressure. The dorsal vagal nuclei contain the parasympathetic preganglionic cell bodies of the vagus nerve which is responsible for the control of the viscera of the thorax and upper abdomen. The Edinger-Westphal nuclei of the midbrain control the reflex changes of the eye. These nuclei receive input from the reticular formation and other sensory inputs, particularly from the hypothalamus (Moffett et al 1993).

It is the sympathetic system that is activated in times of stress, initiating the 'fight or flight' response. The body is made ready for action: there are chemical changes in skeletal muscle which result in the development of tension in the contractile components; in the eyes the pupils dilate; and there is vasoconstriction of the salivary glands, leading to a dry mouth. There is an inhibition of gastric and digestive secretions and a constriction of the sphincters with an increase in sweating. There is also an increase in the rate and force of heart contractions delivering more blood and, therefore, more oxygen to the tissues that need them. Cardiac output is increased and the distribution of blood is adjusted through constrictions of the small blood vessels in the skin and abdominal viscera so that blood is not directed to non-essential tissues. In addition to all this, there is bronchodilation in the lungs and a general increase in metabolism.

These are natural responses to stress but they become inappropriate and possibly pathological when the original reason for stress is removed and the responses remain. Additionally, problems arise when the causes of stress cannot be removed and the individual suffers a high stress response over a prolonged period of time. Stress changes from a natural, transient reaction to a chronic, pathological state. Because so many systems are affected by the normal stress response, it is not surprising that there may be symptoms involving a vast range of body systems in individuals who have abnormal levels of tension or chronic stress. For example, experimental work has shown that abnormally high and prolonged levels of adrenaline and noradrenaline in animals lead to hyperactivity and enlargement of the adrenal cortex, and atrophy of the thymus and lymph nodes (Selye 1984). It has also been shown that prolonged and excessive stress weakens the effectiveness of the immune response and therefore increases vulnerability to disease. At a subjective level, anyone who has experienced high levels of stress will have noticed the general feeling of tiredness which results from sustained high levels of muscular activity.

Relaxation produces the opposite situation and, amongst other things, results in a noticeable reduction in blood pressure, heart and respiratory rates. There is also a reduction in blood cholesterol and blood glucose levels and the activity of the sympathetic nervous system is diminished (Everett et al 1995). Muscle tension is no longer generated and the elastic components of the muscles cause the fibres to return to their resting length – this is muscle relaxation. In complete muscle relaxation there is little or no apparent activity in the contractile components. This is not to say that the motor units are completely inactive as even in a fully relaxed muscle there will be some electrical activity as small groups of motor units are briefly activated. The activation cycles through the motor units so that there is always a degree of tension in the muscle but, under normal circumstances, not sufficient to be seen as a contraction (Tortora & Grabowski 2003).

Case Study 14.1

An executive secretary in her mid-thirties was referred for treatment for unspecified low back pain. On arrival it was noticed that she sat very upright in the chair with her legs tightly wound round each other. Her arms were folded and her shoulder girdle was noticeably elevated. Initially it was thought that she was probably nervous about the impending treatment and that once she realised that the session would be neither painful nor unpleasant, she would relax. This did not happen and it became evident that even undertaking an assessment of her back problem was going to be difficult because of the degree of tension she exhibited. The remainder of the session was spent making her aware of her tension levels and giving her strategies for relaxation. For the next few weeks treatment focused primarily on relaxation and as she became more adept at reducing tension, she was able to report a marked reduction in her back problem, a reduction in the incidence of headaches and an increase in general well-being. She now continues the relaxation on her own at home and has not required further treatment.

WHEN STRESS BECOMES ABNORMAL

At times of either personal or environmental stress there will be challenges and difficulties to face. These lead to a rise in the level of arousal in the brain and the wide range of physical responses discussed earlier. This normal stress response, which is often experienced by the population at large, is usually followed by fatigue, a reduction in the level of arousal and eventually sleep. Selye (1984) defined this form of stress as positive because it is clear that a certain level of arousal is necessary to meet the challenges of life and living efficiently. Problems arise only when the response to stress becomes excessive and out of control, in which circumstances stress can be described as negative or distressful.

The capacity to cope with stressful events varies from person to person. Some people have the ability to recognise excessive stress and deal with these situations or prevent them occurring (Baker 1987). Others fail to recognise excessive stress or are unable to take avoiding action, which inevitably leads to the development of stress symptoms. At a gross level these symptoms include fatigue, loss of sleep and work inefficiency which lead to further muscle tension, causing even greater fatigue. The individual will often attempt to make up for the loss of efficiency by trying to increase their level of arousal, but this is self-defeating as it leads to more physical and emotional tension. If this situation is allowed to continue, a self-perpetuating cycle becomes established which can lead to depression and ill health.

There is no clear dividing point between the experience of positive stress and the change into a clinically recognised anxiety disorder because the duration of stress symptoms varies greatly as does an individual's ability to cope. However, there is no doubt that stress is a major problem which can affect any member of the population and this is evidenced by a review by Durham & Allan (1993) which indicated that at least 30% of the population may be driven to seek professional help for stress-related problems

Pattern of stress

The physical symptoms of stress, which are easily recognised, are often reflected in overactivity of the general body musculature. This excessive muscular tension forms well-recognised patterns that may affect movement or, more commonly, posture. An individual may demonstrate inappropriate muscular tension in any of the major muscle groups, but usually one or two muscle groups may be particularly affected. Because the pattern of tension may manifest itself in a variety of ways, it is important to observe the whole body when looking for signs.

The facial muscles often show abnormal tone; corrugator and frontalis, when not relaxed, will produce vertical and horizontal lines on the forehead. Tension headaches may develop if there is excessive tone in the occipitofrontalis and suboccipital muscle groups. Inappropriate muscle activity in orbicularis oculi and muscles of the eyelids can result either in the eyes being narrowed or held widely open or in tics, particularly of the lower eyelid. Very frequently the masseter muscle responds to stress by contracting to hold the jaws tightly together; on careful observation of the lateral aspect of the cheeks, it is often possible to see the muscle twitching. For some people, tension in the jaw muscles may also manifest itself in grinding of teeth during sleep. The tongue may be held rigidly on the roof of the mouth and the muscles of the throat may contract abnormally, making speech rather harsh and lacking in fluency of pronunciation. There may also be a click as the tongue unsticks itself from the roof of the mouth at the start of each sentence.

The posture of the head at times of stress varies between individuals, but common to all is elevation of the shoulder girdle as a result of abnormal tension in the upper fibres of the trapezius. This is easily recognised because the neck appears shortened and the normally sloping contour of the neck/shoulder region becomes more angular. The upper limbs are often held quite rigidly close to the chest with the elbows flexed. The trunk is generally held stiff and, because of tension in the abdominal musculature, diaphragmatic respiration can be inhibited so that the individual has to breathe using the intercostal and accessory muscles of respiration. In these cases, upper chest movement is observable and the accessory muscles in the neck can be seen contracting.

In general, repeated movements such as finger tapping or swinging the knees from flexion to extension when sitting can be indicators of abnormal muscle tone. Classically, adduction flexion patterns are symptomatic of stress. This may be seen in a seated subject who is tense and will sit rigidly on the edge of the chair with their lower limbs adducted and flexed, while in a standing subject the arms may be folded tightly and the legs crossed at the ankle.

Though there are many ways in which stress or tension can be manifested, it is rare for one person to demonstrate all these symptoms simultaneously and it may be necessary to use careful observation in order to identify the signs. In addition, some people have learnt to hide the signs of tension and will make an effort to slump back in their chair or to stand in a relaxed manner. Despite these efforts it is hard to control tension indicators and an experienced observer will usually be able to notice some abnormal movements or postures.

Task 14.1

Make a list of the symptoms that you manifest when tense. Watch other people carefully and see if you can notice examples of tension in the way in which they move or in their general posture.

Apart from postural symptoms and general feelings of fatigue, increased stress can show in other ways. There may be raised adrenaline production that will result in an increase in heart and respiratory rate. There may also be changes in blood and digestive chemistry that become abnormal if maintained for any length of time. Skilled performance of motor tasks is usually decreased, with a higher incidence of anxiety-induced errors in people who are tense than in people who are more appropriately relaxed (Basmajian & Wolf 1990). This is probably caused by a combination of reduced muscle control in those muscles with abnormal tone and a disruption of concentration. Tension can also lead to emotional changes which may vary from anger to despair, and intellectual performance suffers in these circumstances.

Many students suffer from increased tension, which can interfere with their performance. The stress of study, fear of failure, desire to succeed and pace of work, as well as poor environmental conditions and financial worries, may all contribute to this condition.

RELAXATION THERAPY

There are many specific techniques that can be used to encourage relaxation but it is clear that treating the symptoms alone is not enough and the underlying cause must also be addressed. It is important to seek a solution for the causes of tension as well as learning methods to remove the symptoms. Relaxation techniques can be either physical or behavioural in approach, but there is controversy over which might be the most successful.

In 2002 Huntley et al conducted a systematic review of studies into the effectiveness of relaxation for people with asthma. They found most of the research to be of poor quality but there was stronger evidence for the effectiveness of physical (muscular) techniques than for cognitive approaches. It is likely that the principles of specificity need to be applied when choosing relaxation techniques. Thus cognitive treatment approaches will have most benefit in people whose stress is psychologically based, whereas if a physiological approach is used, most benefits will be seen in the reduction of the physical manifestations of tension (Lehrer et al 1994). If an individual has a generalised response to stress, then a mixed approach to relaxation may be the most appropriate treatment.

The goal of relaxation therapy is primarily to encourage patients to gain physical control so that their response to stress is appropriate rather than destructive. This should then lead to the adoption of normal body posture and normal patterns of movement that will be more energy efficient and will, in turn, lead to a reduction in the feelings of fatigue. Some relaxation techniques require the patient to be rather passive; for example, a sedative massage or a session in a flotation tank may be enjoyable and temporarily effective but overall the improvements are less likely to be long lasting than when a technique which encourages self-control is used (Elton 1993). For the treatment to be effective, patients have to recognise tension in themselves and understand its causes and effects. Once this is achieved and they are aware of their abnormal responses to stress, they can be taught strategies which will lead to more normal reactions and an immediate improvement in physiological function (Elton 1993).

General and local relaxation

Methods of relaxation may involve either learning to relax generally or developing the ability to recognise tension in specific parts of the body and then targeting individual muscles.

General relaxation can be used either as a treatment in its own right or as part of a more extensive treatment plan. Sometimes patients are very tense due to psychological or physical stress, and treatment of a totally unrelated condition may be impossible until general relaxation is gained; in this case relaxation will be preparatory to the main programme.

At other times general relaxation is not appropriate and the treatment objective may be to teach control of abnormal tension in specific muscles. This is often the case where fear of pain leads to protective muscle spasm round a particular joint and in this case local relaxation is often used in conjunction with pain-relieving treatments.

Developing self-awareness

Whatever technique is used, whether for local or general relaxation, the first step is to gain the patient's cooperation and develop their self-awareness. Until patients can recognise the feeling of abnormal muscular activity, they will not be effective in trying to reach a more normal level. They must also learn to recognise the 'feel' of being relaxed so that they can monitor their level of success.

Developing self-awareness can be done using a variety of biofeedback mechanisms. A mirror is an effective means of demonstrating abnormal posture and the success of attempts to reduce increased tone is immediately apparent. Videotape can also be used to record the patient's posture and movement patterns and it can then be viewed and discussed. Repeat filming will demonstrate the success of the intervention process. Patients can also be made aware of the level of activity in their muscles by using electromyography (EMG). Simple EMG biofeedback machines will indicate the level of electrical activity in those muscles underlying the electrodes. Patients are encouraged to try and relax while using the EMG output to measure the degree of success. Electronic blood pressure and pulse rate monitors can also be used as effective biofeedback mechanisms and at a simpler level, patients can take their own pulse or count their own respiratory rate. With the information gained, they can impose conscious control over cardiac or respiratory rate.

The overriding aim is that the patient comes to recognise the feeling of relaxation and that they know what activities will cause a reduction in the symptoms of stress. Emphasis is placed on teaching them to discriminate between abnormal and normal tension so that they can recognise when they have been successful in achieving a relaxed state and are able to produce relaxation at will. The skills of monitoring muscle activity, joint position, respiratory and heart rates have to be learnt and this demands regular practice and concentration.

Associated with the development of self-awareness must be the acceptance that relaxation has to be self-directed. Often when people are stressed and may be upset or frightened by the symptoms produced by their condition, they want to hand over control to the therapist. If relaxation is to be successful in the long term, patients have to take back control and learn to relax independently. It is essential that at the start of the relaxation sessions, the therapist agrees with the patients that they must gradually take over the responsibility for the relaxation process. Once they can do this, they are likely to be able to control the manifestations of stress regardless of their environment.

Preparing for relaxation

In the early stages of teaching total body relaxation, it is advisable to work in a fairly quiet, pleasantly warm environment where the patient can concentrate on the task in hand (Mitchell 1990). The choice of starting position should be left to the patient but it must be one of comfort and full support. Side, supine or prone lying with pillows and blankets for support and comfort are the most likely to be successful but should never be imposed upon the patient. Often during the process of relaxation therapy, the initial starting position may become inappropriate and patients should be reassured that they may change position at any time.

As the ability to relax develops, different positions should be adopted and the environment should be made less protective until the patient is able to relax under any circumstances. It is essential that the treatment sessions proceed beyond the application of a technique and the therapist's goal should be to help patients develop strategies which will allow them to relax in situations which have previously generated stress (Crist & Rickard 1993).

The words used in the treatment session are important. Instructions should be brief, to the point and spoken in a calm, quiet manner so that they give a mental concept of what is required. The same phrases and commands should be used repeatedly so that the words themselves may become a trigger for relaxation. Harsh-sounding words should be avoided and where a command to relax is given, the tone of the voice should reflect the meaning. Therapists should conceal their own personality so that the focus of the session is on the task and not on the individuals involved.

Timing is also important. Patients must be given ample time to assimilate the instructions and monitor their responses, in particular whether they have achieved a release of tension. In the introductory sessions this may take considerably longer than might be expected.

SPECIFIC RELAXATION TECHNIQUES

Apart from teaching patients to develop an increased self-awareness and, through that, a measure of personal control, specific relaxation techniques may also be used. There are many different methods of inducing relaxation but these can all be grouped into two main categories: progressive muscle relaxation, which is based on work reported by Jacobsen in 1929, and cognitive or imaginal techniques.

Progressive muscle relaxation depends on the contraction of a muscle or muscle groups followed by a period of relaxation. Jacobsen was clear that there was a link between mental and physical tension and that if the physiology of the muscles could be altered by reducing tone, there would be a concurrent positive effect on the mind (Everett et al 1995). Whilst Jacobsen advocated contracting the major muscle groups that demonstrated tension, Laura Mitchell, some 30 years later, advised contracting the muscles antagonistic to those in tension. She worked on the principle that it would be better to avoid increasing the tension in an already tense muscle and by contracting the antagonist, reciprocal inhibition of the tense muscle would occur. An alternative approach has been advocated by Carlson in the last two decades. Carlson, like Mitchell, considers that a muscle that is already demonstrating inappropriate tone might get worse if required to contract. Instead it is proposed that the muscles affected by tension should be stretched rather than be required to contract (Carlson et al 1996). This stretching is done utilising the effects of gravity, so for example the patient might allow the head to 'loll' to one side so that the neck muscles are fully stretched. The stretches are held for 10–30 seconds until the full benefit of the manoeuvre is felt.

Apart from any local effect on muscle, these techniques have been shown to have positive systemic effects including reduction in heart and respiratory rate, tonic vasodilation and decreased production of cortisol. They have also been shown to have a positive effect on anxiety states and perceived stress (Bell & Saltikov 2000, Pawlow & Jones 2002).

Cognitive or imaginal techniques require the focusing of thoughts on an activity or place or on a repetitive sound or movement. There are several approaches to these techniques. The individual can practise visualisation, where the stressful situation is imagined as being non-stressful or non-threatening, and this technique is often used in sport or by business people. In guided imagery the patients think about pleasant experiences and by so doing, try to distance themselves from stressful situations. The direction of their thoughts can be towards real events that they found pleasant and are happy to think about or they can be guided to imagine a perfect situation in which they feel little or no stress.

Whilst there is no clear evidence as to which approach is most effective or whether personality type might affect the choice of procedure (Crist & Rickard 1993), the best technique for a specific patient may be that which targets their main manifestations of stress (Lehrer et al 1994). In any event, the therapist needs to be flexible when choosing the relaxation technique and must be prepared to change the approach if success is not being achieved.

Contract–hold–relax or contrast method (Hollis 1988, Ricketts & Cross 1985)

Fox (1996) cites work undertaken by Sherrington in the early part of last century which suggested that a maximal relaxation follows a maximal muscle contraction. This mechanism is mediated through the Golgi tendon organ. When a muscle contracts hard, considerable tension is placed on the Golgi tendon organs in that muscle and this stimulates the inverse stretch reflex. Impulses from the Golgi tendon organs in the contracting muscle pass to the spinal cord and synapse through to alpha motor neurones which transmit the impulses to the same muscle. These are inhibitory impulses and, if the original contraction was strong enough, will result in inhibition of contraction and therefore relaxation (Fox 1996). It is possible that this reflex is utilised in some relaxation techniques.

The contract-hold-relax relaxation technique requires the patient to undertake, in sequence, strong isometric contractions of all major muscle groups and in particular those which are manifesting abnormal tone. The contraction is held and it is then followed by a period of relaxation which should be at least as long as the contraction. The patient should be asked to concentrate on the feeling of relaxation in order to learn to reproduce it. It is usual to work distal to proximal and to begin with one limb and teach contraction of each individual muscle group. When each major muscle group in a limb has been taken through this process, a total limb isometric contraction is undertaken before the process is repeated on the next limb. This process is repeated for all four limbs and the trunk and face. Interspersed at regular intervals through the session should be relaxed diaphragmatic breathing with the emphasis on the expiratory phase.

Commands

- Tighten (a muscle) – hold – let go.
- Breathe deeply in – hold – let the air sigh out of your mouth.

The speed of progression through this technique depends on the patient. It may be necessary to repeat each of the stages many times before relaxation is obtained and it may take many weeks before the whole body is involved.

The physiological or Mitchell's technique (Hollis 1988, Mitchell 1990)

The patient is required to contract the muscles antagonistic to those in tension. This moves the nearby joints out of the position of tension and simultaneously induces reciprocal relaxation in the previously tense muscle groups. After each contraction the patient should be asked to concentrate on the feeling of the new, relaxed position.

It is thought that this technique utilises the mechanism of reciprocal innervation. As a muscle contracts, impulses from the muscle spindle will pass via the spinal cord to the antagonistic muscle group, causing inhibition (Kandel et al 1991). For example, if the trapezius muscle is exhibiting abnormal tone, the patient will be encouraged to contract the shoulder girdle depressor muscles to cause reciprocal inhibition of trapezius.

It is usual to work proximal to distal and to start with the upper limbs followed by the lower limbs, trunk and finally the head. Relaxed diaphragmatic breathing exercises are interspersed throughout the programme. As with the previous technique, groups of muscles are worked individually after which these movements are summated before moving on to the next limb. The starting position is not important as it will change as the patient relaxes.

Commands

- Move in a given direction – stop – let go.
- Feel the new position.
- Breathe deeply in – hold – let the air sigh out of your mouth.

Visualisation or the suggestion method (Hollis 1988)

The aim of this method is to distract patients from negative thoughts and to help them to concentrate on something that is non-threatening and pleasurable. It is a form of autohypnosis and rather similar to techniques used in certain types of meditation. Whereas the previous two techniques concentrated on reducing muscle tone with the presumption that mental relaxation would follow, this technique tries to reduce the mental activity and replace worrying thoughts with something

---

Case Study 14.2

Mr P held a very senior position in a university. His job was stressful and he worked excessively long hours. He often found that when he went to bed at night many of the work issues that worried him would suddenly come to the front of his mind and once this had happened, sleep became impossible. He also found that he would wake in the early hours of the morning sweating with fear, often about small issues that in the day time were of little consequence. He found that the physiological approaches to relaxation did not work well for him but that cognitive methods were usually successful. He used a technique that involved 'confining' his worries. At particularly stressful times, before he tried to go to sleep, he would spend some time imagining that he could physically wrap his worries in a thick piece of plastic. He would then imagine putting the parcel of worries in a large metal box and wrapping round the box a heavy metal chain with a big padlock. Finally, he imagined throwing the box into the river near his house and watching it being swept away. On getting into bed he would consciously remind himself that the worries were no longer in the house and that they therefore could not prevent him sleeping. Finally, as he prepared to sleep, he would think about being in the garden of a holiday cottage he went to each year. He found this garden a place of great peace and happiness and by concentrating on what it felt like to be there, he usually found he went to sleep immediately.

---

pleasant. If the technique works, then a reduction in muscle tone should follow automatically. Ricketts and Cross (1985) suggest that this method is most successful with individuals who may be able to relax physically but find it difficult to stop thinking.

The room must be quiet and warm and the patient comfortable and well supported. It may help to cover them with a blanket. In hypnotic tones the therapist guides the patient to think about pleasurable, non-threatening experiences or objects. Patients are encouraged to absorb themselves in what is being said, fully concentrating on the word picture being painted by the therapist. The therapist should persuade the patient to think about repetitive movements or sounds such as waves gently lapping on the shore or the gentle rustle of a breeze in the trees. The therapist should speak slowly and in low tones. No harsh-sounding words should be used and long vowel sounds should be drawn out.

Interspersed in this technique can be the suggestion that the patient's limbs feel heavy or that they feel as if they are gently floating. As before, this technique is improved by the inclusion of deep relaxed breathing exercises.

Before starting this technique, it is important to explore the types of experiences that have given patients pleasure or the nature of the object on which they wish to focus. In this way the technique will be appropriate and meaningful. Individuals who find this technique particularly helpful can learn to trigger relaxation when alone by thinking about their chosen subject. It is also helpful to concentrate on repetitive sounds or actions such as breathing.

Meditation

Meditation induces a state similar to resting and appears to be as effective as other methods of relaxation (Shapiro 1982). Research has shown that during meditation there are hormonal changes, including an increase in the production of melatonin (Tooley et al 2000) and dopamine (Kjaer et al 2002). The former has a health-promoting effect and the latter acts as a modulator of excitatory synapses in the brain. As meditation is not an easily acquired skill, it is unlikely to be a technique of choice for many therapists, but it would be worthwhile recommending patients to join meditation classes.

Sedative massage

Currently there is no evidence to show that massage has more than a short-term effect on reducing tension but slow, rhythmical stroking, effleurage and kneading can feel very relaxing. As such, massage can be used as a way of introducing the patient to the concept of relaxation. The combination of massage with aromatherapy is popular but research has yet to show convincing evidence that the aromatherapy component contributes to the relaxation effect (Jorm et al 2002).

For massage to be effective, it is essential that the therapist's hands are relaxed and remain so throughout the treatment. The strokes should initially be light but the depth can be increased as the patient adapts to the feel of the massage. For some people, being asked to undress or being touched can be stressful and where this is the case it is possible to allow the patient to remain clothed. Once they are suitably positioned for the massage, a large blanket is tucked firmly round them and stroking is applied through the material. As the aim of all relaxation therapies is to enable patients to take control over their own bodies, massage should only be seen as an interim step before more active methods are introduced.

EMG biofeedback (Basmajian & Wolf 1990, Elton 1993)

This method has been shown to be successful, particularly when used in conjunction with other approaches (Elton 1993, Middaugh & Pawlick 2002). Biofeedback gives specific information about the state of tension in individual muscle groups, enabling patients to take control of the reduction of their muscle tone. There is instant feedback of success and the impartiality of the machine's response is often seen as reassuring.

The electrodes are attached over muscle groups known to be in tension and the patient is placed in a variety of starting positions and encouraged to reduce the electrical activity in the muscles. Once sufficient self-awareness has been developed, the patient is able to reduce inappropriate muscle tone without the help of the machine. Where there is a generalised response to stress, the electrodes are often placed over the frontalis muscle and patients can be taught to control their stress using input from this muscle.

Low-frequency breathing exercises (Leuner 1991)

Low-frequency diaphragmatic breathing exercises induce relaxation and can be used alone or in conjunction with other techniques. In order to breathe diaphragmatically, the abdominal muscles must relax to let the diaphragm descend. In the expiratory phase a sighing action is encouraged so that the air is expired through elastic recoil of soft tissue whilst the respiratory muscles and muscles of the throat and mouth relax. The frequency of respiration should be low in order to avoid hyperventilation. As the patient is resting whilst being asked to undertake deep breathing, it is necessary to reduce the respiratory rate to less than the normal resting rate in order not to disrupt the normal blood chemistry. Eight or ten breaths a minute is often successful and pauses may be incorporated at the end of the inspiratory and the expiratory phases.

This technique results in a reduction in muscle tone as well as a reduction in blood pressure, heart rate and electrical activity in the brain (Bell & Saltikov 2000, Leuner 1991). The mental relaxation which most patients feel with this method results from both the physiological changes and the concentration needed to maintain a low-frequency respiratory pattern. This is a repetitive, non-stressful activity which leads to mental relaxation in much the same way as some meditative techniques.

Case Study 14.3

Mrs V was an asthmatic patient with serious social problems. Her husband was in prison and she was trying to bring up three teenaged children in a small flat on the 13th floor of an ageing tower block. She was unable to work and had to cope on a very limited income. She was deeply concerned that her children should not follow the example of her husband and turn to crime, but she found it very hard to exert control over them. A major problem was that the lift in the block of flats was frequently out of action and her asthma made it impossible for her to tackle the stairs. Consequently, she felt a prisoner in her home and her children were aware that she had no control over them once they were out of the flat. She was experiencing frequent, serious asthma attacks which were resulting in repeated periods of hospitalisation.

It was decided to try low-frequency breathing exercises and general relaxation with this patient and the results were quite dramatic. The incidence of asthma attacks serious enough to warrant hospitalisation dropped to approximately one per year and with the improvement in her health, she felt slightly more able to cope with her life in general.

Pendular exercises (Hollis 1988)

Relaxed swinging of a limb is a repetitive rhythmical movement which probably causes relaxation through two mechanisms. First, it raises the threshold of transmission of impulses from sensory receptors in the moving joint and surrounding soft tissues, leading to a reciprocal inhibition of the afferent impulses from the same spinal segment and a reduction in local muscle tone. Second, the repetitive nature of the movement tends to reduce mental tension. Any starting position which allows a limb to swing with a minimum amount of muscular effort can be used. Pendular exercises in suspension are particularly effective but whatever position is chosen, the exercise should start with small-range movements and never move beyond what is comfortable.

Rhythmical passive movements

These are similar to pendular exercises in that the limb is subjected to gentle repetitive movements until the threshold of sensory receptors is raised. In this technique the patient should attempt to relax whilst the physiotherapist moves the limb. It is important to undertake this technique with constant velocity and range of movement of the joints as any variation in these factors will disrupt the rhythmicity of the procedure.

Physical activity

There is an increasing body of knowledge to show that physical activity reduces stress levels and a thorough review of the current state of knowledge has been presented by Paluska and Schwenk (2000). It has also been shown that when a relatively high level of physical fitness is developed, the responses to acute stress are improved (Brandon & Loftin 1991, Roth & Holmes 1987, Wilfley & Kunce 1986). The type of physical activity is not crucial to the technique and swimming, running, ball sports and fast walking have all been shown to be successful. In recent years t'ai chi has become increasingly popular as it often combines breathing exercises with the movements. There is no evidence as to whether aerobic exercise or anaerobic exercise is the most effective.

There are a number of hypotheses to explain how physical activity can cause relaxation, with some authorities believing it is psychological and others physiological. It is possible that exercise may provide a distraction from the sources of stress or, on the other hand, it may improve the individual's feelings of self-efficacy so that confidence increases and feelings of anxiety decrease. Many physical activities can be quite challenging, both in the physical demands they make but also in the level of skill required to perform the activity well. If stress has arisen through lack of confidence, then success in a non-threatening physical activity may help to restore the patient's feelings of self-worth and control. There is also conflicting evidence about the possible physiological benefits of exercise on tension. A well-popularised theory is that exercise increases the production of endorphins which can induce feelings of mild euphoria and a positively altered mood state. It has also been suggested that exercise improves brain synaptic transmission which, it is hypothesised, can be impaired in stress situations (Paluska & Schwenk 2000).

Despite the conflicting and often poor-quality evidence to support exercise as a means of relaxation, the balance of research indicates that exercise will have a positive effect (Jorm et al 2002). A note of caution has to be sounded as there is also evidence that physical activity is only effective if undertaken in moderation and that if it is taken to extreme levels then the activity in itself will induce stress. People who become fixated on the need to exercise and who push their bodies to the limit run the risk of going beyond the beneficial effects of exercise and introducing stress, with all its unwanted side effects.

Although it is possible to teach relaxation, the initial cause of any excessive tension should not be ignored and the patient should be encouraged to seek solutions for the original cause of stress. This is likely to involve other members of the health-care team or the social or welfare services. While the original cause of stress continues, the ability to move with an economy of effort and therefore less fatigue will be reduced.

REFERENCES

Baker GH 1987 Psychological factors and immunity. Journal of Psychosomatic Research 31: 1–10

Basmajian JV, Wolf SL 1990 Therapeutic exercise, 5th edn. Williams and Wilkins, Baltimore

Bell JA, Saltikov JB 2000 Mitchell's relaxation technique: is it effective? Physiotherapy. 86(9): 473–478

Brandon JE, Loftin MJ 1991 The role of fitness in mediating stress: a correlational exploration of stress reactivity. Perceptual and Motor Skills 73: 1171–1180

Carlson CR, Collins FL, Nitz AJ, Sturges ET, Rogers JL 1996 Muscle stretching as an alternative relaxation training procedure. Journal of Behaviour Therapy and Experimental Psychiatry 21(1): 29–38

Crist DA, Rickard HC 1993 A fair comparison of progressive and imaginal relaxation. Perceptual and Motor Skills 76: 691–700

Durham RC, Allan T 1993 Psychological treatment of generalised anxiety disorder: a review of the clinical significance of results in outcome studies since 1980. British Journal of Psychiatry 163: 19–26

Elton D 1993 Combined use of hypnosis and EMG biofeedback in the treatment of stress-induced conditions. Stress Medicine 9: 25–35

Everett T, Dennis M, Rickett E 1995 Physiotherapy in mental health: a practical approach. Butterworth Heinemann, Oxford

Fox S I 1996 Human physiology, 5th edn. WC Brown, Boston, Massachussetts

Hollis M 1988 Practical exercise therapy, 3rd edn. Blackwell Scientific Publications, Oxford

Huntley A, White AR, Ernst E 2002 Relaxation therapies for asthma: a systematic review. Thorax 57(2): 127–131

Jacobsen E 1929 Progressive relaxation, 2nd edn. University of Chicago Press, Chicago, Illinois

Jorm AF, Christensen H, Griffiths KM, Rodgers B 2002 Effectiveness of complementary and self-help treatments for depression. Medical Journal of Australia 176(5): S84–96

Kandel ER, Schwartz JH, Jessell TM 1991 Principles of neural science, 3rd edn. Elsevier Science Publishing, New York

Kjaer TW, Bertelsen C, Piccini P, Brooks D, Alving J, Lou HC 2002 Increased dopamine tone during meditation-induced change of consciousness. Cognitive Brain Research 13(2): 255–259

Lehrer P, Carr R, Sargunaraj D, Woolfolk RL 1994 Stress management techniques: are they all equivalent, or do they have specific effects? Biofeedback and Self Regulation 19: 353–401

Leuner H 1991 Ein neuer weg sur tiefenentspannung: das respiratorisch feedback. Kranken Gymnastik 43: 246–253

Middaugh SJ, Pawlick K 2002 Biofeedback and behavioural treatment of persistent pain in the older adult. Applied Psychophysiology and Biofeedback 27(3): 185–202

Mitchell L 1990 Simple relaxation: the physiological method for relieving tension. John Murray, London

Moffett DF, Moffett SB, Schauf CL 1993 Human physiology and foundation frontiers. Mosby Year Book, St Louis, Missouri

Paluska AA, Schwenk TL 2000 Physical activity and mental health, current concepts. Sports Medicine 29(3): 167–180

Pawlow LA, Jones GE 2002 The impact of abbreviated progressive muscle relaxation on salivary cortisol. Biological Psychology 60(1): 1–16

Ricketts E, Cross E 1985 The Whitchurch method of stress management by relaxation exercises. Physiotherapy 71: 262–264

Roth DL, Holmes DS 1987 Influence of aerobic exercise training and relaxation training on physical and psychological health following stressful life events. Psychosomatic Medicine 49: 357–365

Selye H 1984 The stress of life. McGraw-Hill, New York

Shapiro DH 1982 Clinical and physiological comparison of meditation with other self control strategies. American Journal of Psychology 139: 267–273

Tooley GA, Armstrong SM, Norman TR, Sali A 2000 Acute increases in night-time plasma melatonin levels following a period of meditation. Biological Psychology 53(1): 69–78

Tortora GJ, Grabowski SR 2003 Principles of anatomy and physiology, 10th edn. John Wiley, New York

Wilfley D, Kunce J 1986 Differential physical and psychological effects of exercise. Journal of Counselling Psychology 33: 337–342

Chapter 15

Human movement through the life span

Marion Trew

LEARNING OUTCOMES

When you have completed this chapter you should:

1. Understand how human movement changes from birth to extreme old age

2. Be aware of the importance of reflexes in developing controlled movement capabilities

3. Have a basic knowledge of the stages involved in developing hand control and walking

4. Understand why physical ability may deteriorate with increasing years

5. Understand the basic physiological changes that can occur with age

6. Understand the concept of the threshold of ability

7. Recognise age-induced changes in posture and gait

8. Understand the importance of recognising that some age changes are reversible.

INTRODUCTION

This chapter is about the changes that occur in human movement throughout the life span. Whilst it is appropriate to consider people as individuals, the reality is that most of us follow a common pattern as we develop, and later lose, movement abilities. These common patterns are very obvious in childhood and equally common patterns of loss of movement ability are seen in older people.

Newborn children are helpless and totally dependent on others until they have developed the basic skills and quality of movement needed to cope with normal life. There is rapid acquisition of motor skills in the first few years of life, after which the developmental process slows down. From the late teens until late middle age there is a period of stability where changes in movement ability are not particularly noticeable and then from the sixth decade onwards there is measurable change that leads towards a decline in ability.

The age at which different motor skills are acquired in childhood is remarkably similar between children, most children developing the same skills within one or two months of each other. At the other end of the life span, the onset and timing of deterioration of abilities vary greatly between individuals because they are dependent on variables such as lifestyle, disease, trauma and personality. The similarity in the developmental sequence in children has made it possible to identify milestones of achievement and to provide guides to the approximate age at which these milestones are likely to occur. Delay or failure in achieving a number of these milestones may be indicative of abnormality but such information must be treated with great caution as there are many examples of children who followed an atypical development sequence and went on to be exceptional adults. Similarly, in old age the loss of movement ability should not be automatically categorised as irreversible age changes because the reversible effects of inactivity can present a similar pattern of movement loss.

Task 15.1

If you know someone with a baby, ask if you may go and observe. When the baby is awake and moving, compare what you see with the suggested milestones given in the first three tables in this chapter. If you don't know anyone with a baby, ask your parents or someone you know who has had a child if they can remember when the major milestones occurred. Most parents will remember when their baby first stood and walked. Compare what you find out with the suggested average milestones in the tables.

THE FETUS AND NEONATE

In the uterus the fetus starts to make jerky movements from the age of about 3 months when it is approximately 3 cm long. The tiny size of the fetus and the fact that these movements mainly involve the mouth and fingers leave the mother unaware of the activity. By the start of the fifth month, the fetus is about 20–26 cm long and fully formed, it moves frequently and it is at this time that the mother becomes aware of what is happening. Movement becomes less jerky as the months pass but the activity appears to be without purpose and is probably stimulated by reflexes. The increase in fetal activity does not continue in a linear manner and at about the sixth month there is a quiescent period when movement is reduced. Why this should be is not clear; however, it is known that at this time the higher centres in the brain are developing and as they are responsible for control of purposeful movement, the quiet period may represent a transition between primitive and more purposeful activity. In the eighth and ninth months of pregnancy the fetus is very active. It is now 48–53 cm long and quite cramped within the uterus yet it moves frequently, turning and changing position and 'kicking' and 'punching' with its arms and legs (Cole & Cole 1993, Gallahue & Ozmun 1998).

The reasons for fetal movement are not clear. Some animal studies have led to the belief that movement in the uterus is necessary if normal development of bones, joints, muscles and the peripheral nervous system is to occur, but the evidence to support this in humans does not exist. It is clear that some fetal activity is a response to external stimuli and it has been shown that a loud noise outside the uterus will stimulate the fetus to move. It is also speculated that the increasing levels of activity are part of the preparation for life after birth. The movements in the uterus may be establishing motor pathways and developing some level of coordination in preparation for the neonatal period. They may also be having a strengthening effect on the muscles.

The full-term neonate has a predominantly flexed posture, has few movement skills and is helpless when considered alongside most other newborn animals. In the early days of life most

Table 15.1 Some primitive and developmental reflexes seen in the first year of life

Reflex	Stimulus	Response
Rooting	Light touch on the cheek or corner of lip.	Head turns to stimulus, tongue moves towards stimulus.
Grasp	Pressure on the ulnar side of the palm.	Strong finger flexion to make a grip.
Moro	Either a sudden noise or allowing the baby's head to drop slightly when held in supine.	Abduction and elevation of the upper limbs with abduction and some extension of the fingers. This is followed by a flexion pattern of upper limb movement.
Placing	Touch on the anterior tibia or dorsum of the foot.	Flexion of the hips, knees and dorsiflexion, as if to move the limb so the foot can be placed on the object it touched.
Walking	When held upright, pressure on the soles of the feet.	Reciprocal flexion and extension of the lower limbs in a pseudo-walking pattern.
Leg extension	Pressure on the sole of the foot.	Extension of the trunk, hips and knees.
Asymmetrical tonic neck	Rotation of the head to one side.	Ipsilateral shoulder abduction and elbow extension. Response is often mild and may only show as an increase in muscle tone.
Symmetrical tonic neck	a) Flexion of the neck. b) Extension of the neck.	An increase in flexor tone in the trunk, upper and lower limbs which may result in movement. An increase in extensor tone in the trunk, upper and lower limbs which may result in movement.
Righting reflexes (labyrinthine, neck and body)	Rotation of the head in relation to the trunk.	Repositioning of the head or trunk either to maintain the correct relationship of the head with the trunk or to position the head correctly in relation to gravity.

Sources: Illingworth 1990, Bee 1999

movements are under the influence of reflexes although infants also demonstrate some purposeful activity. At birth children can hear and see and can turn their heads to follow sounds or the shape of a face, but many of the other movements they make at this stage are clearly the result of primitive reflexes (Illingworth 1990).

Reflex activity

A reflex is a prompt, stereotyped reaction to a stimulus and in the early days of life, most of the movements made by children are reflex responses to stimulus. The reflexes can be divided into categories: some of these reflexes are protective and some are for survival but others appear to

have the role of establishing the movement patterns needed in later months. Thus the rooting reflex is an example of a survival reflex as it helps the infant find the nipple and nourishment, whereas the blink and cough reflexes have obvious protective functions. The walking reflex is thought to play a part in establishing the patterns needed for true walking (Gallahue & Ozmun 1998).

Table 15.1 lists some of the primitive reflexes which are commonly seen or which may have value in the development of mature human movement patterns. Many of these reflexes are present at birth and then fade after a few months; for example, the grasp reflex usually disappears at about 4 months. It has been speculated that the ability to grasp strongly may be protective as it enables the infant to cling to an adult's hair or clothes when being carried or picked up. The grasp reflex is so strong that children have been seen to hold their whole body weight with one hand. It is important that this reflex does not persist beyond a few months, as it would be undesirable to grip everything that touched the palm of the hand. Other reflexes such as the labyrinthine righting reflex appear later, in this case at about 2 months after birth. This reflex causes the infant to position its head with the vertex uppermost and the plane of the face vertical. Thus when the infant is placed in prone or supine the reflex will cause the head to lift and this is the foundation stage for developing the movement patterns to sit upright, stand or walk.

During the normal developmental process most of the primitive reflexes seen in the young child are suppressed or modified as movement maturity develops (Gallahue & Ozmun 1998). However, these reflexes are never totally lost and may be seen again under conditions of stress or following brain damage.

DEVELOPING MATURE MOVEMENT PATTERNS

The amount of physical, cognitive and social development that occurs in the first 2 years of life is phenomenal. As part of the process of physical development, the infant has to gain voluntary control of movement. Whilst it is necessary to retain those reflexes that maintain posture and cause reactions to the effects of gravity and disturbances of balance, it is also necessary for the infant to develop the ability to override most of the primitive reflexes. If this does not happen, movement will remain stereotyped and not necessarily be appropriate to all situations. Movement that remains under the control of primitive reflexes will not become specialised or individualised and there will be no scope for adaptation to different situations.

There are many excellent textbooks that deal in detail with all aspects of the development of the infant and child and it is beyond the remit of this chapter to consider how all the body systems mature. In this chapter a few examples have been used to show how the infant develops hand control, learns to move purposefully, sits, stands and walks. This will convey a flavour of the early, age-related changes in human movement but will not provide a comprehensive review.

The development of hand control

For the human being the ability to use the hand is very important. Approximately 6 months before birth the fetus is able to move its fingers and a month later can open and close its hand but by the time the child is born little further progression in hand ability has been achieved and the hand is relatively useless (Rosenbaum 1991). At this stage the grasp reflex predominates and for most of the time, the hand is held closed. It takes approximately 6 years for good hand control to be developed and children continue to learn new skills and to develop greater speed and precision in increasingly complex hand activities throughout their school days. Table 15.2 shows the main milestones of the development of hand control.

The development of walking ability

In order to be able to walk the infant first needs to achieve a number of related physical milestones. For example, it would be difficult to walk without a stable relationship between the trunk and the head or between the trunk and the lower limbs. Consequently one of the early motor skills to develop is the control of trunk and head position. Most children crawl before they walk, this activity utilising reciprocal movements of the upper and lower limbs in patterns somewhat similar to walking. Crawling starts the development of the motor patterns needed to walk but in the safe environment of a large base of support. Crawling is not essential and there are some children who never crawl but shuffle on their bottoms before they stand and walk. There do not seem to be any adverse effects from not progressing through the crawling stage. Standing and balancing unaided is the final stage before true walking can occur. The achievement of walking occurs around one year after birth though at this stage it is not performed in a skilful manner. It takes several more years before walking and running become fluent and

Table 15.2   Milestones in the development of manipulative skills

Age	Skill acquisition
Birth	Grasp reflex dominant. Hands mostly held closed.
3 months	The grasp reflex is almost gone and the hands are usually held open. Can hold an object between both hands. May try to hit objects.
4 months	Reaches for objects. Plays with objects held in both hands. Grasps at many things but has no precision or eye–hand coordination.
5 months	Can grasp objects voluntarily in one or both hands, but the object is held on the ulnar side of the hand in a crude grip and the thumb is not involved. Starts to show the ability to estimate where to position the hand in order to intercept a moving object.
7–9 months	Passes object from one hand to the other and holds the object on the radial side of the hand. Towards the end of this period may demonstrate the beginnings of a precision grip. May be able to hold and eat a biscuit. Points. Voluntarily lets go and can place objects in containers.
9–12 months	Is able to grip between the pads of the fingers and thumb but the grip is not strong and cannot be sustained. Holds a spoon in a primitive grip. Has limited precision but can hold objects as small as a pea. Waves.
15 months	Has the precision to place one cube on top of another and can, rather clumsily, drink from a cup. Can remove shoes.
18 months	Eye–hand coordination improving but can't turn over individual pages of a book. Can scribble with a pencil and may be able to imitate simple shapes. Can build a cube tower of three cubes. Removes gloves or socks and unzips clothes. Handedness becomes apparent.
2 years	Can put on shoes and socks. Can unscrew a lid. Starts to use scissors. Has the precision to draw a circle. Copies activities of parents and other children.
2 ¹/₂ years	Can build a tower of 8 cubes. Has more precision in using a pencil and can draw horizontal and vertical lines.
3 years	Can undertake most dressing tasks except buttons and laces. Can draw a man. Can catch a large ball between arms and body.
4 years	Can manage buttons. Can draw a square.
5 years	Can tie shoelaces. Drawings are neater, more controlled.
6 years	Can draw a diamond. Is able to undertake hand activities quickly. Has a fairly mature throwing and catching pattern. Can manipulate a needle and thread.
7 years and beyond	All the basic motor skills for the upper limb have been developed and from now on, the child and adult learns new and more complex skills or develops greater precision in existing skills.

Sources: Bee 1999, Brierley 1993, Holt 1991, Illingworth 1990, Rosenbaum 1991

precise. Table 15.3 shows the major milestones leading to the ability to walk well.

Adolescence onwards

By adolescence motor ability is very well developed, to the extent that 'children' in their teens are able to compete in international sporting events such as gymnastics. Improvement in motor ability continues to be seen and as children move through adolescence to adulthood, they show improvements in their balance, strength and speed (Gallahue & Ozmun 1998). Learning motor skills does not end with the onset of adulthood and the

Table 15.3 Milestones in the development of sitting, standing and walking

Age	Skill acquisition
Birth	No head control, hips and knees flexed in lying, unable to extend spine at all. Walking reflex present in supported standing.
3 months	Head control developing, able to raise head against gravity. In prone lying can take weight on forearms. When supported in sitting, is able to keep head up, though not able to hold it still. Rapidly developing control of the head on trunk movement. Walking reflex has disappeared and the baby is unable to bear weight when held in standing.
5 months	Head no longer wobbles when held in sitting and control of the head position in relationship to the moving trunk is quite good. Is able to hold the spine in extension when placed in sitting or supported standing. Can bear weight in standing, when supported by an adult.
7–9 months	In prone, can take weight on one or both hands. Can sit supported in a chair and briefly sit unsupported. Can roll from supine to prone and prone to supine. Has sufficient trunk control to hold the spine straight when reaching for objects. Develops ability to pull into standing. When held in standing, likes to bounce.
9–12 months	Now crawling, initially by pulling body forwards with arms. Has sufficient trunk control to sit unaided without losing balance. Able to stand holding on to furniture, progresses to lifting one leg and then walking whilst holding on. Is not able to sit down with any control.
12 months	Crawling has developed so that weight is borne on feet rather than knees. When sitting, can rotate trunk or head to look round. Walks holding the hand of an adult.
13 months	Walks unaided, but with a wide base and has little control.
15 months	Climbs stairs on hands and knees. Walking improving but unable to stop or turn with control.
18 months	Can carry object whilst walking. May be able to run. Can get on to a chair. Ascends and descends stairs providing there is a handrail. Jumps from both feet.
2 years	Can walk backwards. Is able to run and kick with limited control. Can manage stairs unaided but places both feet on each step.
2 1/2 years	May be able to walk on tiptoes.
3 years	Can balance briefly on one leg, Goes up stairs normally but finds stair descent difficult. Can jump off a low step.
4 years	Goes down stairs normally.
5 years	Can skip normally.
6 years and beyond	Development now takes the form of increases in speed and strength and the ability to combine movements in complex patterns. By 8 years should be able to ride a bicycle.

Sources: Bee 1999, Brierley 1993, Holt 1991, Illingworth 1990

ability to perform complex, precision tasks such as playing a musical instrument can continue to develop through adult life. However, for many young adults, their motor ability levels off fairly quickly and then starts a gradual decline into middle age and a more rapid decline in the sixth or seventh decade. The key to maintaining or developing motor skills throughout life is repetitive practice of activities that challenge existing abilities. Even very old people can develop new motor skills as is seen in elderly people who lose their sight and subsequently learn Braille.

Task 15.2

Before reading the next section of this chapter, make a list of what you think an elderly person in the eighth or ninth decade would be like. Use the headings of 'appearance', 'functional abilities', 'physical abilities' and 'mental capacities' to help you. Make a second list using the same headings but now applying the criteria to someone in their 30s.

Compare your thoughts with other students to see if you are in agreement and then keep a note of the results of this task. When you have reached the end of this chapter, return to this task and see if you have altered your opinions in any way.

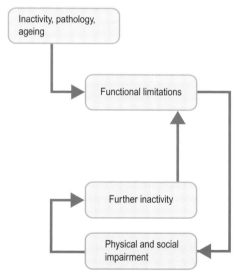

Figure 15.1   The effect of inactivity, pathology and ageing on functional ability.

THE TRANSITION INTO OLD AGE

The loss of the ability to move easily and freely can start to become a problem at any time from middle age onwards, but is most commonly associated with old age. The onset is often insidious and it is sometimes difficult to decide whether a reduction in movement ability is caused by age or disease or whether it is a consequence of an increasingly sedentary lifestyle (Fig. 15.1).

There are many reasons why older people are usually less active than their younger counterparts. Elderly people tend to avoid or have no need to undertake activities that require strength, speed or full ranges of joint movement. Older women, in particular, spend increasing periods of time in sedentary pursuits that make no major physical demands and are therefore vulnerable to the adverse effects of disuse atrophy (Fiatarone 1990). Added to this, cultural expectations tend to constrain physical activity in the later years of life. In a number of cultures there is an expectation that life should slow down with the passage of years and that old people deserve to take life easy. Where these social expectations exist it is inevitable that many older people's lifestyles will become increasingly sedentary and the development of disuse atrophy will eventually contribute to physical deterioration. Not only will a sedentary lifestyle result in a gradual decline in physiological function but it can also have an adverse effect on psychological function. A sedentary lifestyle combined with those physical changes that are an inevitable consequence of ageing will eventually result in a reduced ability to perform even the most basic physical and cognitive tasks associated with activities of daily living. These circumstances lead inexorably to a reduction in quality of life and a substantial dependence on carers.

Although the general population usually accepts a slower pace of life and a loss of ability with the passage of years, the changes caused by inactivity are both preventable and reversible (Williams et al 2002). Good health education and health promotion schemes that explain the importance of maintaining a reasonably active lifestyle in the middle and later years are clearly important. Elderly individuals who exercise regularly are less likely to suffer from movement problems but even those who take up exercise late in life can benefit from an improvement in a number of body systems (Cavani et al 2002, Cress et al 1999, Grimby 1988, McArdle et al 2001, Pereira et al 1998). Being old chronologically is not necessarily the same as being old physically. A 70 year old with good health, the right temperament and social opportunities can demonstrate better motor skills and abilities than a sedentary 30 year old.

However, a reduction in movement capability will directly affect the ability to perform functional activities and can have a catastrophic effect on the quality of life. It is therefore essential not to lose sight of the fact that a number of physical changes associated with growing old can be prevented, slowed down or even reversed. The rest of this chapter considers how ageing can have a direct effect on movement and the ability to undertake everyday activities. Age-induced changes in posture and gait are used as examples and the final part explores how exercise can benefit older people who wish to remain fully active and self-sufficient.

PHYSIOLOGICAL CHANGES ASSOCIATED WITH AGEING

Human movement in elderly people can be compromised in three main ways:

1. Through structural changes which are a direct result of the ageing process. This might include changes in the structure of the eye, leading to deteriorating vision, or the loss of muscle fibres leading to reduced strength and endurance.
2. Changes related to the effects of disease or trauma which may or may not be associated with growing old. In this category can be found diseases such as osteoarthritis or osteoporosis. The most common trauma associated with the ageing process is a fractured neck of femur following a fall.
3. As a consequence of the effects of inactivity.

Cardiovascular changes

The function of the cardiovascular system is significantly reduced in older people and this has a negative effect on both the intensity and duration of physical activity. Resting heart rate changes little with age but the maximum heart rate attainable on activity drops significantly, causing a concurrent reduction in exercise tolerance. The expected maximum heart rate for older people can be obtained by using the formula: 220 minus the age in years = maximum heart rate.

This is an approximate guide that must be used with caution as actual values vary greatly between individuals.

By the age of 85, resting stroke volume is reduced by about 30% and the myocardium is noticeably hypertrophied. Also, at this age, resting cardiac output may be less than half the value it was in the third decade (Fitzgerald 1985).

These changes impair the ability of the heart to deliver blood to the tissues; oxygen uptake in the muscles is also reduced, not because of a loss of muscle oxidative enzymes but as a consequence of the actual loss of muscle fibres. It seems likely that the oxidative enzymes are little affected by age, though there may be a reduction in the resynthesis of ATP due to a reduction in phosphogens (Grimby 1986). With both a reduced delivery of blood to the muscles and also a reduction in the number of muscle fibres available to utilise oxygen, there is a general reduction in movement capacity, particularly in endurance activities. A further adverse effect of ageing on the cardiovascular system is the loss of elasticity in the arterial walls. This leads to an undesirable increase in blood pressure on strenuous activity due to the arteries' inability to accommodate the increase in blood flow.

These cardiovascular changes make activity more difficult with advancing years but in themselves do not have too serious an effect on the ability to perform normal, everyday functions. However, if the natural age changes are combined with a long-term loss of fitness due to an increasingly sedentary lifestyle, then the consequences may start to become serious and essential functional activities may require so much energy that they take an unacceptable length of time to complete or become impossible.

Respiratory system changes

Increasing age may result in degenerative changes in the costovertebral and costosternal joints and may be combined with calcification of the costal cartilages. Eventually these changes will lead to a reduction in thoracic mobility in both the anteroposterior and lateral directions. Elastic recoil of the chest wall, which is necessary for expiration, becomes reduced as a consequence of a generalised loss of elastic tissue and this puts major emphasis on movements of the diaphragm as a means of changing thoracic diameter and lung capacity. All these changes mean that a disproportionate amount of effort is needed for the process of respiration during strenuous activity and these age changes can eventually lead to a 20% increase in respiratory energy requirements (Fitzgerald 1985). By the age of 70, vital capacity can also have decreased by 50% yet, despite all these changes, it appears that a decrease in respiratory function is not a major factor in the limitation of exercise tolerance in elderly people, particularly if they have habitually maintained a fairly active lifestyle. The changes in the heart, the peripheral circulation and the muscles appear to be far more significant in reducing movement capabilities than age-related changes in the respiratory system.

Muscle changes

With increasing age there is a reduction in both aerobic and anaerobic capacity affecting the endurance, strength and speed attributes of muscle. As with the other body systems, the most marked changes occur in extreme old age, particularly after the eighth decade (Fiatarone 1990, Grimby 1986, Young 1986). The rate of loss of strength has been extensively studied but the results are inconclusive. It appears that age-related loss of strength may be dependent on the genetic make-up of the individual but it also varies between muscles, some appearing to be more affected than others. Gender is also a factor, with the menopause being responsible for a marked loss of strength in women (Grabiner & Enoka 1995).

In elderly people beyond their eighth or ninth decade there is a noticeable reduction in muscle bulk. This is mainly a consequence of loss of muscle fibres, though there may also be a reduction in size of the type II fibres (fast twitch), the latter probably caused by disuse atrophy. Although the visible signs of loss of muscle bulk are not always apparent until old age, computer tomography shows that muscle fibres are being lost from at least the age of 30 when they start to be replaced with intramuscular fat. The fat masks visual signs of muscle fibre loss until a substantial number of fibres have disappeared (Williams et al 2002). The

Task 15.3

Start observing children, young adults, middle-aged and elderly people. Watch the speed with which they tackle everyday tasks and the ranges of joint movement that they employ. Are you able to note any differences between these age groups?

replacement of contractile muscle tissue with fat also affects elasticity as the muscle becomes stiffer and movement becomes more difficult.

Despite the significant loss of muscle fibres, there is normally sufficient spare capacity for this not to be a major constraint on function until extreme old age is reached. Once again, it is the combination of age changes and disuse atrophy that is likely to be the cause of the 'weakness' exhibited by many old people.

The lifestyle of many middle-aged and elderly individuals puts little demand on the type II fibres that are responsible for power and speed activities and this inevitably leads to disuse atrophy. Fitness training programmes for middle-aged and older people also tend to concentrate on activities which will not stimulate type II muscle fibre activity. Rapid muscle contractions, in particular, are rarely included in therapeutic or recreational activity sessions.

Interestingly, the pattern of atrophy of type II fibres is not constant throughout all regions of the body. The quadriceps appear to be more subject to atrophy than muscle groups in the upper limb, though this may be a reflection of a reduction in lower limb activities rather than an age-induced change in muscle structure (Grimby 1988). It is hypothesised that the muscles of the upper limb remain in constant use even when the individual has lost the ability to walk and are often used in fairly rapid movements. This continued use probably contributes to the retention of a greater proportion of type II fibres in upper limb muscle groups when compared with lower limb muscles.

Most authorities feel that the decrease in muscle function and muscle mass is mainly due to the loss of muscle fibres and a reduction in oxygen delivery. There may also be changes in cellular structure leading to abnormal cell chemistry

(Williams et al 2002). Whilst there may be a reduction in the enzymic capacity of muscle, this is not a necessary consequence of old age and therefore can be slowed down by the use of exercise (Fitzgerald 1985, Grimby 1986, McArdle et al 2001). However, many muscle fibres in older people are structurally and functionally similar to those seen in younger people and will therefore respond to physical demands and training.

Neurological changes

The neurological system is not protected against age-induced changes although in the absence of disease or trauma it can, in some individuals, continue to function remarkably well into extreme old age. Commonly, ageing can cause a reduction in the effectiveness of the neurotransmitters, a change in nerve cells, especially in the number and effectiveness of synaptic connections, and a reduction in the number of nerve cells (Pickles et al 1995). Reaction times are significantly increased with age, probably due to the reduction in nerve conduction velocity which can be altered by up to 15% (Fitzgerald 1985). The number of motor units decreases and activation of muscle may become more difficult, though the remaining motor units may become larger as axonal sprouting occurs. There will eventually be a reduction in sensory capacity as the number of sensory nerve endings declines and thresholds for transmission of sensory information increase. All these factors may lead to the control and quality of performance of human movement being reduced (Fitzgerald 1985, Grimby 1986).

Skeletal changes

With increasing age there is often a significant loss of bone mass, particularly in elderly women, which may be due to the ageing process or caused by disease. The situation can be exacerbated by lack of exercise, a reduction in dietary calcium, poor diet and also genetic factors (Pickles et al 1995). This osteoporosis and the increased incidence of falls in older people make them particularly vulnerable to fractures. Skeletal changes usually manifest in alterations in posture, particularly in the development of thoracic kyphosis, which is

---

Task 15.4

Look through your grandparents' photograph album. Can you identify the physical changes that have occurred through their lives? Can you work out which structures have changed as they have got older?

Ask your grandparents about the lifestyle they were leading when the photographs were taken and evaluate whether their answers support the theories of ageing discussed in this chapter. When your grandparents talk about their lifestyle, do you notice that they have become progressively inactive?

---

very common in older people. Skeletal changes in the hands and feet are also noticeable in most elderly people and may eventually lead to a reduction in functional ability.

Reduced range or quality of movement in joints is a common problem associated with age. In older people, connective tissue and muscle become less elastic, altering the quality of joint movement. Individuals who adopt a sedentary lifestyle are vulnerable to soft tissue contractures. Any loss of range of movement in the major joints will inevitably reduce the ability to move normally and undertake functional activities with the same efficiency as a younger person. Arthritis starts to develop from an early age and after the sixth decade it is a common cause of movement problems. Research indicates that there is a gender effect on the incidence of musculoskeletal disorders, with women being more likely to have joint problems than men (Arber & Ginn 1994). This, coupled with the fact that in most countries women live longer than men, inevitably leads to musculoskeletal problems being a significant factor in reducing movement capabilities in older people. Joint disease, combined with a reduction in function of other body systems, greatly reduces the functional ability of older people and has an adverse effect on their quality of life. Providing there are no serious degenerative changes, appropriate exercise can increase the range of movement and a small improvement in joint range may cause a disproportionately large functional improvement (Fitzgerald 1985).

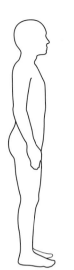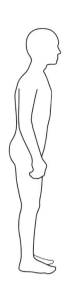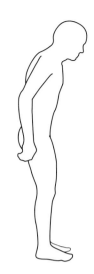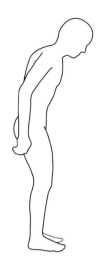

Figure 15.2 The typical development of postural changes associated with ageing.

Postural changes with age

With increasing years most elderly people show some common deviations from normal posture. These deviations occur at different times for different people but are most usual in the eighth and ninth decades. Static standing posture shows typical changes that probably originate in the spine. These cause an alteration in the resting position of the centre of gravity, leading to other body segments readjusting to compensate (Fig. 15.2). In many elderly people there is an increase in the thoracic kyphosis and either a flattening of the lumbar curve with posterior pelvic tilt or a compensatory increase in lumbar lordosis.

Many older people, when standing, adopt a posture of hip and knee joint flexion and ankle joint dorsiflexion. This is in contrast to the more extended joint positions seen in younger adults. With the thoracic spine in a position of kyphosis, the upper limbs will no longer rest by the sides but hang in front of the body when the individual is relaxed. This displaces the centre of gravity even further anteriorly and can stretch the individual's balance ability to the limit. To compensate, the older person may extend both shoulder joints in order to position the upper limbs posteriorly in relation to the trunk. This has the effect of favourably readjusting the centre of gravity in relation to the base of support, making the maintenance of equilibrium less of a challenge. A

negative effect of holding the upper limbs posteriorly is that shoulder joint muscles have to contract to maintain this position and this inevitably increases energy expenditure and leads to sensations of fatigue. In order to reduce the energy requirements of this upper limb posture, the older person may clasp fingers behind the back.

There are a number of reasons why postural changes occur in older people. In the spine it is common to find degenerative changes in the intervertebral discs, osteoporosis of the vertebrae and trunk muscle weakness. Structural changes in the discs and vertebral bodies lead to an increasingly flexed posture which weak trunk musculature and poor postural habits fail to correct. The changes in the lower limb alignment in standing may be a compensatory mechanism for the alteration in spinal posture and the alteration in position of the centre of gravity (Kauffman 1987, Pickles et al 1995). They are also likely to be associated with shortening of the soft tissues anterior to the hip joint which makes the achievement of full hip extension impossible. If the hip cannot fully extend in standing then compensatory repositioning of the knee and ankle joints is necessary if a relatively upright posture is to be maintained. The abnormal pattern of flexion in the lower limbs in standing may also be a reaction to the deterioration in balance ability seen in older people. By adopting a flexed posture of the hip and knee joints in standing, the overall length of the lower limbs is reduced, thus lowering the centre of gravity in relation to the base and somewhat increasing stability.

Gait changes with age

It is easy to observe the differences in gait between old and young people but in line with other age changes, the age at which they occur varies between individuals. Gait, in itself, is highly variable but despite this, as people get older a typical pattern of gait changes can be seen. The gait pattern is not grossly different from the gait of younger people, but most aspects show modifications.

All studies investigating age-related changes in gait have reported that preferred walking velocity drops with age (Finley et al 1969, Hageman & Blanke 1986, Murray et al 1969). Walking velocity is dependent on stride length and cadence, both of which are also reduced in older people, though the main difference occurs in stride length. Murray et al (1969) found that the mean stride length of young men was 89% of their height and that it reduced to 79% of body height in men over 80 years; a similar reduction was also found in women. Minor hip flexion contractures have been found in many elderly people and these appear to affect gait adversely by reducing the stride length and, through that, by reducing walking velocity (Kerrigan et al 1998). The reductions in cadence are not found to be as great as stride length reductions and have variously been reported as reducing by only one or two steps per minute.

It is well documented that balance ability reduces as people grow older and it is therefore logical to expect increases in stride width and foot angle in order to provide a larger base of support. Murray et al (1969) found a small increase of about 2 cm in the stride width of elderly men and an increase in foot angle from an average of 8° in men under 25 years to 13° in men over 80. Double stance is the most stable phase of the gait cycle and in older people approximately 10% more time is spent in this phase than in younger people. The swing phase, which is a time of great vulnerability when only one foot is in contact with the ground, is reciprocally shortened. If the swing phase is reduced in time and the cadence is barely increased then it is inevitable that the stride length

will be reduced. As mentioned earlier, there is usually a loss in spinal rotation and arm swing. This contributes to the reduction in walking velocity as it causes a reduction in step length and, in some cases, a reduction in the cadence.

As joint range has been shown to diminish in older people it has led some scientists to study the range of movement of dorsiflexion during gait. A reduction of 5–10° in ankle joint excursion in older women has been identified in the early swing phase (Finley et al 1969, Hageman & Blanke 1986) and this might be a contributing factor to falls in this age group. If the older person is not able to fully dorsiflex the foot at the start of the swing phase then there is an increasing risk of catching the toe on the floor and stumbling. To compensate, there is a slight increase in flexion at the hip and knee joints which shortens the swing limb during the swing phase. In the younger age range minimum toe clearance during the swing phase is about 1 cm but in men over 80 it has been shown to be 2.6 cm. The ground reaction forces generated in the gait of older people have also been studied and a reduction in the propulsive force generated at the push-off phase has been identified (Kerrigan et al 1998, Murray et al 1969, Whittle 1991, Winter et al 1990). Weakness of the plantar-flexors in older people reduces the ability to propel the body forwards and this may be another factor contributing to a reduction in walking velocity. The main changes in gait of older people are given in Table 15.4.

When gait changes associated with age are considered as a whole it can be seen that they are all interrelated and it is difficult to identify which factors have caused gait changes and which are responsive to gait changes. On the whole, changes in gait are probably due to altered posture, a reduction in joint and, in particular, spinal movement, muscle weakness and a loss in balance ability which is rooted in neurological changes (Pickles et al 1995, Winter et al 1990).

IMPROVING MOVEMENT AND FUNCTION IN OLDER PEOPLE

Ideally people should approach old age with a good level of physical fitness and an expectation

Table 15.4   Age-related changes in gait

Factor	Effect of ageing
Step length	Decreases
Stride length	Decreases
Stride width	Increases
Cadence (steps/min)	Little change or a decrease
Single-stance period	Decreases
Double-stance period	Increases
Velocity	Decreases
Trunk rotation	Decreases
Anterior/posterior pelvic tilt	Decreases
Range of ankle movement	Decreases
Hip lateral rotation	Increases
Toe clearance	Decreases

Task 15.5

Go onto the Internet and search for the results of 'senior', 'masters' and 'veterans' athletics meetings. Look at the performances and the ages of the athletes. Do they conform to your original ideas about the abilities of older people?

As not all older people enjoy competitive sport, you need to be aware of the other sorts of activities that people undertake to maintain or improve their physical ability. Talk to a range of middle-aged and older people about their leisure activities. Evaluate their activities in terms of whether they will be effective in producing a beneficial physical effect.

that they will continue to be physically active. To a certain extent an individual's expectations of old age will be based on cultural norms and financial constraints. All cultures ascribe certain roles to old people and in many cases these carry expectations of a reduction in involvement in society and a general reduction in activity levels. If changes in expectations are to take place, then they will have to occur from childhood onwards. There is a tendency for it to be thought unusual for an elderly person to be active and adventurous and such individuals are often labelled as 'super gran' or 'super grandad'. There needs to be a change in society so that younger people are brought up recognising that it is normal for their grandparents to be active and take a full and interested part in life. Good health education can establish and reinforce these expectations so that there is a greater likelihood of older people maintaining physical well-being and, hopefully, a concurrent good quality of life.

Financial constraints also influence lifestyle and those with low incomes are more likely to have poor diets and limited access to a range of enjoyable physical activities. In the major industrialised countries, women are more likely than men to have an income near to the poverty line

and also a greater level of physical impairment (Arber & Ginn 1994). As women live longer than men, these factors are clearly significant but the solution is not easy to find and changes in society may be necessary.

For those individuals who reach old age in poor physical condition and who live a sedentary lifestyle, intervention from the health-care team is likely to be necessary. The combination of inactivity and ageing has been shown to lead to poor balance, a loss of muscle mass, poor exercise tolerance and some limitation in joint movement. If the worst circumstances prevail, then by the eighth decade many sedentary people may be so frail that the limit of their physical ability is reached simply by the performance of normal activities of daily living. This leaves them with little or no physical capacity in reserve and it takes only the slightest deterioration for their level of ability to drop below the requirements of daily life. Such a drop, which can be caused by a minor illness requiring a few days' bed rest, often proves catastrophic and results in loss of independence. Young (1986) describes a threshold of ability that is necessary for the performance of activities of daily living; if an individual falls below that threshold then self-care becomes impossible. Many very old people live on the border of that threshold because of the debilitating effects of age changes, disease and inactivity. For them, generating sufficient torque in their quadriceps and hip extensor muscles to rise from a low chair or toilet may be the equivalent of a 1 repetition maximum load and getting dressed may well cause the heart rate to rise to its age-predicted maximum. Under these circumstances it is no wonder that frail elderly people find the simplest activities difficult and take an inordinately long time to complete even the most basic of daily tasks.

For those old people living at the threshold of their ability, their frailty usually results in increasing dependency on the help of others and also a greater likelihood of accidents. The quality of life for these frail, old people is often poor and their dependency places a consequent strain on their relatives and carers (Fiatarone 1990).

For their own self-respect and for the benefit of their carers, elderly people need to be able to undertake, at the very least, the basic activities of daily living. They need the physical attributes to be able to move around their living area unassisted and to attend to their eating and toileting needs.

The beneficial effects of exercise for young people are well known and it is generally accepted that older people can experience the same positive changes. Even at an extreme age, there is evidence that training can induce positive changes and a small strength gain may represent a very large improvement in the quality of life. Effective exercise programmes given to people in the older age range will, at the very least, maintain their existing condition, if not improve the function of all major body systems. This should include the heart, lungs, musculoskeletal, metabolic and central and peripheral nervous systems. Some authors have additionally noted that the progress of vascular disease, diabetes, hypertension, chronic obstructive airways disease, osteoporosis and arthritic conditions is retarded in subjects who undertake exercise programmes (Fisher & Pendergast 1995, Fitzgerald 1985, Thompson et al 1988).

The majority of evidence seems to show that exercise for old people is beneficial regardless of whether it is aerobic, mixed or anaerobic. For example, Westhoff et al (2000) asked elderly participants to undertake a 10-week programme of low-intensity (aerobic) exercises and they were able to show a significant improvement in knee extension function, rising from a chair and the timed up and go test. Cavani et al (2002) found that training elderly people three times a week for 6 weeks using a mixed programme of stretching and moderate-intensity exercise produced significant increases in upper and lower limb function and strength. A large number of studies have investigated the effects of anaerobic exercise for older people and the majority have shown that high-intensity resistance training increases strength (O'Neill et al 2000, Porter et al 2002, Tracy et al 1999). Most researchers advise that exercise programmes of at least 12 weeks' duration will produce statistically significant improvements in the strength of muscles, providing an exercise intensity of between 5 and 12 repetition maximum is used. The level of improvement can be substantial, Porter et al (2002) reporting approximately 100% increase in quadriceps and latissimus dorsi strength over 1 year. There is less strong evidence that exercise can result in functional improvement, but again the trend seems to suggest it is possible (Worm et al 2001). Consensus of opinion therefore suggests that exercise is beneficial to older people and that following a programme of exercises, an increased feeling of well-being and an enthusiasm for maintaining an adequate level of physical activity can be expected (James et al 2001, McArdle et al 2001).

Endurance exercises have been shown to increase the maximum oxygen uptake and reduce the heart rate, blood pressure and blood lactate in elderly people (Coggan et al 1992, Hurley & Hagberg 1998). With appropriate, long-duration training, muscle strength and endurance can increase with the same order of magnitude as that seen in younger people on an identical training programme. Obviously no amount of exercise can replace lost muscle fibres, but for those that remain it is possible to induce hypertrophy, better recruitment of motor units and improved delivery and uptake of oxygen (Grimby 1986).

If frail or very old people are to see a substantial improvement in their physical capacity, they may need exercises of an intensity that they are unable to tolerate. It is important to achieve a balance between exercise which is so gentle as to be ineffective and exercise which might be effective but which will place a dangerous stress on the heart or musculoskeletal system (Hauer et al 2002). There is increasing evidence that, providing there are no disease processes that would contraindicate exercise, resistance training can be safe, desirable and effective. Such exercise can be safely undertaken at 70–90% of the older person's maximum work capacity (Hauer et al 2002, Pickles et al 1995). However, it is important to be aware that older people may be more susceptible to injury than the young and any injuries that occur will probably take longer to recover. Exercise programmes must be carefully supervised but a gradual build-up of the intensity of exercise should be sufficient to ensure the safety of the participants (Williams et al 2002).

Ideally, as people age they should be encouraged to develop the habit of exercise so that the age changes that might reduce their ability to perform everyday activities may be avoided or delayed. Unfortunately, this is often not the case and older people may become dependent following a long period of inactivity. Under these circumstances, motivation to exercise is often low, but if the exercise programme is specifically planned for the individual's needs and if achievable goals are set, significant improvements may be seen. Older people should be made aware of the exercise goals and should, where possible, take an active part in their setting. They should be taught how to monitor their own progress and records should be kept so that improvements can be seen and used as motivators.

Exercises for very frail people who have a history of falls or who have significant lower limb problems may initially have to be non-weight bearing, chair based. But the principles of exercise are the same whether for young people, fit elderly people or people who are old and frail. The exercise programme should include exercises which will increase:

- joint range
- muscle strength
- muscle endurance
- heart and respiratory rate
- the ability to move groups of muscles and joints quickly
- coordination
- balance
- the ability to perform functional activities.

For those elderly people who are more fit, encouragement to take part in any physical activity is important: brisk walking, jogging and dancing are excellent methods of undertaking weight-bearing exercise. In all three examples the participant will be using major muscle groups and joints and there will be some beneficial stress placed on their balance mechanisms and their cardiovascular and respiratory systems. Swimming utilises major muscle groups in both the upper and lower limbs and moves the joints through a wide range of movement and stresses the heart and lungs satisfactorily, but it is non-weight bearing. Non-weight bearing activity can be beneficial if the individual has joint pain but swimming does not require or stimulate balance reactions and the effects of weight bearing through the spine and long bones are lost. As such it should be seen as an adjunct and not an alternative to other weight-bearing activities.

Very little research has been undertaken into the most effective duration of exercise programmes for elderly people. Presumptions must be made that the rules that apply to the design of exercise programmes for the young population will be appropriate across the age range. Exercises should be undertaken not less than twice a week. Initially, the duration of the exercises will depend on the ability of the individual and may have to start at a very low level of perhaps a few minutes per day. The exercises, whether for the power or endurance capacity of muscle, should show progression and, if possible, the level of endurance exercises should take the heart rate into the cardiac training zone (60–80% of the predicted maximum heart rate for the individual). Exercise programmes to improve the development of strength in older people should follow the same rules as for younger people and the load should aim to be between 6 and 10 repetition maximum for each individual. Providing there are no pathological reasons why an older person should not work at this level, it is essential to ensure that the principle of 'overload' is followed.

THE FEAR OF FALLING

In addition to those factors already considered in this chapter, it is necessary to address the effect of the fear of falling on human movement and the ability to perform functional activities. With ageing can come an increase in falling frequency and this phenomenon presents a major problem to the patient, their carers and the rehabilitation team. With every fall is the possibility of musculoskeletal damage and this may lead to the faller being placed on bed rest. For those people with an already reduced threshold of physical ability, any period of inactivity can prove very serious and may lead to dependency. Falling also leads to a loss of confidence when undertaking weight-bearing activities and this in turn leads to a reduction in those activities.

Currently, there is no consensus on why elderly people fall, but it is probably a consequence of a number of factors, some of which are intrinsic to the individual and some of which are related to their environment (Pickles et al 1995). A thorough assessment of the individual and their environment may reveal potential contributing factors on which a rehabilitation programme may be built. If not, then a programme which improves lower limb joint range and muscle function, especially around the ankle joint, combined with exercises to improve postural stability, may be successful.

CONCLUSION

The future for old people, in terms of their ability to move and function normally, can be excellent. The maintenance of a reasonable level of physical activity into old age is important and, where fitness levels have dropped significantly, hope should be encouraged because there is always capacity for improvement.

Task 15.6

Reconsider your earlier thoughts about older people. Having read this chapter, have your opinions and expectations of older people changed? What sort of an old age do you want for yourself? Is there anything you might do that would help you achieve your wishes?

REFERENCES

Arber S, Ginn J 1994 Women and aging. Reviews in Clinical Gerontology 4: 349–358

Bee H 1999 The growing child, an applied approach, 2nd edn. Longman, New York

Brierley J 1993 Growth in children. Cassell Education, London

Cavani V, Mier CM, Musto AA, Tummers N 2002 Effects of a 6 week resistance training program on functional fitness of older adults. Journal of Ageing and Physical Activity 10: 443–452

Coggan AR, Spina RJ, King DS 1992 Skeletal muscle adaptations to endurance training in 60-70 yr old men and women. Journal of Applied Physiology 72: 1780–1786

Cole M, Cole SR 1993 The development of children, 2nd edn. Scientific American Books, New York

Cress ME, Buchner DM, Questad KA, Esselman PC, de Lateur BJ, Schwartz RS 1999 Exercise: effects on physical functional performance in independent older adults. Journal of Gerontology. Series A, Biological Sciences and Medical Sciences 54(5): 242–248

Fiatarone MA 1990 Exercise in the oldest old. Topics in Geriatric Rehabilitation 5(2): 63–77

Finley FR, Cody KA, Finizie RV 1969 Locomotion patterns in elderly women. Archives of Physical Medicine 50: 140–146

Fisher NM, Pendergast DR 1995 Application of quantitative and progressive exercise rehabilitation to patients with osteoarthritis of the knee. Journal of Back and Musculoskeletal Rehabilitation 5: 33–53

Fitzgerald PL 1985 Exercise for the elderly. Medical Clinics of North America 69: 189–196

Gallahue DL, Ozmun JC 1998 Understanding motor development. Infants, children, adolescents, adults, 4th edn. McGraw-Hill, Boston

Grabiner MD, Enoka RM 1995 Changes in movement capabilities with aging. In: Holloszy JO (ed) Exercise and sport sciences reviews. Williams and Wilkins, Baltimore

Grimby G 1986 Physical activity and muscle training in the elderly. Acta Medica Scandinavica 711(suppl): 233–237

Grimby G 1988 Physical activity and effects of muscle training in the elderly. Annals of Clinical Research 20: 62–66

Hageman PA, Blanke DJ 1986 Comparison of gait of young women and elderly women. Physical Therapy 66(9): 1382–1387

Hauer K, Specht N, Schuler M, Bartsch P, Oster P 2002 Intensive physical training in geriatric patients after severe falls and hip surgery. Age and Ageing 31: 49–57

Holt KS 1991 Child development. Diagnosis and assessment. Butterworth Heinemann, Oxford

Hurley BF, Hagberg JM 1998 Optimising health in older persons: aerobic or strength training? Exercise and Sport Sciences Reviews 26: 61–89

Illingworth RS 1990 The development of the infant and young child, normal and abnormal, 9th edn. Churchill Livingstone, Edinburgh

James PK, Blumenthal A, Babyak A et al 2001 Effects of exercise training on cognitive functioning among depressed older men and women. Journal of Ageing and Physical Activity 9: 43–57

Kauffman T 1987 Posture and age. Topics in Geriatric Rehabilitation 2: 13–28

Kerrigan DC, Todd MK, Della Croce U, Lipsitz LA, Collins JJ 1998 Biomechanical gait alterations independent of speed in the healthy elderly: evidence for specific limiting impairments. Archives of Physical Medicine and Rehabilitation 79(3): 317–322

McArdle WD, Katch FI, Katch VL 2001 Exercise physiology, energy, nutrition and human performance, 5th edn. Lea and Febiger, Philadelphia

Murray MP, Kory RC, Clarkson BH 1969 Walking patterns in healthy old men. Journal of Gerontology 24: 169–178

O'Neill DOT, Thayer RE, Taylor AW, Dzialoszynski TM, Noble EG 2000 Effects of short-term resistance training on muscle strength and morphology in the elderly. Journal of Ageing and Physical Activity 8: 312–324

Pereira MA, Kriska AM, Dat RD, Cauley JA, LaPorte RE, Kuller LH 1998 A randomised walking trial in post menopausal women. Archives of Internal Medicine 158: 1695–1701

Pickles B, Compton A, Cott C, Simpson J, Vandervoort A 1995 Physiotherapy with older people. WB Saunders, London

Porter MM, Nelson ME, Fiatarone MA et al 2002 Effects of long-term resistance training and detraining on strength and physical activity in older women. Journal of Ageing and Physical Activity 10: 260–270

Rosenbaum DA 1991 Human motor control. Harcourt Brace, San Diego

Thompson RF, Crist DM, Marsh M, Rosenthal M 1988 Effects of physical exercise for elderly patients with physical impairments. Journal of the American Geriatrics Society 36: 130–135

Tracy BL, Ivey FM, Hurlbut D et al 1999 Muscle quality. II Effects of strength training in 65 to 75 year old men and women. Journal of Applied Physiology 86(1): 195–201

Westhoff MH, Stemmerik L, Boshuizen HC 2000 Effects of a low-intensity strength-training programme on knee extensor strength and functional ability in frail older people. Journal of Ageing and Physical Activity 8: 325–342

Whittle M 1991 Gait analysis, an introduction. Butterworth Heinemann, Oxford

Williams GN, Higgins MJ, Lewek MD 2002 Ageing skeletal muscle: physiologic changes and the effects of training. Physical Therapy 82(1): 62–68

Winter DA, Patla AE, Frank JS, Walt SE 1990 Biomechanical walking pattern changes in the fit and healthy elderly. Physical Therapy 70: 340–347

Worm CH, Vad E, Puggaard L, Stovring H, Lauritsen J, Kragstrup J 2001 Effects of a multi component exercise program on functional ability in community dwelling, frail older adults. Journal of Ageing and Physical Activity 9: 412–424

Young A 1986 Exercise physiology in geriatric practice. Acta Medica Scandinavica 711(suppl): 227–232

Index